Advances in Respiratory Care of the Newborn

Guest Editors

JUDY L. ASCHNER, MD
RICHARD A. POLIN, MD

CLINICS IN PERINATOLOGY

www.perinatology.theclinics.com

Consulting Editor

LUCKY JAIN, MD, MBA

September 2012 • Volume 39 • Number 3

SAUNDERS an imprint of ELSEVIER, Inc.

W.B. SAUNDERS COMPANY
A Division of Elsevier Inc.

Elsevier, Inc. • 1600 John F. Kennedy Blvd. • Suite 1800 • Philadelphia, PA 19103-2899

http://www.theclinics.com

CLINICS IN PERINATOLOGY Volume 39, Number 3
September 2012 ISSN 0095-5108, ISBN-13: 978-1-4557-4920-1

Editor: Kerry Holland
Developmental Editor: Donald Mumford

Photocopying
Single photocopies of single articles may be made for personal use as allowed by national copyright laws. Permission of the Publisher and payment of a fee is required for all other photocopying, including multiple or systematic copying, copying for advertising or promotional purposes, resale, and all forms of document delivery. Special rates are available for educational institutions that wish to make photocopies for non-profit educational classroom use. For information on how to seek permission visit www.elsevier.com/permissions or call: (+44) 1865 843830 (UK)/(+1) 215 239 3804 (USA).

Derivative Works
Subscribers may reproduce tables of contents or prepare lists of articles including abstracts for internal circulation within their institutions. Permission of the Publisher is required for resale or distribution outside the institution. Permission of the Publisher is required for all other derivative works, including compilations and translations (please consult www.elsevier.com/permissions).

Electronic Storage or Usage
Permission of the Publisher is required to store or use electronically any material contained in this journal, including any article or part of an article (please consult www.elsevier.com/permissions). Except as outlined above, no part of this publication may be reproduced, stored in a retrieval system or transmitted in any form or by any means, electronic, mechanical, photocopying, recording or otherwise, without prior written permission of the Publisher.

Notice
No responsibility is assumed by the Publisher for any injury and/or damage to persons or property as a matter of products liability, negligence or otherwise, or from any use or operation of any methods, products, instructions or ideas contained in the material herein. Because of rapid advances in the medical sciences, in particular, independent verification of diagnoses and drug dosages should be made. Although all advertising material is expected to conform to ethical (medical) standards, inclusion in this publication does not constitute a guarantee or endorsement of the quality or value of such product or of the claims made of it by its manufacturer.

Clinics in Perinatology (ISSN 0095-5108) is published quarterly by Elsevier Inc., 360 Park Avenue South, New York, NY 10010-1710. Months of issue are March, June, September, and December. Business and Editorial Offices: 1600 John F. Kennedy Blvd., Ste. 1800, Philadelphia, PA 19103-2899. Customer Service Office: 3251 Riverport Lane, Maryland Heights, MO 63043. Periodicals postage paid at New York, NY and additional mailing offices. Subscription prices are $273.00 per year (US individuals), $401.00 per year (US institutions), $326.00 per year (Canadian individuals), $509.00 per year (Canadian institutions), $400.00 per year (foreign individuals), $509.00 per year (foreign institutions), $130.00 per year (US students), and $187.00 per year (Canadian and foreign students). Foreign air speed delivery is included in all Clinics subscription prices. All prices are subject to change without notice. **POSTMASTER:** Send address changes to *Clinics in Perinatology*, Elsevier Health Sciences Division, Subscription Customer Service, 3251 Riverport Lane, Maryland Heights, MO 63043. **Customer Service: Telephone: 1-800-654-2452** (U.S. and Canada); **1-314-447-8871** (outside U.S. and Canada). **Fax: 1-314-447-8029. E-mail: journalscustomerservice-usa@elsevier.com** (for print support); **journalsonlinesupport-usa@elsevier.com** (for online support).

Reprints. For copies of 100 or more, of articles in this publication, please contact the Commercial Reprints Department, Elsevier Inc., 360 Park Avenue South, New York, NY 10010-1710. Tel. (212) 633-3812; Fax: (212) 482-1935; E-mail: reprints@elsevier.com.

Clinics in Perinatology is also publishhed in Spanish by McGraw-Hill Interamericana Editores S.A., P.O. Box 5-237, 06500 Mexico D.F., Mexico.

Clinics in Perinatology is covered in *MEDLINE/PubMed (Index Medicus) Current Contents, Excepta Medica, BIOSIS and ISI/BIOMED.*

Printed and bound by CPI Group (UK) Ltd, Croydon, CR0 4YY

Transferred to Digital Print 2012

Contributors

CONSULTING EDITOR

LUCKY JAIN, MD, MBA
Richard W. Blumberg Professor and Executive Vice Chairman, Department of Pediatrics,
Emory University School of Medicine, Atlanta, Georgia

GUEST EDITORS

JUDY L. ASCHNER, MD
Julia Carell Stadler Professor of Pediatrics, Vanderbilt University School of Medicine;
Director, Mildred Stahlman Division of Neonatology, Monroe Carell Jr. Children's Hospital
at Vanderbilt, Nashville, Tennessee

RICHARD A. POLIN, MD
Director, Division of Neonatology, Professor of Pediatrics, College of Physicians and
Surgeons, Columbia University, New York, New York

AUTHORS

KURT H. ALBERTINE, PhD
Professor and Editor-in-Chief, The Anatomical Record, Departments of Pediatrics,
Medicine, Neurobiology & Anatomy, University of Utah School of Medicine,
Salt Lake City, Utah

EDUARDO BANCALARI, MD
Professor, Division of Neonatology, Department of Pediatrics, University of Miami Miller
School of Medicine, University of Miami, Miami, Florida

VINEET BHANDARI, MD, DM
Associate Professor of Pediatrics, Obstetrics, Gynecology and Reproductive Sciences;
Director, Program in Perinatal Research, Division of Perinatal Medicine, Department
of Pediatrics, Yale University School of Medicine, Yale Child Health Research Center,
New Haven, Connecticut

WALDEMAR A. CARLO, MD
Professor of Pediatrics, Division of Neonatology, Department of Pediatrics, Women and
Infants Center, University of Alabama at Birmingham, Birmingham, Alabama

NELSON CLAURE, MSc, PhD
Associate Research Professor, Division of Neonatology, Department of Pediatrics,
University of Miami Miller School of Medicine, University of Miami, Miami, Florida

NEIL N. FINER, MD
Professor of Pediatrics, Director, Division of Neonatology, Department of Pediatrics, University of California San Diego School of Medicine, University of California San Diego Medical Center, San Diego, California

KIMBERLY FIRESTONE, BS, RRT
Neonatal Outreach Educator, Neonatal ICU, Department of Neonatology, Akron Children's Hospital, Akron, Ohio

GABRIEL HADDAD, MD
Professor of Pediatrics, Department of Pediatrics, Rady Children's Hospital, University of California San Diego, La Jolla, California

AARON HAMVAS, MD
James P. Keating, M.D. Professor of Pediatrics, Department of Pediatrics, Washington University School of Medicine, St Louis, Missouri

MARK R. HOLLAND, PhD
Research Associate Professor of Physics and Pediatrics, Department of Physics, Washington University, St Louis, Missouri

SUDARSHAN R. JADCHERLA, MD, FRCPI, DCH, AGAF
The Neonatal and Infant Feeding Disorders Program; Professor of Pediatrics, Divisions of Neonatology, Pediatric Gastroenterology and Nutrition, Center for Perinatal Research, Department of Pediatrics, The Research Institute at Nationwide Children's Hospital, The Ohio State University Wexner College of Medicine, Columbus, Ohio

ALAN H. JOBE, MD, PhD
Division of Pulmonary Biology, Cincinnati Children's Hospital Medical Center, University of Cincinnati, Cincinnati, Ohio

MARTIN KESZLER, MD
Associate Director of NICU, Director of Respiratory Services, Professor of Pediatrics, Women and Infants Hospital of Rhode Island, Warren Alpert Medical School, Brown University, Providence, Rhode Island

SATYAN LAKSHMINRUSIMHA, MD
Associate Professor of Pediatrics, Chief, Division of Neonatology, Women and Children's Hospital of Buffalo; Director, Center for Developmental Biology of the Lung, State University of New York at Buffalo, Buffalo, New York

MATTHEW M. LAUGHON, MD, MPH
Division of Neonatal-Perinatal Medicine, The University of North Carolina at Chapel Hill, Chapel Hill, North Carolina

TINA A. LEONE, MD
Associate Clinical Professor of Pediatrics, University of California San Diego School of Medicine, University of California San Diego Medical Center, San Diego, California

PHILIP T. LEVY, MD
Fellow in Pediatrics, Department of Pediatrics, Washington University School of Medicine, St Louis, Missouri

RICHARD J. MARTIN, MD
Drusinsky-Fanaroff Chair in Neonatology, Division of Neonatology, Department of Pediatrics, Rainbow Babies & Children's Hospital, Case Medical Center/University Hospitals; Professor of Pediatrics, Case Western Reserve University, Cleveland, Ohio

COLIN J. MORLEY, MD, FRCPCH, FRACP
Professor, Neonatal Research, The Royal Women's Hospital, Melbourne, Australia; Great Shelford, Cambridge, United Kingdom

MEGAN O'REILLY, PhD, BBiomedSc(Hons)
Department of Pediatrics, Women and Children Health Research Institute, University of Alberta, Edmonton, Alberta, Canada

ROBERT H. PFISTER, MD
Associate Professor of Pediatrics, University of Vermont, Burlington, Vermont

PROF. J. JANE PILLOW, BMedSci (Dist), MBBS, FRACP, PhD (Dist)
The Centre for Neonatal Research and Education; School of Women's and Infants' Health, The University of Western Australia, Perth; Neonatal Clinical Care Unit, King Edward Memorial Hospital, Western Australia, Australia

THOMAS M. RAFFAY, MD
Division of Neonatology, Department of Pediatrics, Rainbow Babies & Children's Hospital, Case Medical Center/University Hospitals, Cleveland, Ohio

JAMES D. REYNOLDS, PhD
Department of Anesthesia and Perioperative Medicine, Case Medical Center/University Hospitals; Institute for Transformative Molecular Medicine, Case Western Reserve University, Cleveland, Ohio

WADE RICH, RRT, CCRC
Clinical Research Coordinator, Division of Neonatology, Department of Pediatrics, University of California San Diego Medical Center, San Diego, California

PETER C. RIMENSBERGER, MD
Professor of Pediatrics, Pediatric and Neonatal ICU, Department of Pediatrics, University Hospital of Geneva, Geneva, Switzerland

JULIE RYU, MD
Assistant Professor, Department of Pediatrics, Rady Children's Hospital, University of California San Diego, La Jolla, California

RAKESH SAHNI, MD
Professor of Clinical Pediatrics, Division of Neonatal-Perinatal Medicine, Department of Pediatrics, College of Physicians and Surgeons, Columbia University, New York, New York

G.M. SANT'ANNA, MD, PhD, FRCPC
Associate Professor of Pediatrics, McGill University Health Center, Montreal, Québec, Canada

GAUTAM K. SINGH, MD
Professor of Pediatrics, Department of Pediatrics, Washington University School of Medicine, St Louis, Missouri

ROGER F. SOLL, MD
Professor of Pediatrics, University of Vermont, Burlington, Vermont

HOWARD STEIN, MD
Director of Neonatology, Clinical Associate Professor of Pediatrics, Department of Neonatology, Toledo Children's Hospital, Toledo, Ohio

BERNARD THÉBAUD, MSc, MD, PhD
Department of Pediatrics, Women and Children Health Research Institute, Cardiovascular Research Center, Department of Physiology, University of Alberta, Edmonton, Alberta, Canada

ANDREA TREMBATH, MD, MPH
Division of Neonatology, Rainbow Babies & Children's Hospital, Case Western Reserve University, Cleveland, Ohio

Contents

The immediate newborn transition is a time of great physiologic adjustments and many infants need assistance to make a successful transition to newborn life. Assisted ventilation is the most important intervention performed during this transitional period. Noninvasive ventilation is a necessary skill for all pediatric providers because it is the most frequently required life-saving measure provided in the delivery room. Providing ventilation in the least injurious manner is also necessary and many aspects of how this can best be done are still unknown. Following the normal physiology of fetal to neonatal transition continues to be a logical, but challenging, approach to initial ventilatory support of the newborn in the delivery room.

Very preterm infants are commonly exposed to a chronic, often asymptomatic, chorioamnionitis that is diagnosed by histologic evaluation of the placenta only after delivery. The reported effects of these exposures on fetal lungs are inconsistent because exposure to different organisms, durations of exposure, and fetal/maternal responses affect outcomes. In experimental models, chorioamnionitis can both injure and mature the fetal lung and cause immune nodulation. Postnatal care strategies also change how chorioamnionitis relates to clinical outcomes such as bronchopulmonary dysplasia.

This article explores the potential benefits and risks for the various approaches to the initial respiratory management of preterm infants. The authors focus on the evidence for the increasingly used strategies of initial respiratory support of preterm infants with continuous positive airway pressure (CPAP) beginning in the delivery room or very early in the hospital course and blended strategies involving the early administration of surfactant replacement followed by immediate extubation and stabilization on CPAP. Where possible, the evidence referenced in this review comes from individual randomized controlled trials or meta-analyses of those trials.

from mechanical ventilation is desirable. Weaning protocols may be help-ful in achieving more rapid reduction in support. There is no clear consen-sus regarding the level of support at which an infant is ready for extubation. An improved ability to predict when a preterm infant has a high likelihood of successful extubation is highly desirable. In this article, available evidence is reviewed and reasonable evidence-based recommendations for expedi-tious weaning and extubation are provided.

ventilation (in conjunction with continuous positive airway pressure), followed by prolonged permissive hypercapnia if mechanical ventilation is needed is an alternative to early ventilation and surfactant. Permissive hypercapnia may improve pulmonary outcomes and survival.

A growing understanding of endogenous nitric oxide (NO) biology is helping to explain how and when exogenous NO may confer benefit or harm; this knowledge is also helping to identify new better-targeted NO-based therapies. In this review, results of the bronchopulmonary dysplasia clinical trials that used inhaled NO in the preterm population are placed in context, the biologic basis for novel NO therapeutics is considered, and possible future directions for NO-focused clinical and basic research in developmental lung disease are identified.

No test can provide a definitive diagnosis of aerodigestive disease. When interpreting tests, one should weigh the benefits and weaknesses of different technologies and methods, scientific appropriateness of the testing conditions, clinicopathologic correlation, and pharmacologic approaches. Gastroesophageal reflux disease (GERD) symptoms and airway symptoms can coexist, and they cannot be distinguished without specific testing and direct observations. Important aerodigestive disorders include dysphagia, GERD, and aggravation of airway injury due to malfunctions of swallowing or airway protection mechanisms. Objective evaluation of aerodigestive reflexes and symptom correlation may provide support for evidence-based personalized management of feeding and airway protection strategies.

The pulmonary circulation rapidly adapts at birth to establish lungs as the site of gas exchange. Abnormal transition at birth and/or parenchymal lung disease can result in neonatal hypoxemic respiratory failure. This article reviews the functional changes in pulmonary hemodynamics and structural changes in pulmonary vasculature secondary to (1) normal and abnormal transition at birth, and (2) diseases associated with neonatal hypoxemic respiratory failure. Various management strategies to correct respiratory failure are also discussed.

Long-term increases in pulmonary vascular resistance and pulmonary arterial pressure resulting from structural alterations and abnormal vasoreactivity of the pulmonary vasculature may lead to right ventricular (RV) remodeling. Conventional methods of assessment of RV structure and function do not provide sensitive markers of RV remodeling for prognostic information. Advances in cardiac imaging have provided the capability to obtain quantitative information on the RV structure and function. This article reviews the clinical conditions that result in PH and discusses the novel and emerging methods for the assessment of right heart structure and function in PH in infants and children.

Recent advances in our understanding of stem/progenitor cells and their potential to repair damaged organs offer the possibility of cell-based treatments for neonatal lung injury. This review summarizes basic concepts of stem/progenitor cell biology and discusses the recent advances and challenges of cell-based therapies for lung diseases, with a particular focus on bronchopulmonary dysplasia (BPD), a form of chronic lung disease that primarily affects very preterm infants. Despite advances in perinatal care, BPD still remains the most common complication of extreme prematurity, and there is no specific treatment.

Brain injury is a frequent comorbidity in chronically ventilated preterm infants. However, the molecular basis of the brain injury remains incompletely understood. This article discusses the subtle (diffuse) form of brain injury that has white matter and gray matter lesions without germinal matrix hemorrhage–intraventricular hemorrhage, posthemorrhagic hydrocephalus, or cystic periventricular leukomalacia. This article synthesizes data that suggest that diffuse lesions to white matter and gray matter are collateral damage related to ventilator strategy. Evidence is introduced from the 2 large-animal, physiologic models of evolving neonatal chronic lung disease that suggest that an epigenetic mechanism may underlie the collateral damage.

GOAL STATEMENT

The goal of *Clinics in Perinatology* is to keep practicing neonatologists and maternal-fetal medicine specialists up to date with current clinical practice in perinatology by providing timely articles reviewing the state of the art in patient care.

ACCREDITATION

The *Clinics in Perinatology* is planned and implemented in accordance with the Essential Areas and Policies of the Accreditation Council for Continuing Medical Education (ACCME) through the joint sponsorship of the University of Virginia School of Medicine and Elsevier. The University of Virginia School of Medicine is accredited by the ACCME to provide continuing medical education for physicians.

The University of Virginia School of Medicine designates this enduring material activity for a maximum of 15 *AMA PRA Category 1 Credit*(s)™ for each issue, 60 credits per year. Physicians should only claim credit commensurate with the extent of their participation in the activity.

The American Medical Association has determined that physicians not licensed in the US who participate in this CME enduring material activity are eligible for a maximum of 15 *AMA PRA Category 1 Credit*(s)™ for each issue, 60 credits per year.

Credit can be earned by reading the text material, taking the CME examination online at http://www.theclinics.com/home/cme, and completing the evaluation. After taking the test, you will be required to review any and all incorrect answers. Following completion of the test and evaluation, your credit will be awarded and you may print your certificate.

FACULTY DISCLOSURE/CONFLICT OF INTEREST

The University of Virginia School of Medicine, as an ACCME accredited provider, endorses and strives to comply with the Accreditation Council for Continuing Medical Education (ACCME) Standards of Commercial Support, Commonwealth of Virginia statutes, University of Virginia policies and procedures, and associated federal and private regulations and guidelines on the need for disclosure and monitoring of proprietary and financial interests that may affect the scientific integrity and balance of content delivered in continuing medical education activities under our auspices.

The University of Virginia School of Medicine requires that all CME activities accredited through this institution be developed independently and be scientifically rigorous, balanced and objective in the presentation/discussion of its content, theories and practices.

All authors/editors participating in an accredited CME activity are expected to disclose to the readers relevant financial relationships with commercial entities occurring within the past 12 months (such as grants or research support, employee, consultant, stock holder, member of speakers bureau, etc.). The University of Virginia School of Medicine will employ appropriate mechanisms to resolve potential conflicts of interest to maintain the standards of fair and balanced education to the reader. Questions about specific strategies can be directed to the Office of Continuing Medical Education, University of Virginia School of Medicine, Charlottesville, Virginia.

The faculty and staff of the University of Virginia Office of Continuing Medical Education have no financial affiliations to disclose.

The authors/editors listed below have identified no professional or financial affiliations for themselves or their spouse/partner:

Kurt H. Albertine, PhD; Vineet Bhandari, MD, DM; Robert Boyle, MD (Test Author); Neil N. Finer, MD; Gabriel Haddad, MD; Aaron Hamvas, MD; Kerry Holland, (Acquisitions Editor); Mark R. Holland, PhD; Sudarshan R. Jadcherla, MD, FRCPI, DCH, AGAF; Lucky Jain, MD, MBA (Consulting Editor); Alan H. Jobe, MD, PhD; Tina A. Leone, MD; Philip T. Levy, MD; Richard J. Martin, MD; Megan O'Reilly, PhD; Robert H. Pfister, MD; Richard Polin, MD (Guest Editor); Thomas M. Raffay, MD; Wade Rich, RRT, CCRC; Peter C. Rimensberger, MD; Julie Ryu, MD; Rakesh Sahni, MD; G.M. Sant'Anna, MD, PhD, FRCPC; Gautam K. Singh, MD; Bernard Thébaud, MSc, MD, PhD; and Andrea Trembath, MD, MPH.

The authors/editors listed below identified the following professional or financial affiliations for themselves or their spouse/partner:

Judy L. Aschner, MD (Guest Editor) owns stock in Gilead Sciences.
Eduardo Bancalari, MD has a patent with CareFusion.
Waldemar A. Carlo, MD is on the Board of Directors for MEDNAX.
Nelson Claure, MSc, PhD receives research support and has a patent with CareFusion.
Kimberly Firestone, BS, RRT is on the Speakers' Bureau for Maquet Getinge Group.
Martin Keszler, MD is on the Advisory Board for Discovery Laboratories and Ikaria, Inc, is on the Speakers' Bureau for Ikaria, Inc. and Draeger Medical, Inc., and receives research support and is a consultant for Draeger Medical, Inc.
Satyan Lakshminrusimha, MD receives research support, is a consultant, and is on the Speakers' Bureau for Ikaria LLC.
Matthew M. Laughon, MD, MPH is a consultant (DSMB member) for Astellas and Pfizer, Inc.
Colin J. Morley, MD, FRCPCH, FRACP is a consultant and is on the Speakers' Bureau for Fisher and Paykel Healthcare and Drager Medical, and is a consultant for Laerdal Global Health.
J. Jane Pillow, BMedSci (Dist), MBBS, FRACP, PhD (Dist) receives research support from Fisher & Paykel Healthcare, Drager Medical, Care Fusion, Chiesi Farmaceutici, and Pari; is on the Speakers' Bureau for Drager Medical, SLE Pty Ltd, Ikaria, and Chiesi Farmaceutici; and is a consultant for Drager Medical.
James D. Reynolds, PhD owns stock in N30 Pharmaceuticals and Miach Medical Innovations.
Roger F. Soll, MD is employed by Vermont Oxford Network.
Howard Stein, MD is on the Speakers' Bureau for MAQUET.

TO ENROLL

CLINICS IN PERINATOLOGY

RELATED INTEREST

Obstetrics and Gynecology Clinics of North America, Volume 39, Issue 1 (March 2012)
Management of Preterm Birth: Best Practices in Prediction, Prevention, and Treatment
Alice Reeves Goepfert, MD, *Guest Editor*

DOWNLOAD
Free App!

Review Articles
THE CLINICS

NOW AVAILABLE FOR YOUR iPhone and iPad

Foreword

Respiratory Care of the Newborn: What Does the Future Hold?

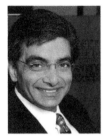

Lucky Jain, MD, MBA
Consulting Editor

Some of the most notable gains in neonatology since its origin as a subspecialty have come from advances in respiratory care. A sound understanding of the pathophysiology of lung disorders fueled the evolution of cutting-edge new therapies, many of which have withstood the test of time. Indeed, physiology of the developing lung was an essential element in any neonatology training curriculum and one could not pass the Neonatal-Perinatal Board exams in the United States without a flawless knowledge of LaPlace's Law, Poiseuille's Law, Bohr and Haldane equations, and various nerve-wracking calculations of dead space, ventilation/perfusion mismatch, etc. Continuous positive airway pressure,[1] surfactant,[2] nitric oxide,[3] and extracorporeal membrane oxygenation,[4] to name a few, all owe their origin to diligent observations in the laboratory with rigorous clinical trials to show safety and efficacy. Add to these antenatal steroids,[5] better perinatal management of the at-risk fetus, and a consistent approach to neonatal resuscitation: the gains in preventing neonatal deaths are truly outstanding[6] (**Fig. 1**). This is not to say that other areas of neonatal care have not contributed to the drop in mortality. Indeed, from elements of basic neonatal care such as temperature regulation and cord care to advances in anesthesia and surgical care, it would be impossible to create a rank list of winning interventions.

This discussion is relevant though, since significant gaps still persist in our knowledge of physiology and have surely contributed to shortfalls in our therapeutic armamentarium. For example, more than 50 years after the initial recognition of retinopathy of prematurity (and its relationship to high ambient oxygen), we are still grappling with what hemoglobin saturations to shoot for and how much oxygen to give to our tiniest neonates.[7] Chronic lung disease has found a permanent home in our NICUs and we still deal with ventilator-dependent infants who are several months old and refuse to wean off support. Steroids came and left with a lot of fanfare. The

perinatology.theclinics.com

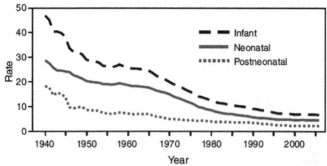

Fig. 1. Infant, neonatal, and postneonatal mortality rates in the United States [Deaths per 1000 live births for each group: infant (aged <1 year), neonatal (aged <28 days), and post-neonatal (aged 28 days to <1 year)].

mortality rate in congenital diaphragmatic hernia remains unacceptably high. Indeed, after the roaring decades of respiratory advances, the pace of new discoveries seems to have slowed down considerably.

This issue of the *Clinics in Perinatology* has done a great job in highlighting these and many other issues as they relate to advances in respiratory care of the newborn. Drs Aschner and Polin are to be congratulated to putting together a remarkable set of articles by thought-leaders in the field. Collectively, these writings issue a call for us to return to the basics: a rigorous pursuit of the underlying pathophysiologic processes is essential to uncover new frontiers of pulmonary biology that will yield the next set of enduring therapies.

Lucky Jain, MD, MBA
Department of Pediatrics
Emory University School of Medicine
2015 Uppergate Drive
Atlanta, GA 30322, USA

E-mail address:
ljain@emory.edu

REFERENCES

1. Gregory GA, Edmunds LH Jr, Kitterman JA, et al. Continuous positive airway pressure and pulmonary and circulatory function after cardiac surgery in infants less than three months of age. Anesthesiology 1975;43(4):426–31.
2. Avery ME. Surfactant deficiency in hyaline membrane disease: the story of discovery. Am J Respir Crit Care Med 2000;161(4 Pt 1):1074–5.
3. Ignarro LJ. Nitric oxide as a unique signaling molecule in the vascular system: a historical overview. J Physiol Pharmacol 2002;53(4 Pt 1):503–14.
4. Bartlett RH. Extracorporeal life support: history and new directions. ASAIO J 2005; 51(5):487–9.
5. Liggins GC, Howie RN. A controlled trial of antepartum glucocorticoid treatment for prevention of the respiratory distress syndrome in premature infants. Pediatrics 1972;50(4):515–25.
6. Heron M, Hoyert DL, Murphy SL, et al. Deaths: final data for 2006. Natl Vital Stat Rep 2009;57(14):1–134.
7. Carlo WA, Finer NN, Walsh MC, et al. Target ranges of oxygen saturation in extremely preterm infants. N Engl J Med 2010;362(21):1959–69.

Preface

Advances in Respiratory Care of the Newborn

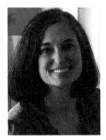 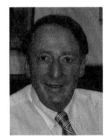

Judy L. Aschner, MD   Richard A. Polin, MD
Guest Editors

Advances in respiratory care defined the early decades of neonatology and drove improvements in neonatal morbidity and mortality. Surfactant replacement therapy, the culmination of years of basic and translational research, changed the management and outcomes for preterm infants with respiratory distress and set a very high bar for the introduction of new evidenced-based therapies in the NICU. More recent advances in respiratory care have been driven by technological developments and bioengineering tours de force. Yet, more than 60 years after the discovery of surfactant, we are still struggling to define the optimal approach to the respiratory management of our patients. In this edition of *Clinics in Perinatology* we have chosen cutting-edge topics in the diagnosis and management of respiratory diseases spanning the full spectrum of neonatal care. The topics have been carefully chosen with the goal of presenting both the current state of the art and a glimpse into what the future may hold for "advances in respiratory care of the newborn." It is clear there is still much more work to be done.

We want to thank all of the authors for their comprehensive contributions to this volume. The invited authors for this edition of *Clinics in Perinatology* are trailblazers in their respective fields of investigation and the thought-leaders in our subspecialty. They have summarized the literature and identified gaps in our knowledge. In many cases, they have shared their views on the most promising future therapies and approaches, based on their own innovative investigations in human infants and animal models of neonatal respiratory disease. We hope you will agree that this edition serves

Clin Perinatol 39 (2012) xvii–xviii
http://dx.doi.org/10.1016/j.clp.2012.07.002   **perinatology.theclinics.com**

as an indispensible resource for trainees, advance practice nurses, respiratory therapists, and neonatologists at all stages of their careers.

Judy L. Aschner, MD
Vanderbilt University School of Medicine
11111 Doctor's Office Tower
2200 Children's Way
Nashville, TN 37232-9544, USA

Richard A. Polin, MD
Morgan Stanley Children's Hospital of New York
3959 Broadway
CHN 1201
New York, NY 10032, USA

E-mail addresses:
judy.aschner@vanderbilt.edu (J.L. Aschner)
rap32@columbia.edu (R.A. Polin)

Delivery Room Respiratory Management of the Term and Preterm Infant

Tina A. Leone, MD[b], Neil N. Finer, MD[a],*, Wade Rich, RRT, CCRC[c]

KEYWORDS

- Neonatal resuscitation • Ventilation • CPAP • Oxygen

KEY POINTS

- The immediate newborn transition is a time of great physiologic adjustments and many infants need assistance to make a successful transition to newborn life.
- Assisted ventilation is the most important intervention performed during this transitional period.
- Noninvasive ventilation is a necessary skill for all pediatric providers because it is the most frequently required lifesaving measure provided in the delivery room.
- Providing ventilation in the least injurious manner is also necessary and many aspects of how this can best be done are still unknown.
- Following the normal physiology of fetal to neonatal transition continues to be a logical, but challenging, approach to initial ventilatory support of the newborn in the delivery room.

Establishing adequate ventilation is the most important step in neonatal resuscitation. Most newborn infants initiate spontaneous breathing without intervention shortly after birth. Those who do not begin breathing on their own can require a significant amount of support from their care providers. Many preterm infants need additional support to allow adequate oxygenation and ventilation even if they are breathing spontaneously. During the transition from fetal to newborn life, the infant must replace fetal lung fluid with air, establishing functional residual capacity (FRC) in the lung, and increase pulmonary blood flow, transitioning from placental to pulmonary gas exchange. The infant initiates this process by taking the first breaths after birth. When care providers need to assist ventilation, it is often difficult to mimic the natural process. The goals of

Disclosures: The authors have no financial relationships conflicts of interest to disclose.
[a] Division of Neonatology, Department of Pediatrics, University of California San Diego School of Medicine, University of California San Diego Medical Center, 402 Dickinson Street, MPF 1-140, San Diego, CA 92103, USA; [b] University of California San Diego School of Medicine, University of California San Diego Medical Center, 402 Dickinson Street, MPF 1-140, San Diego, CA 92103, USA; [c] Division of Neonatology, Department of Pediatrics, University of California San Diego Medical Center, 402 Dickinson Street, MPF 1-140, San Diego, CA 92103, USA
* Corresponding author.
E-mail address: nfiner@ucsd.edu

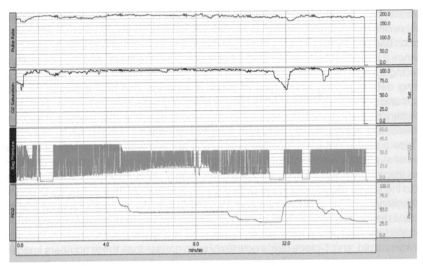

Fig. 1. Inadvertent increase in PEEP using a T-piece resuscitator.

Pressure and Volume

Lung injury occurs as a consequence of assisted ventilation. Providing the amount of ventilation that is needed to help a baby transition after birth while causing the least amount of lung injury is a major goal of resuscitation. Lung injury is thought to be caused by excessive pressure or excessive volume delivery to diseased or immature lungs. Repeated opening followed by complete closing of lung units is an important mechanism of lung injury. Therefore, maintaining FRC is critical to minimizing lung injury. Animal models have shown that PEEP helps develop and maintain FRC.[23] It is likely that the rapid development and maintenance of FRC will prevent the need for excessive PIPs. In spontaneously breathing infants, CPAP can similarly help maintain FRC. Most ventilation in newborn resuscitation continues to be provided with pressure targeting. Pressure targets are chosen arbitrarily. Infants spontaneously breathing after birth generate high pressures on the first breaths after birth. Many infants have some spontaneous breathing but still need additional support. The spontaneous breaths are important in helping clear lung fluid and develop FRC. In infants who do not breathe at all, the level of support necessary to achieve physiologic stability is often much more than the level of support needed for spontaneously breathing infants. Our resuscitation practice includes the use of sustained inflations up to 5 seconds in duration, followed by an increase in PIP early in the ventilation algorithm if the heart rate is less than 100 beats per minute (bpm) and is not responding, especially if a good indication of end-tidal CO_2 is not seen. Others have described providing ventilation based on tidal volume targets. Similar to pressure targeting, the best tidal volume to target immediately after delivery is not known. The normal term spontaneously breathing infant takes breaths of varying tidal volumes, with the first breaths taken up to an average of 10 to 12 mL/kg.[24] In a randomized controlled trial of tidal volume monitoring for management of ventilation, Schmölzer and colleagues[25] found that use of a tidal volume monitor allowed the number of breaths with very high tidal volumes to be limited.

Oxygen

The period following delivery is unique in that it is the only time during life when it is normal to have SpO_2 values as low as 30%. These values then increase over the next

7 to 10 minutes of life to values of 85% to 95%. Fetal development occurs in a low-oxygen environment, with intrauterine PaO_2 levels of 15 to 30 mm Hg, resulting in fetal SpO_2 levels of 45% to 55%, and, following delivery, these levels may initially decrease before gradually increasing to between 50 and 80 mm Hg ($SpO_2 > 90\%$) depending on the status of the lungs, the pulmonary circulation, and the presence of other stressors at delivery. During resuscitation with 100% oxygen, the PaO_2 may increase to greater than 80 mm Hg within 5 minutes of birth. Vento and colleagues[26] reported that infants resuscitated with pure oxygen had PaO_2 levels of more than 100 mm Hg by 5 to 6 min, whereas infants resuscitated with air did not exceed 80 to 90 mm Hg.

Preterm infants have lower antioxidant capacities consistent with their expected low-oxygen fetal environment. Multiple morbid conditions associated with extreme immaturity may be potentiated by an excess of oxygen free radicals in infants intrinsically deficient in antioxidants.[27–30] The fetus and premature infant are susceptible to inflammation and infections that lead to an increased oxidative stress. Silvers and colleagues[31,32] reported that low plasma antioxidant activity at birth in premature infants was an independent risk factor for mortality.

Assisted ventilation with 100% oxygen immediately after birth has been associated with increased risk of childhood lymphatic leukemia.[33–35] The risk was higher if the manual ventilation lasted for 3 minutes or more. Spector and colleagues,[36] using the Collaborative Perinatal Project, also reported an association between oxygen use for 3 minutes or longer following delivery and later cancer in childhood.

Several studies have compared the use of pure oxygen with air for the initial resuscitation of depressed term newborn infants.[37,38] The Resair 2 study reported that death within 7 days and/or moderate or severe hypoxic-ischemic encephalopathy was not significantly different between the groups. In a meta-analysis including 10 studies, of which 6 were randomized trials, the risk of neonatal mortality was reduced in the air group compared with the 100% O_2 group, both in the analysis of all studies and in the analysis of strictly randomized studies.[39] Similar results were published by Davis and colleagues[40] and Tan and colleagues.[41]

Few randomized studies have compared fraction of inspired oxygen (FiO_2) concentrations for the resuscitation of the preterm infant. Harling and colleagues[42] performed the first resuscitation trial of infants of less than 31 weeks' gestation with either 50% or 100% oxygen for the resuscitation period and found no significant differences in cytokines, death, or survival without bronchopulmonary dysplacia (BPD). All subsequent trials in preterm infants comparing a high versus low oxygen concentration used a targeted oxygen saturation strategy. These studies showed that initiating resuscitation with lower oxygen concentrations can decrease the total oxygen exposure, decrease the level of oxidative stress measured during the first month of life, and may be associated with less chronic lung disease.[43] However, the prospective studies and experiential data suggest that preterm infants frequently need some oxygen during resuscitation to achieve expected oxygen saturation levels or clinical stability. As noted in our review, there is a need for large prospective trials to compare room air with a higher initial FiO_2, and to report the important long-term outcomes of such infants.

Oxygen Saturation Targets

It is not known how to adjust the oxygen concentration during neonatal resuscitation. The currently suggested strategies are based on observed oxygen saturation values recorded from infants who transitioned without any interventions. The most extensive compilation of these normal data was published by Dawson and colleagues[44] as curves composed of 3rd to 97th percentile values. It has been presumed that maintaining SpO_2 levels within these normal curves is a safe practice. Whether maintaining levels near the lower percentiles versus higher percentiles would be more or less safe is not known at this time. Because these normal values change over the first 15 minutes of life, it is not easy to target these levels without some aid. Our group has used a computer-assisted device that plots an infant's SpO_2 level on the normal curve and allows the resuscitation team to adjust FiO_2 if the infant's values move outside the curve (**Fig. 2**). We chose to use the 10th and 50th percentiles as the outer limits of the curves for our target SpO_2 levels. This Transitional Oxygen Targeting System (TOTS) has been effective at decreasing the amount of time that infants spend outside the targeted range.[45]

The most appropriate response of the resuscitation team to SpO_2 values less than the normal range is not known. Providing assisted ventilation, increasing the level of assisted ventilation, or increasing the inspired oxygen concentration are all possible responses to a low SpO_2 level. Providing assisted ventilation should be the first response if the infant is not breathing or the heart rate is low. However, increasing the FiO_2 is an important intervention if SpO_2 values remain low.

CPAP

CPAP has been used as the initial respiratory support for preterm infants for many years by many centers. However, the early use of CPAP has only recently been tested in randomized trials compared with early surfactant. The largest of these trials, SUPPORT (Surfactant Positive Airway Pressure and Pulse Oximetry Trial), showed that infants of 24 to 25 weeks' gestation randomized to CPAP in the delivery room with a limited ventilator strategy had 8% less death than infants treated with surfactant administered within an hour of birth and conventional ventilator management. The subsequent follow-up of these infants did not show any increase in neurodevelopmental disabilities with the use of early CPAP.[46]

Several trials have compared early CPAP with early surfactant or ventilation[47–49] and have shown no benefit to routine intubation and surfactant administration. A small number of infants require intubation for resuscitation in the delivery room. For those who do not require intubation for resuscitation, we recommend the continuing use

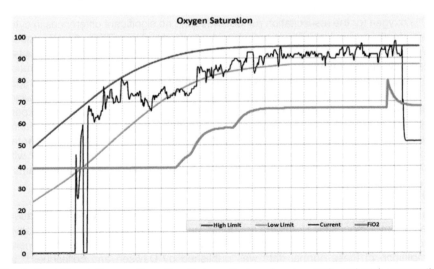

Fig. 2. Transitional Oxygen Targeting System display, showing 10th and 50th percentile curves, real-time oxygen saturation, and FiO_2.

of CPAP and intermittent PPV until it is clear that the infant cannot maintain adequate ventilation, at which time intubation is recommended. With the increasing use of CPAP, we have now observed that some very immature infants on CPAP alone can experience significant hypercarbia. It is now our practice for such very immature infants on CPAP to administer minimum positive pressure breaths via bag/mask until a blood gas or CO_2 monitoring is available. Infants not requiring intubation for resuscitation are most effectively treated with CPAP until criteria are met for surfactant therapy.

Intubation

Ventilation can most often be delivered effectively during the immediate neonatal transition using noninvasive devices. Endotracheal intubation is indicated when the infant remains apneic despite adequate noninvasive ventilation, when the heart rate remains less than 100 bpm despite adequate attempts to provide noninvasive ventilation, or when desired SpO_2 levels cannot be achieved with noninvasive ventilation and supplemental oxygen. Appropriate responses to insufficient noninvasive ventilation include adjusting the head and mask positioning to ensure an open airway, increasing the inspiratory pressure, and possibly providing a sustained inflation. If there is an indication of end-tidal CO_2 presence with these maneuvers, it is worth continuing to deliver ventilation in that mode without interruption as the infant is beginning to improve. The endotracheal intubation procedure is often destabilizing to the baby, leading to bradycardia and desaturation. During the intubation procedure, the infant does not receive any assisted ventilation and can therefore lose FRC. Intubation attempts of greater than 30 seconds are associated with increased frequency of bradycardia and desaturation. It is therefore our practice to limit all attempts to 30 seconds and to stop to provide mask ventilation to reestablish acceptable heart rate and SpO_2 in between attempts.[50] O'Donnell and colleagues[51] reviewed videos of intubations performed during neonatal resuscitation and found that decreases in heart rate and SpO_2 occurred more commonly when these parameters were low before the procedure. It is therefore beneficial to begin the procedure with the infant in the most stable condition possible. In the NICU, the American Academy of Pediatrics has recommended use of premedication before intubation. Many infants can be stabilized with noninvasive ventilation and then intubated at a later time, if necessary, for surfactant or invasive ventilation. The team can then perform the intubation in a more controlled manner. An intravenous line can then be placed and premedication can be given before intubation. Using regular video review of all newborn resuscitations, we have seen infants with severe hydrops fetalis stabilized with mask ventilation and drainage of body cavities, allowing an increase in heart rate to normal levels before intubation. We are currently giving premedication in the delivery room for selected cases, and our initial experience suggests that this approach is feasible and can most often be done using a peripherally inserted intravenous line without the need for a central line. Training in neonatal intubation is not easy and requires many experiences to achieve consistent success. In the current training framework in the United States, general pediatricians are not given an adequate exposure to neonatal intubation during training to develop competence. The most recent proposed training guidelines will eliminate the requirement for pediatric residents to become competent at endotracheal intubation. If implemented, this further emphasizes the need to develop excellent skills for providing noninvasive ventilation.

SUMMARY

The immediate newborn transition is a time of great physiologic adjustments and many infants need assistance to make a successful transition to newborn life. Assisted ventilation is the most important intervention performed during this transitional period. Noninvasive ventilation is a necessary skill for all pediatric providers because it is the most frequently required lifesaving measure provided in the delivery room. Providing ventilation in the least injurious manner is also necessary and many aspects of how this can best be done are still unknown. Following the normal physiology of fetal to neonatal transition continues to be a logical, but challenging, approach to initial ventilatory support of the newborn in the delivery room.

REFERENCES

1. Katheria A, Rich W, Finer N. Obtaining a continuous heart rate during neonatal resuscitation: EKG versus pulse oximetry. E-PAS2012:2855.4. Proceedings of the 2012 Pediatric Academic Society Meeting, Boston MA.
2. Poulton DA, Schmolzer GM, Morley CJ, et al. Assessment of chest rise during mask ventilation of preterm infants in the delivery room. Resuscitation 2011;82:175–9.
3. Brugada M, Schilleman K, Witlox RS, et al. Variability in the assessment of 'adequate' chest excursion during simulated neonatal resuscitation. Neonatology 2011;100:99–104.
4. Tracy M, Downe L, Holberton J. How safe is intermittent positive pressure ventilation in preterm babies ventilated from delivery room to newborn intensive care unit? Arch Dis Child Fetal Neonatal Ed 2004;89:F84–7.
5. Finer NN, Rich W, Wang C, et al. Airway obstruction during mask ventilation of very low birth weight infants during neonatal resuscitation. Pediatrics 2009;123:865–9.
6. Leone TA, Lange A, Rich W, et al. Disposable colorimetric carbon dioxide detector use as an indicator of a patent airway during noninvasive mask ventilation. Pediatrics 2006;118:e202–4.
7. Aziz HF, Martin JB, Moore JJ. The pediatric disposable end-tidal carbon dioxide detector role in endotracheal intubation in newborns. J Perinatol 1999;19:110–3.
8. Repetto JE, Donohue PA-C PK, Baker SF, et al. Use of capnography in the delivery room for assessment of endotracheal tube placement. J Perinatol 2001;21:284–7.
9. Wood FE, Morley CJ, Dawson JA, et al. Improved techniques reduce face mask leak during simulated neonatal resuscitation: study 2. Arch Dis Child Fetal Neonatal 2008;93:F230–4.
10. O'Donnell CP, Davis PG, Morley CJ. Positive pressure ventilation at neonatal resuscitation: review of equipment and survey of practice. Acta Paediatr 2004; 93:583–8.
11. O'Donnell CP, Davis PG, Morley CJ. Neonatal resuscitation: review of ventilation equipment and survey of practice in Australia and New Zealand. J Paediatr Child Health 2004;40:208–12.
12. Roehr CC, Grobe S, Rudiger M, et al. Delivery room management of very low birth weight infants in Germany, Austria and Switzerland—a comparison of protocols. Eur J Med Res 2010;15:493–503.
13. Iriondo M, Thio M, Buron E, et al. A survey of neonatal resuscitation in Spain: gaps between guidelines and practice. Acta Paediatr 2009;98:786–91.
14. Finer N, Rich W, Craft A, et al. Comparison of methods of bag and mask ventilation for neonatal resuscitation. Resuscitation 2001;49(3):299–305.
15. Bennett S, Finer N, Rich W, et al. A comparison of three neonatal resuscitation devices. Resuscitation 2005;67(1):113–8.
16. Finer NN, Rich W. Unintentional variation in positive end expiratory pressure during resuscitation with a T-piece resuscitator. Resuscitation 2011;82:717–9.

17. Hoskyns EW, Milner AD, Hopkin IE. A simple method of face mask resuscitation at birth. Arch Dis Child 1987;62:376–8.
18. Klingenberg C, Dawson JA, Gerber A, et al. Sustained inflations: comparing three neonatal resuscitation devices. Neonatology 2011;100:78–84.
19. te Pas AB, Siew M, Wallace MJ, et al. Establishing functional residual capacity at birth: the effect of sustained inflation and positive end-expiratory pressure in a preterm rabbit model. Pediatr Res 2009;65:537–41.
20. Sobotka KS, Hooper SB, Allison BJ, et al. An initial sustained inflation improves the respiratory and cardiovascular transition at birth in preterm lambs. Pediatr Res 2011;70:56–60.
21. Klingenberg C, Sobotka KS, Ong T, et al. Effect of sustained inflation duration; resuscitation of near-term asphyxiated lambs. Arch Dis Child Fetal Neonatal Ed 2012 July 10. [Epub ahead of print].
22. Lindner W, Hogel J, Pohlandt F. Sustained pressure-controlled inflation or intermittent mandatory ventilation in preterm infants in the delivery room? A randomized controlled trial on initial respiratory support via nasopharyngeal tube. Acta Paediatr 2005;94:303–9.
23. Siew ML, te Pas AB, Wallace MJ, et al. Positive end-expiratory pressure enhances development of a functional residual capacity in preterm rabbits ventilated from birth. J Appl Physiol 2009;106:1487–93.
24. Vyas H, Milner AD, Hopkins IE. Intrathoracic pressure and volume changes during the spontaneous onset of respiration in babies born by cesarean section and by vaginal delivery. J Pediatr 1981;99:787–91.
25. Schmölzer GM, Morley CJ, Wong C, et al. Respiratory function monitor guidance of mask ventilation in the delivery room: a feasibility study. J Pediatr 2012;160: 377–381.e2.
26. Vento M, Asensi M, Sastre J, et al. Oxidative stress in asphyxiated term infants resuscitated with 100% oxygen. J Pediatr 2003;142:240–6.
27. Vento M, Aguar M, Escobar J, et al. Antenatal steroids and antioxidant enzyme activity in preterm infants: influence of gender and timing. Antioxid Redox Signal 2009;11(12):2945–55.
28. Smith CV, Hansen TN, Martin NE, et al. Oxidant stress responses in premature infants during exposure to hyperoxia. Pediatr Res 1993;34:360–5.
29. Frank L, Sosenko IR. Development of lung antioxidant enzyme system in late gestation: possible implications for the prematurely born infant. J Pediatr 1987;110:9–14.
30. Walther FJ, Wade AB, Warburton D, et al. Ontogeny of antioxidant enzymes in the fetal lamb lung. Exp Lung Res 1991;17:39–45.
31. Silvers KM, Gibson AT, Russell JM, et al. Antioxidant activity, packed cell transfusions, and outcome in premature infants. Arch Dis Child 1998;78(3):F214–9.
32. Kumar VH, Swartz D, Nielsen LC, et al. Resuscitation in room air compared to 100% oxygen lowers oxidative stress without increasing metabolic acidosis in term newborn lambs. PAS 2005;57:37.
33. Paneth N. The evidence mounts against use of pure oxygen in newborn resuscitation. J Pediatr 2005;147(1):4–6.
34. Naumburg E. Results of recent research on perinatal risk factors: resuscitation using oxygen increases the risk of childhood leukemia. Lakartidningen 2002; 99(24):2745–7.
35. Naumburg E, Bellocco R, Cnattingius S, et al. Supplementary oxygen and risk of childhood lymphatic leukaemia. Acta Paediatr 2002;91(12):1328–33.
36. Spector LG, Klebanoff MA, Feusner JH, et al. Childhood cancer following neonatal oxygen supplementation. J Pediatr 2005;147(1):27–31.

37. Ramji S, Ahuja S, Thirupuram S, et al. Resuscitation of asphyxic newborn infants with room air or 100% oxygen. Pediatr Res 1993;34(6):809–12.

38. Saugstad OD, Rootwelt T, Aalen O. Resuscitation of asphyxiated newborn infants with room air or oxygen: an international controlled trial: the Resair 2 study. Pediatrics 1998;102(1):E11–7.

39. Saugstad OD, Ramji S, Soll RF, et al. Resuscitation of newborn infants with 21% or 100% oxygen: an updated systematic review and meta-analysis. Neonatology 2008;94(3):176–82.

40. Davis PG, Tan A, O'Donnell CP, et al. Resuscitation of newborn infants with 100% oxygen or air: a systematic review and meta-analysis. Lancet 2004;364(9442): 1329–33.

41. Tan A, Schulze A, O'Donnell CP, et al. Air versus oxygen for resuscitation of infants at birth. Cochrane Database Syst Rev 2005;2:CD002273.

42. Harling AE, Beresford MW, Vince GS, et al. Does use of 50% oxygen at birth in preterm infants reduce lung injury? Arch Dis Child Fetal Neonatal Ed 2005;90: F401–5.

43. Finer N, Saugstad O, Vento M, et al. Use of oxygen for resuscitation of the extremely low birth weight infant. Pediatrics 2010 Feb;125(2):389–91.

44. Dawson JA, Kamlin CO, Wong C, et al. Defining the reference range for oxygen saturation for infants after birth. Pediatrics 2010;125:e1340–7.

45. Gandhi BB, Rich WD, Finer NN. Improving oxygen saturation targeting during neonatal resuscitation. E-PAS2012:2855.6. Proceedings of the 2012 Pediatric Academic Society Meeting, Boston MA.

46. Finer NN, Carlo WA, Walsh M, et al. Early CPAP versus surfactant in extremely preterm infants. N Engl J Med 2010;362(21):1970–9.

47. Morley CJ, Davis PG, Doyle LW, et al. Nasal CPAP or intubation at birth for very preterm infants. N Engl J Med 2008;358:700–8.

48. Dunn MS, Kaempf J, de Klerk A, et al. Randomized trial comparing 3 approaches to the initial respiratory management of preterm neonates. Pediatrics 2011;128: e1069.

49. Sandri F, Plavka R, Ancora G, et al. Prophylactic or early selective surfactant combined with nCPAP in very preterm infants. Pediatrics 2010 Jun;125(6): e1402–9.

50. Lane B, Finer N, Rich W. Duration of intubation attempts during neonatal resuscitation. J Pediatr 2004 Jul;145(1):67–70.

51. O'Donnell CP, Kamlin CO, Davis PG, et al. Endotracheal intubation attempts during neonatal resuscitation: success rates, duration and adverse effects. Pediatrics 2006;117:e16–21.

Effects of Chorioamnionitis on the Fetal Lung

Alan H. Jobe, MD, PhD

KEYWORDS

- Respiratory distress syndrome • Bronchopulmonary dysplasia • Lung development
- Lung maturation • Lung injury

KEY POINTS

- Very preterm infants are commonly exposed to a chronic, often asymptomatic, chorioamnionitis that is diagnosed by histologic evaluation of the placenta only after delivery.
- The reported effects of these exposures on fetal lungs are inconsistent because exposure to different organisms, durations of exposure, and fetal/maternal responses affect outcomes.
- In experimental models, chorioamnionitis can both injure and mature the fetal lung and cause immune nodulation.
- Postnatal care strategies also change how chorioamnionitis relates to clinical outcomes such as bronchopulmonary dysplasia.

CHORIOAMNIONITIS: A MULTIFACETED FETAL EXPOSURE

Overview

There is no consensus about the relationships between chorioamnionitis and 3 pulmonary outcomes of concern for preterm infants: respiratory distress syndrome (RDS), pneumonia/sepsis, and bronchopulmonary dysplasia (BPD). The difficulty in defining clear relationships results from the multiple variables contributing to the antenatal exposures, the postnatal exposures, and care strategies that contribute to the diagnoses of the short-term outcomes of RDS and pneumonia/sepsis, and the longer term outcome of BPD. Multivariate analyses of large data sets are imperfect tools to define relationships because of the inter-related nature of the variables, the poorly defined fetal exposures, and the imprecision of diagnosis of diseases such as RDS and BPD. This article discusses these problems based on the clinical data. In contrast, research with animal models provides solid information about how experimental chorioamnionitis can affect the fetal lung. The combination of an appreciation of the clinical complexity and the experimental effects of chorioamnionitis provides insight into

Division of Pulmonary Biology, Cincinnati Children's Hospital Medical Center, University of Cincinnati, 3333 Burnet Avenue, ML#7029, Cincinnati, OH 45229-3039, USA
E-mail address: alan.jobe@cchmc.org

Clin Perinatol 39 (2012) 441–457
http://dx.doi.org/10.1016/j.clp.2012.06.010
0095-5108/12/$ – see front matter © 2012 Elsevier Inc. All rights reserved.
perinatology.theclinics.com

how individual preterm infants present and respond to therapy. The focus of this article is the lungs of preterm infants born at less than 32 weeks' gestation, during the period of saccular expansion and before alveolarization.

Diagnosis

Chorioamnionitis can be diagnosed before the infant is born by findings such as maternal fever, increased white blood cell count, tender uterus, and by amniotic fluid analyses for bacteria, inflammatory mediators, or inflammatory cells. Histologic chorioamnionitis is a postdelivery diagnosis that is graded by the amount of inflammatory cells and the amount of necrosis in the chorioamnion.[1] The diagnosis of clinical chorioamnionitis does not reliably predict the presence or severity of histologic chorioamnionitis, which is more common following very preterm birth. Furthermore, the diagnosis of histologic chorioamnionitis is not reproducible between pathologists.[1]

The diagnosis of chorioamnionitis correlates with the clinical presentation of a pregnancy at risk for very preterm delivery. Preterm premature rupture of membranes is a surrogate for chorioamnionitis with a high concordance. Preterm labor of unknown cause or with a short cervix is frequently associated with chorioamnionitis.[2] In various populations, 50% to 70% of women delivering very preterm infants have chorioamnionitis, with the incidence increasing as gestation at delivery decreases.[2,3]

The Organisms

The organisms associated with early gestational delivery can be single species or polymicrobial aerobic and anabolic isolates that generally are vaginal flora (**Table 1**).[4] More than 50% of amniotic fluids collected by amniocentesis or at cesarean delivery from women with preterm premature rupture of membranes were positive for *Ureaplasma*.[5] These organisms are not usually considered to be pathogens. The generally accepted pathway to the subclinical histologic chorioamnionitis associated with very preterm birth is a diffuse ascending colonization of the endometrial-chorionic space with extension into the fetal membranes, the amniotic fluid, and ultimately the fetus.[6] Recent pathologic analyses suggest that another route may be more common. A localized epithelial colonization of the endometrium may breach the chorioamnion locally, contaminating the amniotic fluid with subsequent extension to the fetal membranes and fetus.[7] The identification of organisms associated with chorioamnionitis by culture does not capture the entire population of organisms; more noncultivable organisms can be identified by polymerase chain reaction (PCR).[8]

Table 1
Organisms cultured from chorion in association with preterm deliveries[a]

Organism Type			
Ureaplasma/Mycoplasma	Aerobes	Anaerobes	% of Culture-Positive Placentas[a]
+	−	−	9
−	+	−	30
−	−	+	21
+	+	−	3
+	−	+	4
−	+	+	28
+	+	+	6

[a] 51% of 1365 placentas were culture positive.
Data from Onderdonk AB, Delaney ML, DuBois AM, et al. Detection of bacteria in placental tissues obtained from extremely low gestational age neonates. Am J Obstet Gynecol 2008; 198:110.e1–7.

Duration of Fetal Exposure

Ureaplasma parvum and *Mycoplasma hominis* are the organisms most frequently associated with very early gestation deliveries (**Box 1**).[4,5] These organisms are normal vaginal flora in 67% of women of reproductive age.[9] However, *Ureaplasma* was also identified in about 12% of 433 amniotic fluids collected for genetic analysis from normal pregnancies before 20 weeks' gestation.[10,11] Only 7% of the *Ureaplasma*-positive amniotic fluids were associated with preterm delivery. This behavior of *Ureaplasma* in human pregnancy is similar to experimental infection in fetal sheep. Fetal sheep exposed to intra-amniotic *Ureaplasma* at 50 days' gestation have high titers of organisms continuously for 100 days to term, with a 20% fetal loss.[12] Some animals have chorioamnionitis and others do not despite persistence of the organism. There is no information about the potential for the multiple other organisms associated with prematurity to cause prolonged fetal exposures. Women with preterm labors that progress to ruptured membranes and then delayed delivery presumably carry fetuses with bacterial exposures for days to months.

The Fetal Exposure

The fetal response to chorioamnionitis should, intuitively, depend on the organisms and the duration of the exposure. However, for early gestation deliveries, there is little clinical information correlating organism or duration of exposure with fetal response. The exposure is complex because both the bacteria and products of the inflammation bathe the chorioamnion (fetal tissue) and the fetal skin. The fetal gut is exposed from swallowed amniotic fluid.[6] Amniotic fluid also mixes with fetal lung fluid by fetal breathing causing a lung exposure.[13] Thus, the fetal lung is just 1 organ that can respond to chorioamnionitis. Funisitis is an infiltration of fetal inflammatory cells around the vessels of the cord, indicating a systemic fetal response and perhaps a longer duration of fetal exposure or more pathogenic organisms.[14]

RESPONSES OF THE FETAL LUNG TO CHORIOAMNIONITIS: CLINICAL RESPONSES
An Overview

The instinctive response of the clinician to a diffuse lung exposure to bacteria and inflammatory products is to assume that the outcome will be an acute pneumonia. In the preterm, pneumonia caused by pathogens often is accompanied by sepsis because of immature innate immune defenses. However, for the 9595 infants with birth gestations of 22 to 28 weeks cared for in the National Institute of Child Health and Human Development Neonatal Research Network between 2003 and 2007, only 2% had early onset sepsis diagnosed by positive blood culture.[15] The diagnosis of pneumonia was so infrequent that it was not reported. Nevertheless, 25% of the population had rupture of membranes more than 24 hours before delivery and 48%

Box 1
Variables contributing to chorioamnionitis

- Organisms: single microbes and polymicrobial organisms
- Duration of exposure in utero
- Intensity of maternal and fetal inflammatory responses
- Rupture of membranes
- Therapies that modulate infection: antibiotics and antenatal corticosteroids

had a pathologic diagnosis of chorioamnionitis. Although many of these infants must have had a fetal pulmonary exposure, no clinical syndrome of lung infection was recognized. However, tracheal aspirates from infants exposed to chorioamnionitis and collected at intubation shortly after birth contain increased proinflammatory cells, cytokines, and prostaglandins as indicators of a fetal lung response.[16,17] *Ureaplasma* of antenatal origin can be cultured or identified by PCR from 20% to 45% of these preterm infants.[18,19] Thus, these very preterm infants have frequent but generally silent lung exposures to infection/inflammation.

Chorioamnionitis and RDS

A decreased incidence of RDS was associated in 1974 with preterm prolonged rupture of the membranes, a surrogate marker for chorioamnionitis.[20] Watterberg and colleagues[16] then reported that ventilated preterm infants exposed to histologic chorioamnionitis had a lower incidence of RDS, but a higher incidence of BPD, than infants not exposed to chorioamnionitis. The exposure to histologic chorioamnionitis decreased the incidence of RDS for a consecutive series of 446 preterm births of less than 32 weeks' gestational age, but histologic chorioamnionitis with isolation of *Ureaplasma* or *Mycoplasma* from cord blood did not correlate with a decreased risk of RDS.[14,21] Lahra and colleagues[22] also noted in a population of 724 preterm infants that RDS was decreased for infants exposed to histologic chorioamnionitis (odds ratio [OR] 0.49, 95% confidence interval [CI] 0.31–0.78) or chorioamnionitis plus funisitis (OR 0.23, 95% CI 0.15–0.35) relative to no chorioamnionitis. This group also reported their 13-year experience that histologic chorioamnionitis (with or without funisitis) was associated with a decreased risk of BPD (OR 0.58, 95% CI 0.51–0.67).[3]

In contrast, there are other reports associating chorioamnionitis with poor pulmonary and other outcomes. Hitti and colleagues[23] reported that high levels of tumor necrosis factor α in amniotic fluid predicted prolonged postnatal ventilation, suggesting early and persistent lung injury from chorioamnionitis. Ramsey and colleagues[24] also showed that chorioamnionitis increased neonatal morbidities. Laughon and colleagues[25] cultured 1340 placentas of infants born before 28 weeks of gestation and found no association between histologic chorioamnionitis, funisitis, or specific organisms and the initial oxygen requirements of the infants. They did not report the diagnosis of RDS specifically. The Canadian Neonatal Network also reported that clinical chorioamnionitis did not predict RDS.[26]

These discrepant RDS outcomes for very preterm infants exposed to chorioamnionitis need to be understood within the context of the following complexities:

1. The diagnosis of chorioamnionitis was imprecise and did not include information about the duration, intensity, or organisms contributing to the exposure.
2. No attempt was made to make a specific diagnosis of surfactant deficiency as a cause of the respiratory distress.
3. The diagnosis of RDS was imprecise in very preterm infants because most of the infants have some respiratory adaptation problems soon after birth.
4. The severity of the respiratory distress was not calibrated, and there are important differences between severe and mild RDS.
5. Surfactant treatment and mechanical ventilation at birth interfere with assigning a diagnosis of RDS.

A clinical indicator for how chorioamnionitis may confound outcomes is found in the report by Been and colleagues,[27] in which infants with RDS and exposed to chorioamnionitis have good responses to surfactant treatment, whereas infants exposed to chorioamnionitis and with funisitis have poor responses to surfactant. The major confounder for a comparison of the incidence of an outcome such as RDS between groups of very low birth weight (VLBW) infants is the comparison group. Because all VLBW deliveries are associated with abnormalities, there is no normal comparison group. **Fig. 1** shows the problem of correlation of chorioamnionitis with an outcome such as RDS. Chorioamnionitis can be associated with severe RDS; likely the combination of surfactant deficiency and a diffuse pneumonia/inflammation with a nonculturable organism. Chorioamnionitis can also result in an infant without RDS, in which case the signature of the chorioamnionitis could be detected only by analysis of tracheal aspirate collected shortly after birth.

Chorioamnionitis and BPD

The relationship between chorioamnionitis and BPD is as obscure as the relationship of chorioamnionitis with RDS, and for similar reasons. Following the seminal article by Watterberg and colleagues[16] in 1996 that associated chorioamnionitis with a decrease in RDS and an increase in BPD in ventilated infants, multiple reports showed that chorioamnionitis increased the risk of BPD. Schelonka and colleagues[19] reported a meta-analysis in 2005 showing that Ureaplasma in association with chorioamnionitis increased the risk of BPD in infants (OR 1.6, 95% CI 1.1–2.3), but the effect was greater in smaller than larger studies. A recent systematic review of 59 studies including more than 15,000 infants concluded that BPD was increased by chorioamnionitis (OR 1.89, 95% CI 1.56–2.3).[28] However, this estimate decreased to an OR of 1.58 and 95% CI 1.11 to 2.24 with adjustments for birth weight differences. The relationship was significant only for histologic chorioamnionitis.

In contrast, Laughon and colleagues[25] found no relationship between BPD and histologic chorioamnionitis for 1340 infants born before 28 weeks' gestational age. A report from the Canadian Neonatal Network also found no association between clinical chorioamnionitis and BPD.[26] BPD is caused primarily by mechanical ventilation and oxygen exposure, with potent modulators being other occurrences during postnatal care such as a patent ductus arteriosus and postnatal sepsis.[29,30] Three reports highlight the complexities of these associations. Van Marter and colleagues[31] reported

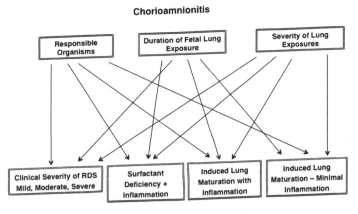

Chorioamnionitis

| Responsible Organisms | Duration of Fetal Lung Exposure | Severity of Lung Exposures |

| Clinical Severity of RDS Mild, Moderate, Severe | Surfactant Deficiency + Inflammation | Induced Lung Maturation with Inflammation | Induced Lung Maturation – Minimal Inflammation |

Spectrum of RDS/No RDS Diagnoses in VLBW Infants

1. Pathways from several of the variables contributing to chorioamnionitis and the clinical severity of RDS, lung maturation, and inflammation.

that chorioamnionitis decreased BPD (OR 0.2) in ventilated preterm infants unless they were ventilated for more than 7 days or had postnatal sepsis, which increased the risk of BPD (ORs of about 3.0). Lahra and colleagues[3] also found that BPD was decreased in a population of 761 infants by histologic chorioamnionitis, but chorioamnionitis plus postnatal sepsis increased the risk. The characteristics of the chorioamnionitis also altered the association. For example, in a cohort of 446 singleton deliveries, there was no increase in BPD with histologic chorioamnionitis, but a cord blood culture positive for *Ureaplasma* or *Mycoplasma* increased the BPD rate almost 3-fold in the same cohort.[14,21] BPD is a complicated lung development/injury/repair syndrome with multiple postnatal factors contributing to its occurrence and progression. Some chorioamnionitis exposures may protect the infant from BPD by decreasing the severity of RDS (lung maturation), whereas other types of exposures may promote BPD by initiating a progressive inflammatory response. Some of these possibilities are shown in **Fig. 2**.

PROOF OF PRINCIPAL: LUNG EFFECTS OF CHORIOAMNIONITIS IN ANIMAL MODELS
Chorioamnionitis and Lung Inflammation

Intra-amniotic injections of proinflammatory mediators such as *Escherichia coli* lipopolysaccharide (LPS; an endotoxin), interleukin (IL)-1 or single live organisms such as *Ureaplasma* are used to create chorioamnionitis; generally defined as inflammation of the fetal membranes.[12,32] Intra-amniotic injections of LPS or proinflammatory mediators cause an acute lung inflammation in fetal sheep and mouse lungs.[33,34] This lung inflammation is characterized by:

1. A mediator dose-dependent recruitment of primarily neutrophils to the lung parenchyma that can be detected within hours of the intra-amniotic exposure.[35]
2. A large increase in expression of proinflammatory cytokines such as IL-1β, IL-6, IL-8, and monocyte chemotactic protein-1 (MCP-1).[33,34]
3. The mediator must have direct contact with the fetal lung, as shown by surgical isolation of the lung from the amniotic fluid.[13]

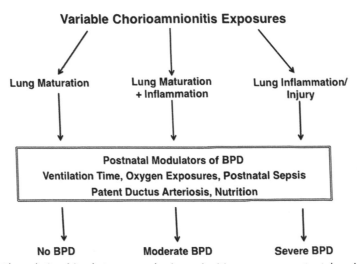

Fig. 2. The relationships between a chorioamnionitis exposure, postnatal variables that modulate the risk of BPD, and the BPD outcome.

4. A sequence of early injury that includes apoptosis, proliferation, and microvascular injury.[36,37]
5. The inflammatory response is signaled via nuclear factor κB (NFκB) activation in lung monocytes in fetal mouse lungs.[38]

In the fetal sheep, the inflammation from intra-amniotic LPS does not cause a severe pneumonia or consolidation, even with repetitive or direct applications of LPS via the fetal trachea.[13,39] The initial inflammatory response to intra-amniotic injection of live *Ureaplasma* induces less neutrophil recruitment and cytokine expression than does LPS in the fetal sheep lung.[40] Inflammation is substantial following *Ureaplasma* exposure of fetal mouse and monkey lungs, based on the limited information available.[41,42] *Ureaplasma* are readily recoverable from the fetal lungs and fetal lung fluid.[43] Although chorioamnionitis causes lung inflammation in experimental models, that inflammation does not progress to severe pneumonia, consistent with the infrequent diagnosis of pneumonia in VLBW infants shortly after birth.[15] The fetus has a well-developed ability to suppress and modulate inflammation.

Consequences of Lung Inflammation

Induced lung maturation
Bry and colleagues[44,45] showed that intra-amniotic injection of IL-1 or LPS induced early lung maturation in rabbits, as indicated by increased mRNA for the surfactant proteins and increases in pressure-volume curves. Intra-amniotic LPS increases the numbers of type II cells and the expression of mRNA for surfactant proteins via NFkB-dependent pathways in fetal mouse lungs.[46] In fetal sheep, the lung maturation response is characterized by:

1. An increase in the mRNA for the surfactant proteins within 24 hours of the LPS or IL-1 exposure.[47]
2. An increase in surfactant lipids in the airspaces and improved pressure-volume curves after 4 to 5 days, with maximal responses at 7 to 15 days.[48]
3. A maturational response that requires inflammation and contact of the proinflammatory mediator with the fetal airways.[13,49]
4. Inflammation can initiate lung maturation as early as 60 days' gestation (term is 150 days).[50]
5. Lung maturation without an increase in fetal plasma cortisol.[48]
6. Maturation of immature monocytes to alveolar macrophages in the fetal lung via induction of granulocyte-macrophage colony-stimulating factor and the transcription factor PU.1.[51]

These effects of exposure of the fetal lungs to chorioamnionitis and those caused by mediators such as LPS or IL-1 can change postnatal lung function with resultant severe RDS to no RDS.[48] *Ureaplasma* also induces surfactant protein mRNA and more modest and less consistent increases in pressure-volume curves in sheep without maturing monocytes to alveolar macrophages.[40,52] Thus, the lung exposures to clinical chorioamnionitis may result in variable effects on lung maturation, depending on the organism and the duration of the exposure.

Lung injury from chorioamnionitis
Induced lung maturation involves the risk of injury to the developing lung from inflammation. The diffuse, but modest, inflammation followed by the injury responses of apoptosis and proliferation indicates a prototypic injury response.[36] Fetal sheep exposed to intra-amniotic LPS have persistently activated leukocytes in the airways,

recruitment of CD3-positive lymphocytes to lung tissue, increased expression of toll-like receptors (TLRs) 2 and 4, decreased caveolin-1 expression, and changes in multiple other signaling pathways.[53–55] The net effects in the intact fetal sheep are changes in lung collagen and elastin with a transient inhibition of alveolar septation and an increase in vascular wall thickness.[56,57] In mechanistic in vitro studies using explants from mouse lungs, LPS activates NFκB, which interferes with fibroblast growth factor-10 and integrin expression, resulting in decreased airspace branching.[58] Macrophages resident in the fetal lung tissue mediate the activation of NFκB signaling that inhibits multiple genes critical to lung development, with thickening of the lung interstitium and decreased airway branching.[38] Although LPS exposure disrupts alveolar septation and vascular development, the fetal sheep lung can continue to develop and grow through continued LPS exposure.[39]

Short-interval *Ureaplasma* exposures cause acute inflammation in rhesus monkey lungs[42] and fetal exposures of 2 to 3 days caused chorioamnionitis and lung colonization in preterm baboons.[59] Following delivery and ventilation for 14 days, some animals cleared the *Ureaplasma* from the airways with improving lung function, whereas others had persistent colonization and worse lung function. At 14 days, the *Ureaplasma*-infected animals had greater profibrotic responses and fibrosis.[60] In a mouse model, intra-amniotic *Ureaplasma* increased the postnatal oxygen-induced lung injury.[41] Prolonged exposure of fetal sheep to *Ureaplasma* had no demonstrable effect on a 3-hour ventilation–mediated lung injury.[61]

These experiences show inconsistent interactive effects between chorioamnionitis-induced lung injury and postnatal lung function. A reasonable interpretation is that fetal lung inflammation caused by chorioamnionitis can promote progression toward BPD by initiating alveolar simplification and by interfering with multiple signaling pathways involved in lung development. However, the effects depend on the bacterial agent and the other characteristics of the exposure, which are not known in clinical practice.

CHORIOAMNIONITIS AND IMMUNE MODULATION IN THE FETAL LUNG
An Overview

Studies of immune modulation in the fetal lung have been limited to fetal sheep. The advantage of this model is that the fetuses can be repetitively exposed over months and subsequently allowed to deliver for the evaluation of total effects later in life.[62] The fetus is generally considered to have depressed immune/inflammatory responses because of incomplete development of immune defense systems and lack of immune challenges such that response systems are naive. Within the context of the infectious causes of the chronic and indolent chorioamnionitis frequently associated with very preterm delivery, the fetus can respond to proinflammatory mediators such as LPS (a TLR4 agonist), IL-1, and live *Ureaplasma* (**Box 2**). The lung response is a low-grade

---

Box 2
Immune modulation by chorioamnionitis in the fetal sheep lung

- A primary response to LPS that is low grade
- Maturation of monocytes to alveolar macrophages
- No persistent or secondary inflammatory responses to continuous or repeated LPS (endotoxin tolerance)
- A cross-tolerance for a mediator different from the initial mediator
- Increases in innate host defense proteins surfactant protein (SP)-A and SP-D

inflammation (recruitment of granulocytes, cytokine expression) followed by a resolution of the acute inflammation with minimal effects on lung development other than induced lung maturation. However, this lung response cannot be understood in isolation from other fetal responses to chorioamnionitis that are being described in animal models. The fetal gut has injury, developmental, and immunomodulatory responses to intra-amniotic LPS or IL-1.[63] The fetal skin has a diffuse inflammatory response with increased cytokine expression on exposure to intra-amniotic LPS.[64] The systemic effects are modest: the acute-phase reactant serum amyloid A increases in the liver and there are small changes in white blood cell counts and platelets, but no significant increase in plasma cortisol in fetal sheep.[48,65] Fetal humans exposed to chorioamnionitis do have increased cortisol levels in cord blood, perhaps because of stress related to preterm labor.[66] Changes in immune status of the fetal lung probably reflect lung-specific effects from direct contact with the organisms and inflammatory products in the amniotic fluid and systemic responses to skin and gut exposures.

The fetal sheep lung contains few monocytic lineage cells or mature alveolar macrophages,[67] which is in contrast with the fetal mouse lung, which contains more mature monocytes.[38] The human fetal lung is thought to be like the sheep lung with the recruitment and maturation of monocytes to alveolar macrophages after delivery. Intra-amniotic LPS induces granulocyte-macrophage colony-stimulating factor (GM-CSF) mRNA in the fetal lung and increased GM-CSF protein, which is a known inducer of the transcription factor PU.1 and monocyte to macrophage maturation.[51] Mature-appearing alveolar macrophages are induced in the fetal lung at 80% gestation in the fetal sheep. Fetal exposure to live *Ureaplasma* does not mature monocytes to macrophages.[40]

The monocytes/macrophages recovered from fetal lung tissue of control animals have minimal oxidant or IL-6 secretory responses to challenge with LPS in vitro.[68] Seven days after intra-amniotic LPS, the cells produce oxidants and IL-6 comparably with alveolar macrophages from adult sheep. These cells that were minimally responsive to TLR4 and other TLR agonists become responsive to in vitro challenge to multiple TLR agonists after intra-amniotic LPS, a phenomenon referred to as cross-tolerance.[69] Fetal lung monocytes increased their potential to respond to infectious challenges following exposure to LPS/chorioamnionitis.

In vivo, a second fetal exposure to intra-amniotic LPS or IL-1 does not increase inflammatory cells or cytokine expression in the fetal lung; an endotoxin tolerance type response.[70] Monocytes/macrophages recovered after a second intra-amniotic LPS exposure also have severely blunted responses to in vitro exposure to multiple TLR agonists. An example is the effect of chronic fetal *Ureaplasma* colonization on the lung responses to intra-amniotic LPS. Animals exposed to live *Ureaplasma* 70 days before preterm delivery have high titers of *Ureaplasma* in their amniotic fluid and lung, but with a minimal inflammatory response as indicated by cytokine expression or myeloperoxide-positive cells relative to controls (**Fig. 3**).[71] Intra-amniotic LPS given 2 days before delivery induced a large inflammatory response in the lung. The maturational indicator for monocytes, PU.1, increased, as did IL-6 secretion by blood monocytes in vitro. However, the intra-amniotic LPS had no effect on the lungs chronically colonized with *Ureaplasma*. Chorioamnionitis also increases other components of the complex innate immune system. Two examples are the large increases in surfactant A and surfactant D proteins by intra-amniotic LPS.[54]

A Perspective on Immune Modulation

The fetus is capable of complex immune modulation despite the immaturity of the immune system. The fetal lung is a primary organ receiving the signals that result in immune/inflammatory responses in that it is in direct contact with the chorioamnionitis

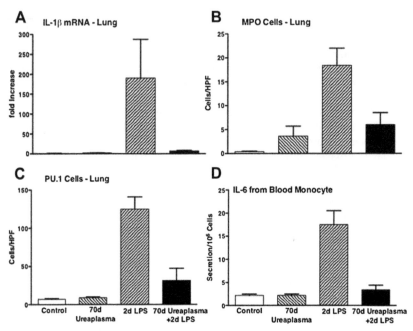

Fig. 3. Intra-amniotic *Ureaplasma* given 70 days before a second intra-amniotic exposure to *E coli* LPS suppressed the LPS responses in lungs of preterm fetal sheep. The chronic fetal exposure to *Ureaplasma* (*A*) suppressed IL-1β mRNA in the fetal lung, (*B*) decreased recruitment of myeloperoxidase positive cells (MPO) to the lung, (*C*) prevented the expression of the macrophage maturation transcription factor PU.1 in lung, and (*D*) decreased the release of IL-6 from blood monocytes challenged in culture with LPS. HPF, high power field. (*Data from* Kallapur SG, Kramer BW, Knox CL, et al. Chronic fetal exposure to *Ureaplasma parvum* suppresses innate immune responses in sheep. J Immunol 2011;187:2688–95.)

via the amniotic fluid. The lung is also an end organ for both beneficial and adverse immune/inflammatory responses because it is the target of ventilation and oxygen-mediated injuries following delivery. The importance of specific fetal immune modulations from chorioamnionitis on lung outcomes such as BPD remain speculative.

CHORIOAMNIONITIS AND ANTENATAL CORTICOSTEROIDS

Antenatal corticosteroids are given to more than 80% of the women at risk of preterm delivery before 30 weeks' gestation, and most of these women have undiagnosed (histologic) chorioamnionitis.[25,72] The current recommendation is to give antenatal corticosteroids with preterm labor or preterm rupture of membranes because the treatment decreases the incidence of RDS, intraventricular hemorrhage, and death.[73] In clinical series, antenatal corticosteroids are of benefit for preterm deliveries that, in retrospect, had associated histologic chorioamnionitis.[74] A recent analysis of observational studies identified the benefit of corticosteroid treatment of women with chorioamnionitis.[75] Antenatal corticosteroids also decrease the fetal inflammatory response syndrome in preterm infants exposed to histologic chorioamnionitis.[74]

Although there is no clinical information about how corticosteroids might influence chorioamnionitis, the corticosteroids could suppress inflammation (a potential benefit) or increase the risk of progressive infection (a potential risk). Maternal treatment with betamethasone initially suppressed the inflammation caused by intra-amniotic endotoxin in the chorioamnion and lungs of fetal sheep.[76,77] Inflammatory cells and proinflammatory cytokine expression were suppressed for about 2 days after the betamethasone treatment, but subsequently inflammation was increased in the lungs of lambs exposed to both maternal betamethasone and intra-amniotic endotoxin

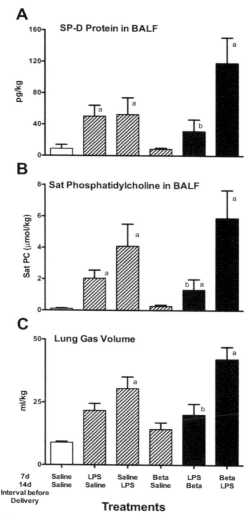

Fig. 4. Indicators of lung maturation following intra-amniotic *E coli* LPS (LPS) and/or maternal betamethasone (Beta) given 7 or 14 days before preterm delivery at 120 days gestational age. (*A, B*) The indicators surfactant protein-D (SP-D), and saturated (Sat) phosphatidylcholine in bronchoalveolar lavage fluid (BALF) increased with LPS exposure, but increased more when the order of exposure was LPS given 14 days and Beta given 7 days before delivery. (*C*) The lung gas volumes measured with air inflation to 40 cm H_2O pressure reflected the amounts of saturated phosphatidylcholine. [a] $P<.05$ relative to control. [b] $P<.05$ LPS/Beta relative to Beta/LPS. (*Data from* Kuypers E, Collins JJ, Kramer BW, et al. Intra-amniotic LPS and antenatal betamethasone: inflammation and maturation in preterm lamb lungs. Am J Physiol Lung Cell Mol Physiol 2012;302:L380–9.)

relative to endotoxin alone 5 and 15 days after the exposures.[77] Lung maturation was greater in lambs exposed to both betamethasone and endotoxin given together than in lambs exposed to either treatment alone.[78] The more likely clinical scenarios are corticosteroid treatments of women with chronic, indolent chorioamnionitis or women who develop chorioamnionitis after corticosteroid treatments. Fetal sheep exposed to maternal betamethasone and/or intra-amniotic LPS 7 and 14 days before preterm delivery have different indicators of lung maturation depending on the order of the exposures (**Fig. 4**).[54] The innate host defense protein SP-D was increased by the LPS, but not betamethasone. The combination of LPS given 7 days before betamethasone caused the largest increase in SP-D. The largest increases in saturated phosphatidylcholine, the major surfactant lipid, occurred if the LPS exposure preceded the maternal betamethasone exposure. This combination also had the greatest effect on the maximal lung gas volume. These results with fetal sheep support the clinical observations that betamethasone can further decrease RDS in the presence of histologic chorioamnionitis.[74] In fetal sheep, the lung maturational response to endotoxin was larger and more uniform than was the response to betamethasone. Betamethasone also augmented the lung maturation induced by chronic fetal *Ureaplasma* colonization.[79]

The increased inflammation in the fetal sheep lungs that occurred 5 to 15 days after simultaneous betamethasone and endotoxin exposures is a potential concern. Such effects have not been apparent clinically, but they have not been carefully evaluated. A potential mechanism to explain the increased inflammation is that both betamethasone and the endotoxin mature an immature inflammatory system. Blood monocytes from fetal sheep have decreased responses in vitro to endotoxin stimulation relative to monocytes from adult sheep.[68] However, 7 days after the fetal exposures, the monocytes respond to endotoxin in vitro similarly to monocytes from adult sheep. Maternal betamethasone initially suppresses the fetal monocyte function, but function is increased 7 days after the maternal treatment.[80] These results show how clinically complex interactions between exposures may be. Repetitive courses of betamethasone treatments may be a concern, particularly when chorioamnionitis is present. The clinical dilemma is that histologic chorioamnionitis is a retrospective diagnosis of a clinically silent process.

REFERENCES

1. Redline RW, Faye-Petersen O, Heller D, et al. Amniotic infection syndrome: nosology and reproducibility of placental reaction patterns. Pediatr Dev Pathol 2003;6:435–48.
2. Goldenberg RL, Culhane JF, Iams JD, et al. Epidemiology and causes of preterm birth. Lancet 2008;371:75–84.
3. Lahra MM, Beeby PJ, Jeffery HE. Intrauterine inflammation, neonatal sepsis, and chronic lung disease: a 13-year hospital cohort study. Pediatrics 2009;123:1314–9.
4. Onderdonk AB, Delaney ML, DuBois AM, et al. Detection of bacteria in placental tissues obtained from extremely low gestational age neonates. Am J Obstet Gynecol 2008;198:110.e1–7.
5. Oh KJ, Lee KA, Sohn YK, et al. Intraamniotic infection with genital mycoplasmas exhibits a more intense inflammatory response than intraamniotic infection with other microorganisms in patients with preterm premature rupture of membranes. Am J Obstet Gynecol 2010;203:211.e1–8.
6. Romero R, Espinoza J, Chaiworapongsa T, et al. Infection and prematurity and the role of preventive strategies. Semin Neonatol 2002;7:259–74.

7. Kim MJ, Romero R, Gervasi MT, et al. Widespread microbial invasion of the chorioamniotic membranes is a consequence and not a cause of intra-amniotic infection. Lab Invest 2009;89:924–36.
8. DiGiulio DB, Romero R, Amogan HP, et al. Microbial prevalence, diversity and abundance in amniotic fluid during preterm labor: a molecular and culture-based investigation. PLoS One 2008;3:e3056.
9. Viscardi RM. *Ureaplasma* species: role in diseases of prematurity. Clin Perinatol 2010;37:393–409.
10. Gerber S, Vial Y, Hohlfeld P, et al. Detection of *Ureaplasma urealyticum* in second-trimester amniotic fluid by polymerase chain reaction correlates with subsequent preterm labor and delivery. J Infect Dis 2003;187:518–21.
11. Perni SC, Vardhana S, Korneeva I, et al. *Mycoplasma hominis* and *Ureaplasma urealyticum* in midtrimester amniotic fluid: association with amniotic fluid cytokine levels and pregnancy outcome. Am J Obstet Gynecol 2004;191:1382–6.
12. Dando SJ, Nitsos I, Kallapur SG, et al. The role of the multiple banded antigen of *Ureaplasma parvum* in intra-amniotic infection: major virulence factor or decoy? PLoS One 2012;7:e29856.
13. Moss TJ, Nitsos I, Kramer BW, et al. Intra-amniotic endotoxin induces lung maturation by direct effects on the developing respiratory tract in preterm sheep. Am J Obstet Gynecol 2002;187:1059–65.
14. Andrews WW, Goldenberg RL, Faye-Petersen O, et al. The Alabama Preterm Birth study: polymorphonuclear and mononuclear cell placental infiltrations, other markers of inflammation, and outcomes in 23- to 32-week preterm newborn infants. Am J Obstet Gynecol 2006;195:803–8.
15. Stoll BJ, Hansen NI, Bell EF, et al. Neonatal outcomes of extremely preterm infants from the NICHD Neonatal Research Network. Pediatrics 2010;126:443–56.
16. Watterberg KL, Demers LM, Scott SM, et al. Chorioamnionitis and early lung inflammation in infants in whom bronchopulmonary dysplasia develops. Pediatrics 1996;97:210–5.
17. De Dooy J, Colpaert C, Schuerwegh A, et al. Relationship between histologic chorioamnionitis and early inflammatory variables in blood, tracheal aspirates, and endotracheal colonization in preterm infants. Pediatr Res 2003;54:113–9.
18. Kasper DC, Mechtler TP, Bohm J, et al. In utero exposure to *Ureaplasma* spp. is associated with increased rate of bronchopulmonary dysplasia and intraventricular hemorrhage in preterm infants. J Perinat Med 2011;39:331–6.
19. Schelonka RL, Katz B, Waites KB, et al. Critical appraisal of the role of *Ureaplasma* in the development of bronchopulmonary dysplasia with metaanalytic techniques. Pediatr Infect Dis J 2005;24:1033–9.
20. Richardson CJ, Pomerance JJ, Cunningham MD, et al. Acceleration of fetal lung maturation following prolonged rupture of the membranes. Am J Obstet Gynecol 1974;118:1115–8.
21. Goldenberg RL, Andrews WW, Goepfert AR, et al. The Alabama Preterm Birth Study: umbilical cord blood *Ureaplasma urealyticum* and *Mycoplasma hominis* cultures in very preterm newborn infants. Am J Obstet Gynecol 2008;198:43.e1–5.
22. Lahra MM, Beeby PJ, Jeffery HE. Maternal versus fetal inflammation and respiratory distress syndrome: a 10-year hospital cohort study. Arch Dis Child Fetal Neonatal Ed 2009;94:F13–6.
23. Hitti J, Krohn MA, Patton DL, et al. Amniotic fluid tumor necrosis factor-alpha and the risk of respiratory distress syndrome among preterm infants. Am J Obstet Gynecol 1997;177:50–6.

24. Ramsey PS, Lieman JM, Brumfield CG, et al. Chorioamnionitis increases neonatal morbidity in pregnancies complicated by preterm premature rupture of membranes. Am J Obstet Gynecol 2005;192:1162–6.
25. Laughon M, Allred EN, Bose C, et al. Patterns of respiratory disease during the first 2 postnatal weeks in extremely premature infants. Pediatrics 2009;123: 1124–31.
26. Soraisham AS, Singhal N, McMillan DD, et al. A multicenter study on the clinical outcome of chorioamnionitis in preterm infants. Am J Obstet Gynecol 2009;200: 372.e1–6.
27. Been JV, Rours IG, Kornelisse RF, et al. Chorioamnionitis alters the response to surfactant in preterm infants. J Pediatr 2010;156:10–15.e1.
28. Hartling L, Liang Y, Lacaze-Masmonteil T. Chorioamnionitis as a risk factor for bronchopulmonary dysplasia: a systematic review and meta-analysis. Arch Dis Child Fetal Neonatal Ed 2012;97:F8–17.
29. Bancalari E, Claure N, Sosenko IR. Bronchopulmonary dysplasia: changes in pathogenesis, epidemiology and definition. Semin Neonatol 2003;8:63–71.
30. Laughon MM, Langer JC, Bose CL, et al. Prediction of bronchopulmonary dysplasia by postnatal age in extremely premature infants. Am J Respir Crit Care Med 2011;183:1715–22.
31. Van Marter LJ, Dammann O, Allred EN, et al. Chorioamnionitis, mechanical ventilation, and postnatal sepsis as modulators of chronic lung disease in preterm infants. J Pediatr 2002;140:171–6.
32. Berry CA, Nitsos I, Hillman NH, et al. Interleukin-1 in lipopolysaccharide induced chorioamnionitis in the fetal sheep. Reprod Sci 2011;18:1092–102.
33. Prince LS, Dieperink HI, Okoh VO, et al. Toll-like receptor signaling inhibits structural development of the distal fetal mouse lung. Dev Dyn 2005;233:553–61.
34. Kallapur SG, Willet KE, Jobe AH, et al. Intra-amniotic endotoxin: chorioamnionitis precedes lung maturation in preterm lambs. Am J Physiol 2001;280: L527–36.
35. Kramer BW, Moss TJ, Willet K, et al. Dose and time response after intra-amniotic endotoxin in preterm lambs. Am J Respir Crit Care Med 2001;164:982–8.
36. Kramer BW, Kramer S, Ikegami M, et al. Injury, inflammation and remodeling in fetal sheep lung after intra-amniotic endotoxin. Am J Physiol Lung Cell Mol Physiol 2002;283:L452–9.
37. Kallapur SG, Bachurski C, Le Cras TD, et al. Vascular injury and remodeling following intra-amniotic endotoxin in the preterm lamb lung. Am J Physiol Lung Cell Mol Physiol 2004;287:L1178–85.
38. Blackwell TS, Hipps AN, Yamamoto Y, et al. NF-kappaB signaling in fetal lung macrophages disrupts airway morphogenesis. J Immunol 2011;187:2740–7.
39. Kallapur SG, Nitsos I, Moss TJM, et al. Chronic endotoxin exposure does not cause sustained structural abnormalities in the fetal sheep lungs. Am J Physiol Lung Cell Mol Physiol 2005;288:L966–74.
40. Collins JJ, Kallapur SG, Knox CL, et al. Inflammation in fetal sheep from intra-amniotic injection of Ureaplasma parvum. Am J Physiol Lung Cell Mol Physiol 2010;299:L852–60.
41. Normann E, Lacaze-Masmonteil T, Eaton F, et al. A novel mouse model of Urea-plasma-induced perinatal inflammation: effects on lung and brain injury. Pediatr Res 2009;65:430–6.
42. Novy MJ, Duffy L, Axthelm MK, et al. Ureaplasma parvum or Mycoplasma hom-inis as sole pathogens cause chorioamnionitis, preterm delivery, and fetal pneumonia in rhesus macaques. Reprod Sci 2009;16:56–70.

43. Knox CL, Dando SJ, Nitsos I, et al. The severity of chorioamnionitis in pregnant sheep is associated with in vivo variation of the surface-exposed multiple-banded antigen/gene of *Ureaplasma parvum*. Biol Reprod 2010;83: 415–26.

44. Bry K, Lappalainen U, Hallman M. Intraamniotic interleukin-1 accelerates surfactant protein synthesis in fetal rabbits and improves lung stability after premature birth. J Clin Invest 1997;99:2992–9.

45. Bry K, Lappalainen U. Intra-amniotic endotoxin accelerates lung maturation in fetal rabbits. Acta Paediatr 2001;90:74–80.

46. Prince LS, Okoh VO, Moninger TO, et al. Lipopolysaccharide increases alveolar type II cell number in fetal mouse lungs through Toll-like receptor 4 and NF-kappaB. Am J Physiol Lung Cell Mol Physiol 2004;287:L999–1006.

47. Bachurski CJ, Ross GF, Ikegami M, et al. Intra-amniotic endotoxin increases pulmonary surfactant components and induces SP-B processing in fetal sheep. Am J Physiol Lung Cell Mol Physiol 2001;280:L279–85.

48. Jobe AH, Newnham JP, Willet KE, et al. Endotoxin induced lung maturation in preterm lambs is not mediated by cortisol. Am J Respir Crit Care Med 2000; 162:1656–61.

49. Kallapur SG, Moss JTM, Newnham JP, et al. Recruited inflammatory cells mediate endotoxin-induced lung maturation in preterm fetal lambs. Am J Respir Crit Care Med 2005;172:1315–21.

50. Moss TM, Newnham J, Willet K, et al. Early gestational intra-amniotic endotoxin: lung function, surfactant and morphometry. Am J Respir Crit Care Med 2002;165: 805–11.

51. Kramer BW, Joshi SN, Moss TJ, et al. Endotoxin-induced maturation of monocytes in preterm fetal sheep lung. Am J Physiol Lung Cell Mol Physiol 2007; 293:L345–53.

52. Moss TJM, Knox CL, Kallapur SG, et al. Experimental amniotic fluid infection in sheep: effects of *Ureaplasma parvum* serovars 3 and 6 on preterm or term fetal sheep. Am J Obstet Gynecol 2008;198:e1–8.

53. Cheah FC, Pillow JJ, Kramer BW, et al. Airway inflammatory cell responses to intra-amniotic lipopolysaccharide in a sheep model of chorioamnionitis. Am J Physiol Lung Cell Mol Physiol 2009;296:L384–93.

54. Kuypers E, Collins JJ, Kramer BW, et al. Intra-amniotic LPS and antenatal betamethasone: inflammation and maturation in preterm lamb lungs. Am J Physiol Lung Cell Mol Physiol 2012;302:L380–9.

55. Kunzmann S, Collins JJ, Yang Y, et al. Antenatal inflammation reduces expression of caveolin-1 and influences multiple signaling pathways in preterm fetal lungs. Am J Respir Cell Mol Biol 2011;45:969–76.

56. Willet KE, Jobe AH, Ikegami M, et al. Lung morphometry after repetitive antenatal glucocorticoid treatment in preterm sheep. Am J Respir Crit Care Med 2001;163: 1437–43.

57. Kallapur SG, Bachurski CJ, Le Cras TD, et al. Vascular changes following intra-amniotic endotoxin in preterm lamb lungs. Am J Physiol Lung Cell Mol Physiol 2004;287:L1178–85.

58. Benjamin JT, Smith RJ, Halloran BA, et al. FGF-10 is decreased in bronchopulmonary dysplasia and suppressed by Toll-like receptor activation. Am J Physiol Lung Cell Mol Physiol 2007;292:L550–8.

59. Yoder BA, Coalson JJ, Winter VT, et al. Effects of antenatal colonization with *Ureaplasma urealyticum* on pulmonary disease in the immature baboon. Pediatr Res 2003;54:797–807.

60. Viscardi RM, Atamas SP, Luzina IG, et al. Antenatal *Ureaplasma urealyticum* respiratory tract infection stimulates proinflammatory, profibrotic responses in the preterm baboon lung. Pediatr Res 2006;60:141–6.

61. Polglase GR, Hillman NH, Pillow JJ, et al. Ventilation mediated injury following preterm delivery of *Ureaplasma* colonized fetal lambs. Pediatr Res 2010;67(6): 630–5.

62. Lee AJX, Lambertmont VAC, Pillow JJ, et al. Fetal responses to lipopolysaccharide-induced chorioamnionitis alter immune and airway responses in 7-week-old sheep. Am J Obstet Gynecol 2011;204(4):364.e17–24.

63. Wolfs TG, Kallapur SG, Polglase GR, et al. IL-1alpha mediated chorioamnionitis induces depletion of FoxP3+ cells and ileal inflammation in the ovine fetal gut. PLoS One 2011;6:e18355.

64. Kemp MW, Saito M, Nitsos I, et al. Exposure to in utero lipopolysaccharide induces inflammation in the fetal ovine skin. Reprod Sci 2010;18:88–98.

65. Wilson TC, Bachurski CJ, Ikegami M, et al. Pulmonary and systemic induction of SAA3 after ventilation and endotoxin in preterm lambs. Pediatr Res 2005;58: 1204–9.

66. Watterberg KL. Adrenocortical function and dysfunction in the fetus and neonate. Semin Neonatol 2004;9:13–21.

67. Kramer BW, Jobe AH, Ikegami M. Monocyte function in preterm, term, and adult sheep. Pediatr Res 2003;54:52–7.

68. Kramer BW, Ikegami M, Moss TJ, et al. Endotoxin-induced chorioamnionitis modulates innate immunity of monocytes in preterm sheep. Am J Respir Crit Care Med 2005;171:73–7.

69. Kramer BW, Kallapur SG, Moss TJ, et al. Intra-amniotic LPS modulation of TLR signaling in lung and blood monocytes of fetal sheep. Innate Immun 2009;15: 101–7.

70. Kallapur SG, Jobe AH, Ball MK, et al. Pulmonary and systemic endotoxin tolerance in preterm fetal sheep exposed to chorioamnionitis. J Immunol 2007;179: 8491–9.

71. Kallapur SG, Kramer BW, Knox CL, et al. Chronic fetal exposure to *Ureaplasma parvum* suppresses innate immune responses in sheep. J Immunol 2011;187: 2688–95.

72. Goldenberg RL, Hauth JC, Andrews WW. Intrauterine infection and preterm delivery. N Engl J Med 2000;342:1500–7.

73. Harding JE, Pang J, Knight DB, et al. Do antenatal corticosteroids help in the setting of preterm rupture of membranes? Am J Obstet Gynecol 2001;184: 131–9.

74. Goldenberg RL, Andrews WW, Faye-Petersen OM, et al. The Alabama Preterm Birth Study: corticosteroids and neonatal outcomes in 23- to 32-week newborns with various markers of intrauterine infection. Am J Obstet Gynecol 2006;195: 1020–4.

75. Been JV, Degraeuwe PL, Kramer BW, et al. Antenatal steroids and neonatal outcome after chorioamnionitis: a meta-analysis. BJOG 2011;118:113–22.

76. Newnham J, Kallapur SG, Kramer BW, et al. Betamethasone effects on chorioamnionitis induced by intra-amniotic endotoxin in sheep. Am J Obstet Gynecol 2003; 189:1458–66.

77. Kallapur SG, Kramer BW, Moss TJ, et al. Maternal glucocorticoids increase endotoxin-induced lung inflammation in preterm lambs. Am J Physiol Lung Cell Mol Physiol 2003;284:L633–42.

78. Newnham JP, Moss TJ, Padbury JF, et al. The interactive effects of endotoxin with prenatal glucocorticoids on short-term lung function in sheep. Am J Obstet Gynecol 2001;185:190–7.

79. Moss TJM, Nitsos I, Knox CL, et al. *Ureaplasma* colonization of amniotic fluid and efficacy of antenatal corticosteroids for preterm lung maturation in sheep. Am J Obstet Gynecol 2008;200:96.e1–6.

80. Kramer BW, Ikegami M, Moss TJ, et al. Antenatal betamethasone changes cord blood monocyte responses to endotoxin in preterm lambs. Pediatr Res 2004;55: 764–8.

Initial Respiratory Support of Preterm Infants

The Role of CPAP, the INSURE Method, and Noninvasive Ventilation

Robert H. Pfister, MD[a],*, Roger F. Soll, MD[b]

KEYWORDS

- Respiratory support • Preterm infants • CPAP • Noninvasive ventilation

KEY POINTS

- Respiratory support of preterm infants is increasingly being achieved through noninvasive methods.
- Nasal continuous positive airway pressure (CPAP) is safe and is at least as effective as management via conventional mechanical ventilation.
- Nasal CPAP is associated with a decreased risk of developing chronic lung disease compared with conventional mechanical ventilation.
- An intubate, surfactant, and extubation (INSURE) strategy has been successfully applied both early and late in the course of respiratory distress syndrome.
- Techniques for administering exogenous surfactant while providing noninvasive respiratory support require further investigation.

INTRODUCTION

This article explores the potential benefits and risks for the various approaches to the initial respiratory management of preterm infants. The authors focus on the evidence for the increasingly used strategies of initial respiratory support of preterm infants with continuous positive airway pressure (CPAP) beginning in the delivery room (DR) or very early in the hospital course and blended strategies involving the early administration of surfactant replacement followed by immediate extubation and stabilization on CPAP. Where possible, the evidence referenced in this review comes from individual randomized controlled trials (RCTs) or meta-analyses of those trials.

[a] Department of Pediatrics, University of Vermont, FAHC - Smith 556, Burlington, VT 05401, USA; [b] Department of Pediatrics, University of Vermont, FAHC - Smith 174, Burlington, VT 05401, USA
* Corresponding author. Department of Pediatrics, University of Vermont, FAHC - Smith 556, Burlington, VT 05401.
E-mail address: Robert.Pfister@vtmednet.org

Clin Perinatol 39 (2012) 459–481
http://dx.doi.org/10.1016/j.clp.2012.06.015   perinatology.theclinics.com
0095-5108/12/$ – see front matter © 2012 Elsevier Inc. All rights reserved.

HISTORICAL PERSPECTIVE

Based on the combined weight of multiple RCTs and their subsequent meta-analyses performed in the 1990s, surfactant was given as part of the initial resuscitation and management of preterm infants either at risk for or with evidence of respiratory distress syndrome (RDS). Available evidence led neonatologists to develop strong convictions that among infants who were intubated for respiratory distress, early surfactant administration was associated with decreased risk of pneumothorax (typical relative risk [RR] 0.63 [95% confidence interval (CI) 0.59–0.82]; typical risk difference [RD] -0.05 [95% CI -0.08 to -0.03]); decreased chronic lung disease (CLD) (typical RR 0.70 [95% CI 0.55–0.88]; typical RD -0.03 [95% CI -0.05 to -0.01]); and decreased mortality (typical RR 0.87 [95% CI 0.77–0.99]; typical RD -0.03 [95% CI -0.06 to -0.00]).[1] Intubation and surfactant administration immediately following birth was thought to be effective and lifesaving in infants thought to be at risk for RDS. On the weight of such sentiment, the proportion of infants receiving surfactant within 2 hours of life became a therapeutic goal, a standard endorsed by the National Quality Forum for infants born less than or equal to 29 weeks' gestation.[2]

However, as the adage goes, things change. Investigators began to more broadly examine the possibility of less-invasive respiratory support with the possibility of alternate approaches that potentially avoid deleterious outcomes of the accepted standards of care. An understanding that the physiology and the severity of illness of RDS were tied closely with the ability to establish a functional residual capacity (FRC)[3] led to treatment involving the administration of continuous distending pressure in lieu of surfactant replacement. Both CPAP and surfactant replacement were seen as leading to the same final goal of establishing and maintaining FRC. As such, the spectrum of respiratory support given to preterm neonates continues to evolve and become increasingly complex.

DRAWBACKS OF THE CONVENTIONAL APPROACH

Despite the well-documented benefits of surfactant replacement therapy, there are several negative aspects related to the way surfactant is administered and the subsequent respiratory management that follows. The act of placing an endotracheal tube (ETT) is invasive and may be traumatic. Laryngoscopy and intratracheal intubation is often unsuccessful[4] and may cause hypoxemia, bradycardia, increased cranial pressure, systemic and pulmonary hypertension, and airway trauma.[5] In part to avoid these complications, the American Academy of Pediatrics has suggested that sedation be offered to all nonemergent intubations; however, this too may be associated with undesirable side effects, such as respiratory depression that could potentially interfere with spontaneous respiration. Surfactant replacement itself is associated with changes in cerebral blood flow, although the impact of these changes is not fully understood.[6] Most relevant to this article, avoidance of mechanical ventilation use altogether may be the best way to avoid or reduce the risk of CLD from volutrauma and barotrauma.[7,8] Additionally, animal data suggest that mechanical ventilation is associated with inflammatory lung injury.[9] As such, reduction of mechanical ventilation by means of noninvasive ventilation has become the most accepted method by which to reduce ventilator-associated lung injury and CLD.

In 1987, a game-changing report by Avery and colleagues[7] suggested that one center's less-invasive approach, namely stabilization with nasal CPAP from birth in preterm infants with respiratory distress, was associated with a decreased risk of CLD when compared with 7 other centers that relied on conventional mechanical ventilator management. In 2001, Van Marter and colleagues[10] noted similar protective findings of CPAP against the development of CLD when compared with conventional ventilator stabilization. Surfactant administration and antenatal corticosteroids are thought to be synergistic, and this report was notable in that it occurred in a period that had high rates of maternal antenatal steroids and surfactant administration. Although observational in design, these studies demonstrated that CPAP may be associated with improved outcomes over surfactant administration even in infants who had the benefits of antenatal steroids and created a need for RCTs to address whether or not preterm infants at risk for surfactant deficiency could be safely managed on CPAP alone.

Linder and colleagues[11] published a retrospective cohort study following the outcomes of extremely low birth weight (ELBW) infants at a single center during a period when the local DR policy changed from one of immediate intubation of any infant at risk to transitional support with a bag and mask and stabilization on CPAP, saving intubation only for infants who did not transition to spontaneous breathing. They noted that by providing an individualized intubation strategy, even in ELBW infants, 25% of these smallest infants were never intubated.

CPAP INTERFACES

CPAP has been successfully administered through a variety of methods. Although first administered for the treatment of RDS via ETT,[12] and later via only one naris through a modified ETT or single nasal prong, other superior interfaces have been developed and adopted. The most common interfaces in use today typically involve a nose mask or, more commonly, short bilateral nasal prongs. Distending pressure is generated either by simply placing the distal end of a CPAP circuit under a known depth of water (bubble CPAP), connecting it to a ventilator (ventilator CPAP), or to a variable-flow nasal continuous positive airway pressure (nCPAP) device (infant flow driver). Each method has its theoretic advantages and proponents. One RCT comparing variable-flow with constant-flow CPAP[13] and one RCT comparing variable-flow to bubble CPAP to a variable-flow device[14] failed to show any significant difference in rates of extubation failure.

CPAP BENEFITS

It is thought that CPAP assists the breathing of preterm infants in several ways. CPAP stents open the airways of preterm infants, which are characterized by their poor muscle tone and compliant structure. This effect reduces obstructive events that may translate to less apnea and less atelectasis.[15] Animal models have demonstrated that CPAP causes a mechanical strain that is associated with accelerated lung protein accretion, lung growth, elastic recoil, and ultimately improved remodeling of lung parenchyma.[16]

If CPAP is successfully applied and intubation is avoided, less trauma to the airway will occur as a result of laryngoscopy, intubation, and from an ETT that is left in place chronically. Early CPAP alone will prevent progression to respiratory failure in many spontaneously breathing preterm infants and in combination with antenatal steroids, the number of infants without clinical symptoms of RDS is further decreased.[17]

CPAP DRAWBACKS

Pragmatically there are few problems with CPAP, mostly directly related to the CPAP interface. Given that the goal of CPAP is to provide continuous distending pressure that extends from the interface through the nasopharynx and the proximal airway and transmitted to the distal airways and alveoli, a tight seal must be maintained throughout. Leakage and the resultant pressure loss may occur at many points: from the CPAP system itself, out the mouth, or at the nasal interface. Chin straps may be used to ensure that the mouth stays shut and may reduce mouth leak.[18] It is vital that caregivers at the bedside ensure that there is a tight seal in the nares. Efforts to maintain the required tight seal, incorrect positioning, or poorly sized nasal prongs can cause serious injury to the inside of the nose and the columella. Constant caregiver vigilance toward developmentally appropriate positioning is vital for the success of nasal CPAP.

CPAP IN THE DR

Following the promising results of these early observational studies, several RCTs have been performed to address the question of whether the conventional approach of intubation and subsequent mechanical ventilation versus nasal CPAP is the superior approach for initial stabilization of the preterm infant at risk for developing RDS. The details of these studies are discussed later.

In 2004, Finer and colleagues[19] reported the results of their feasibility study that examined whether initiating mask CPAP using a T-piece resuscitator in the DR and continuing CPAP therapy via nasal CPAP once in the neonatal intensive care unit (NICU), without intubation for surfactant, was possible in a population of 104 ELBW infants. Despite the intention to avoid intubation in the DR for the purpose of surfactant administration, 27 infants randomized to the DR CPAP arm were intubated as part of their initial resuscitation. After admission to the NICU, all nonintubated infants were placed on CPAP and were to be intubated for surfactant administration only after they met a prespecified definition of hypoxia or respiratory distress. Of the infants initially randomized to stabilization on CPAP, 16 more were subsequently intubated in the NICU by the seventh day of life. Overall, 80% of the studied infants required intubation within the first 7 days of life. This early study was illustrative for several reasons. It showed that trials of CPAP in the DR are feasible and that greater than 90% of the infants in the study received the DR intervention to which they were randomized. It also demonstrated that there are at least 3 circumstances that ultimately lead to intubation: prophylactically for the purpose of surfactant administration (independent of respiratory status), as part of the initial DR resuscitation, and finally as later rescue for infants initially stabilized on CPAP.

Ammari and colleagues[20] made similar observations. They followed a cohort of consecutively born infants with a birthweight less than or equal to 1250 g and noted that they could be divided into 3 groups (termed *ventilator-started*, *CPAP-failure*, and *CPAP-success*) based on their initial respiratory support modality and whether CPAP was able to be continued at 72 hours of age. They noted that CPAP in the DR was progressively less successful in more preterm, smaller infants; about a third of the infants born 23 to 25 weeks' gestation or weighing less than 700 g needed to be intubated as part of their initial resuscitation and about 40% of these infants failed CPAP and required increased support by 72 hours of life.

These observations are important to keep in mind when evaluating the studies of initial respiratory support of preterm infants with CPAP beginning in the DR and the blended strategies of surfactant replacement with subsequent stabilization on CPAP. To understand the results and outcomes of the various trials discussed later, it is important to view their eligibility criteria through the prism that separates out the infants based on whether or not they needed intubation as initial respiratory support. The trials discussed later are characterized accordingly as those that enrolled only infants who had successfully transitioned but had mild to moderate respiratory insufficiency (infants successfully transitioned [ie, not requiring intubation as part of initial resuscitation]) and those that enrolled all infants at high risk for respiratory distress regardless of their initial stabilization.

EARLY CPAP VERSUS STANDARD CARE (INTUBATION IN DR AND MECHANICAL VENTILATION)

There are 3 large trials that examine the strategy of initial stabilization on nasal CPAP versus conventional management of intubation and surfactant administration in preterm infants (**Table 1**).

The CPAP Or nasal INtubation at birth (COIN) trial was a large RCT that compared CPAP versus early intubation among 610 preterm infants born between 25 + 0 and 28 + 6 weeks' gestation.[21] Only infants who exhibited some degree of respiratory distress but were spontaneously breathing at 5 minutes of life were eligible. In essence, the most well and most ill infants were excluded; infants were ineligible if they required intubation by 5 minutes of life or if they did not require any type of respiratory support or supplemental oxygen. Among the infants randomized to receive CPAP, single or binasal prongs delivered 8 cm of H_2O pressure. Infants randomized to the nCPAP group were intubated if they had severe apnea, hypoxia (fraction of inspired oxygen [F_{IO_2}] >0.6), or severe respiratory acidosis. The protocol did not specify that the infants randomized to intubation be given surfactant and there were no discrete extubation criteria. There was no difference between the CPAP group and the intubation group in the primary outcome, death, or oxygen treatment at 36 weeks' postmenstrual age (unadjusted odds ratio [OR] 0.80 [95% CI 0.58–1.12]). As expected, the CPAP group used significantly less surfactant and spent less time on mechanical ventilation. The CPAP group required less postnatal steroids for CLD. Of concern, the group of infants stabilized on CPAP also had significantly more pneumothoraces (9.1% vs 3.0%). This difference is especially notable given that among the intubated infants, only 77% received surfactant (typically as part of a less successful late-rescue strategy), which has been documented to reduce the incidence of all air leaks.[1,22]

The Surfactant Positive Pressure and Oxygen Randomized Trial (SUPPORT) was a large trial sponsored by the National Institute of Child Health and Human Development that compared stabilization on CPAP with early surfactant therapy following intubation and mechanical ventilation according to the Neonatal Resuscitation Program's guidelines.[23] This comparison was one part of a 2 × 2 factorial design that also assigned infants 1 of 2 oxygenation saturation target ranges. The SUPPORT trial enrolled 1316 infants between 24 + 0 and 27 + 6 weeks' gestation. In contrast to the COIN trial, infants were randomized before delivery to eliminate the entry requirement that infants need to be spontaneously breathing. This trial also benefitted by having clear criteria to address both the intubation of infants initially stabilized on CPAP and the extubation of infants initially stabilized following surfactant administration and mechanically ventilated. CPAP was initiated early, in the DR if required, at 5 cm H_2O and could be provided with any CPAP device. The investigators reported no difference in the primary outcome of mortality or CLD (OR 0.95 [95% CI 0.85–1.05]). In keeping with the findings of the COIN trial, infants randomized to CPAP in the delivery room received less surfactant, spent less time on mechanical ventilation, and received less postnatal steroids. The increased rate of pneumothorax observed in the COIN trial was not noted, perhaps because of a lower initial CPAP pressure or possibly because of a lower threshold for designating CPAP failure. Antenatal steroid

Table 1
Early CPAP versus STD care (intubate, surf, mechanical ventilation)

Author, Year	n	Gest Age	Comparison	Status in DR	Primary Outcome	Results of Primary Outcome	Notes
Morley et al,[21] 2008	610	25–28 + 6	CPAP in DR vs STD care	Mild-mod resp distress Spontaneously breathing	CLD @ 36 wk or mortality	OR 0.80 (95% CI 0.58–1.12)	CPAP group spent less time on mechanical vent, less postnatal steroids 9.1% vs 3.0% PTX rate in CPAP group vs in STD care Only 77% of intubated infants received surfactant CPAP failure threshold high (F_{IO_2} >0.6) Initial CPAP at 8 cm H_2O
Finer et al,[23] 2010	1316	24–27 + 6	CPAP in DR vs STD care	All comers independent of respiratory status	CLD @ 36 wk or mortality	OR 0.95 (95% CI 0.85–1.05)	High antenatal steroids rates CPAP group spent less time on ventilator, received less postnatal steroids One part of a 2 × 2 factorial design also investigation 2 oxygenation saturation target ranges
Dunn et al,[25] 2011	648	26–29 + 6	CPAP in DR vs STD care	All comers independent of respiratory status	CLD @ 36 wk or mortality	RR 0.83 (95% CI 0.64–1.09)	High antenatal steroids rates 48% in CPAP group were never intubated Third comparison group received INSURE

Abbreviations: CI, confidence interval; CLD, chronic lung disease; CPAP, continuous positive airway pressure; DR, delivery room; F_{IO_2}, fraction of inspired oxygen; Gest, gestational; INSURE, intubate, surfactant, and extubation; mod, moderate; OR, odds ratio; PTX, pneumothorax; resp, respiratory; RR, relative risk; STD, standard.

administration in both groups was high (>96%). However, these high antenatal steroid rates are much higher than what is typically achievable, drawing concern that the results might not be generalizable to real-world scenarios in which the benefits of antenatal steroids were not administered.[24] Despite these limitations, the investigators of the SUPPORT trial concluded that CPAP in the DR could be considered as an alternate path for consideration in the management of even quite preterm ELBW infants.

The Vermont Oxford Network Delivery Room Management trial (VON DRM) also compared early stabilization on CPAP versus intubation, prophylactic surfactant, and mechanical ventilation.[25] However, a third arm of infants was also included that was intubated, given prophylactic surfactant, and rapidly extubated to CPAP (details of this third arm are discussed later.) The VON DRM trial included 648 infants born between 26 + 0 and 29 + 6 weeks' gestation. Enrollment was stopped early because of declining enrollment rates before the goal sample size was reached. Similar to the SUPPORT trial, the VON DRM featured randomization before delivery and excluded no infants based on their need for immediate intubation secondary to inadequate initial respiratory drive. Accordingly, the antenatal steroid administration rate in this trial was also very high. There was no difference between the primary outcome of mortality or CLD at 36 weeks' postmenstrual age between the CPAP group and those treated with conventional management (RR 0.83 [95% CI 0.64–1.09]). Additionally, there were no statistically significant differences in mortality or other complications of prematurity.

The findings from these 3 studies are remarkably consistent. Although entry criteria and indications for intubation and surfactant administration were different, no single trial was able to demonstrate a statistically significant difference in the risk of death or CLD when infants were managed initially with CPAP. A recent Cochrane systematic review of prophylactic versus selective use of surfactant by Rojas-Reyes and colleagues[26] contained a subgroup that specified that CPAP be used to stabilize infants in the selective-surfactant-use arm. This report included the SUPPORT trial and the comparison arm detailed in the VON DRM trial comparing prophylactic surfactant and subsequent standard care with DR CPAP. The COIN trial was not included because infants at risk in the standard-care arm did not routinely receive prophylactic surfactant. A meta-analysis of these two studies demonstrated a compelling trend toward an increase in the risk of neonatal mortality or CLD associated with the use prophylactic surfactant when compared with early stabilization on CPAP with selective use of surfactant (n = 1744) (typical RR 1.12 [95% CI 1.02–1.24], typical RD 0.06 [95% CI 0.01–0.10]). The investigators concluded that routine stabilization on CPAP was associated with less risk of CLD or death when compared with prophylactic surfactant administration.

A COMBINED STRATEGY: INTUBATE, SURFACTANT, AND EXTUBATION

From the results of the COIN, SUPPORT, and VON DRM trials as well as the Rojas-Reyes meta-analysis, it is clear that initial stabilization on CPAP and provision of rescue surfactant only when necessary is at least as beneficial and quite possibly preferred over the standard therapy of intubation of all infants at risk in the DR and subsequent support with mechanical ventilation. However, the optimal respiratory care of newborns with RDS may involve yet another choice. Because mechanical ventilation before surfactant administration has been associated with decreased dynamic compliance, bronchiolar injury, and less therapeutic benefit,[27–29] an approach that combines the benefits of surfactant administration and the benefits of early CPAP but without the drawbacks associated with mechanical ventilation has great intellectual appeal. Described by Verder and colleagues[30] in 1992 at a Danish hospital that routinely stabilized infants on CPAP, this novel approach has been named INSURE (intubate, surfactant, extubate). Linked to the core concept of INSURE are the observations that a single dose of surfactant was enough to reverse RDS in most cases and that administering surfactant treatment to infants earlier in the course of their disease is more desirable.

In Verder and colleague's initial trial, the infants had severe distress on CPAP and were treated with surfactant at a mean age of 19 hours of life.[30] This same Scandinavian group went on to perform 2 additional unblinded studies in the 1990s, enrolling infants born at less than 30 weeks' gestation and stabilized on CPAP. When the infants exhibited signs of RDS, they were randomized to intubation, surfactant administration, and rapid extubation to CPAP or to continued CPAP with rescue surfactant only if needed as evidenced by clinical deterioration.[31,32] The results were encouraging; the investigators noted a decreased need for repeat dosing of surfactant, oxygen requirement, and subsequent mechanical ventilation in the earlier-treated infants.

The INSURE method has been reported in several different contexts and compared with existing respiratory support strategies. The INSURE method has been evaluated in the DR or shortly after birth (within 1 hour) as the method of initial stabilization and has also been used later in the course of illness to treat established RDS in spontaneously breathing preterm infants already on nasal CPAP. For the purpose of this discussion, the authors refer to INSURE used as the initial stabilization in the DR or during the initial hour of life as *early INSURE* and refer to INSURE used later in the course of established RDS as *late INSURE*. Both early and late INSURE strategies have been compared with the conventional standard approach of intubation, surfactant administration, and continued mechanical ventilation and compared with continued nasal CPAP.

EARLY INSURE VERSUS EARLY CPAP AS INITIAL STABILIZATION

Given that previous studies supported the concept that in preterm infants at risk of RDS prophylactic surfactant was more effective than rescue surfactant, An International Randomized Controlled Trial to Evaluate the Efficacy of Combining Prophylactic Surfactant and Early Nasal Continuous Positive Airway Pressure in Very Preterm Infants (CURPAP) trial was designed to evaluate early CPAP in the DR and early rescue surfactant for CPAP failures versus brief initial intubation, surfactant administration, and extubation to CPAP by 1 hour of life (INSURE) (**Table 2**).[33] CPAP failure was defined as requiring a FIO_2 greater than 0.4, severe apnea requiring bag and mask intervention twice per hour, pH less than 7.2, or PCO_2 greater than 65 mm Hg. Infants that were intubated for insufficient initial respiratory drive or as part of resuscitation were excluded, similar to the COIN exclusion criteria. Unlike the COIN trial, infants intubated and given surfactant initially were extubated back to CPAP at 1 hour of life (INSURE) if satisfactory respiratory drive was present. Two hundred eight infants born between 25 + 0 and 28 + 6 weeks' gestation were enrolled. Unfortunately, this trial did not clarify which approach was superior. Thirty-one percent of infants in the INSURE group needed mechanical ventilation in the first 5 days compared with 33% in the CPAP group (RR 0.95 [95% CI 0.64–1.41]). Almost half (49%) of the infants in the CPAP group ultimately needed rescue surfactant. No statistically significant differences in the primary outcome, need for mechanical ventilation during the first 5 days of life, were reported (RR 0.95 [95% CI 0.64–1.41]). Additionally, no significant differences in mortality, steroid use, or any measure of CLD were reported. Of note, the incidence of pneumothorax was similar between the two groups and much lower than that reported in the COIN trial. Postulated reasons for the lack of effect include that the INSURE group received preintubation sedation, high antenatal

Table 2
Early INSURE versus early CPAP as initial stabilization

Author, Year	n	Gest Age	Comparison	Status at Enrollment	Primary Outcome	Results of Primary Outcome	Notes
Sandri et al,[33] 2010	208	25–28 + 6	Early CPAP (and rescue surfactant if needed) vs INSURE	Spontaneous breathing (intubated infants excluded)	Mechanical ventilation within the first 5 d of life	RR 0.95 (95% CI 0.64–1.41)	No difference in mortality, CLD, or any other outcomes 50% of infants 25–28 wk managed without intubation
Dunn et al,[25] 2011	648	26–29 + 6	Early CPAP vs INSURE	All comers independent of respiratory status			45% of infants in CPAP group intubated 51% of infants in INSURE group intubated No difference in mortality, CLD, or other outcomes
Rojas et al,[34] 2009	279	27–31 + 6	Early CPAP vs INSURE	Spontaneously breathing on CPAP between 15–60 min of life	Subsequent mechanical ventilation	RR 0.69 (0.49–0.97)	Less pneumothorax in INSURE group Trend toward less CLD (RR 0.84 [95% CI 0.66–1.05]) Slightly larger, more mature infants

Abbreviations: CI, confidence interval; CLD, chronic lung disease; CPAP, continuous positive airway pressure; Gest, gestational; INSURE, intubate, surfactant, and extubation; RR, relative risk.

steroid rates, and earlier rescue surfactant administration. The CURPAP trial median rescue surfactant administration time was 4.0 hours compared with 6.6 hours in the COIN trial. The investigators did demonstrate that using these strategies, greater than 50% of infants between 25 and 28 weeks' gestation could be managed without intubation.

The multicenter VON DRM trial discussed in the previous section on stabilization on nCPAP also included an INSURE arm in which infants were intubated, given prophylactic surfactant, and rapidly extubated to CPAP.[25] Termed *ISX* in this study (for intubation, surfactant, extubation), these infants were compared with infants who were intubated, given prophylactic surfactant, and maintained on mechanical ventilation. (Comparison of early stabilization on CPAP vs intubation, prophylactic surfactant, and mechanical ventilation is discussed earlier.) Infants between 26 + 0 and 29 + 6 weeks' gestation were included in this study. Unlike the COIN and CURPAP studies, this trial did not exclude infants based on their need for immediate intubation secondary to inadequate initial respiratory drive during initial resuscitation. Similar to the SUPPORT trial, antenatal steroid administration was nearly universal. The INSURE (ISX) group was intubated 5 to 15 minutes after birth, administered surfactant, and extubated to CPAP 15 to 30 minutes later if their Fio_2 was less than 0.6 without severe respiratory distress or apnea. The early CPAP arm had CPAP applied within 15 minutes of birth and was rescued (intubated for surfactant administration) only for severe apnea, Pco_2 greater than 65 mm Hg, or Fio_2 greater than 0.4. In keeping with the findings of the CURPAP trial, almost half (51% in the INSURE group and 45% in the CPAP group) required intubation during the first week of life, and the rates of pneumothoraces in both groups were much lower than those in the COIN trial. However, this study also failed to demonstrate any difference in the primary outcome of death or CLD at 36 weeks' postmenstrual age between the 3 groups.

Rojas and colleagues performed a trial that examined the INSURE method in slightly larger infants. Rojas and colleagues[34] enrolled 279 infants from 8 centers in Columbia. Infants between 27 + 0 and 31 + 6 weeks' gestation (mean 29 weeks and 1300 g) were eligible if they had evidence of RDS and were spontaneously breathing on nasal CPAP between 15 and 60 minutes of life. The infants were randomized to continued nasal CPAP or to brief intubation, surfactant administration, and extubation to CPAP (INSURE). The primary outcome was the need for subsequent mechanical ventilation using predefined criteria. All of the infants in the INSURE group were successfully extubated to CPAP. The need for intubation and mechanical ventilation was lower in the INSURE group compared with the CPAP group (26% vs 39%). Pneumothorax was noted less frequently in the INSURE group compared with the CPAP group (2% vs 9%). The percentage of patients receiving surfactant after the first hour of life was also significantly less in the INSURE group compared with the CPAP group (12% vs 26%). Importantly, the incidence of CLD at 36 weeks' postmenstrual age was high in both groups: 49% in the INSURE group compared with 59% in the CPAP group (RR: 0.84 [95% CI 0.66–1.05]).

EARLY INSURE VERSUS STANDARD CARE (INTUBATION IN DR AND MECHANICAL VENTILATION)

Little data are available that directly compare the INSURE method to the more conventional approach of intubation, prophylactic surfactant administration, and continued mechanical ventilation (**Table 3**). This lack of data may be partly caused by the observation that centers implementing INSURE strategies are heavily invested in CPAP as

Table 3
Early INSURE versus standard care (intubation in DR and mechanical ventilation)

Author, Year	n	Gest Age	Comparison	Primary Outcome	Results of Primary Outcome	Notes
Tooley et al,[35] 2003	42	25–28 + 6	INSURE vs intubation in DR and mechanical ventilation	Need for mechanical ventilation at 1 h of life	Mechanical ventilation at 1 h of life: CPAP group 62% Standard group 100% ($P = .0034$)	All infants intubated in DR, received surfactant, and caffeine None of STD group intubated by 6 h of life 47% of INSURE infants never needed mechanical ventilation No difference in CLD or mortality
Dunn et al,[25] 2011	1316	24–27 + 6	INSURE vs intubation in DR and mechanical ventilation	CLD @ 36 wk or mortality	RR 0.78 (95% CI 0.59–1.03)	High antenatal steroids rates INSURE group extubated by 6 h of life Third arm of this study on CPAP

Abbreviations: CI, confidence interval; CLD, chronic lung disease; CPAP, continuous positive airway pressure; DR, delivery room; Gest, gestational; INSURE, intubate, surfactant, and extubation; RR, relative risk; STD, standard.

primary stabilization and have lost equipoise toward continued management on mechanical ventilation.

Tooley and Dyke[35] performed a pilot RCT that enrolled 42 infants born between 25 + 0 and 28 + 6 weeks' gestation. All infants in the study were electively intubated at delivery, received one dose of prophylactic surfactant, and a loading dose of caffeine. Infants randomized to the standard therapy arm were managed on conventional ventilation and weaned toward extubation using a predefined guideline. These infants were also routinely given morphine as an analgesic. Infants randomized to an INSURE strategy were extubated to CPAP following surfactant administration within 1 hour of birth. Strict criteria for increasing CPAP support and CPAP failure (F_{IO_2} >0.70, pH <7.2, hypoxia, and significant apnea) were followed. However, the treatment of CPAP failures with rescue surfactant or repeat dosing surfactant for the standard group was not part of the study protocol. The primary outcome in this study was the need for continued mechanical ventilation after 1 hour from birth for the INSURE group versus 6 hours of life for the standard care group. Of the infants who were extubated to CPAP by 1 hour of life, 47% never required reintubation. None of the infants in the standard therapy group were extubated within 6 hours from birth. This study was limited by its small sample size and failed to show any difference in outcomes of interest (CLD at 36 weeks or mortality); however, it did confirm that a significant number of preterm infants treated with the INSURE strategy can be successfully extubated and avoid continued ventilation.

The 3-armed VON DRM trial contained the comparison of intubation, prophylactic surfactant, and mechanical ventilation (standard care) versus an early INSURE strategy.[25] This trial is described in detail earlier. The INSURE (ISX) group was intubated 5 to 15 minutes after birth, administered surfactant, and extubated to CPAP 15 to 30 minutes later if their F_{IO_2} was less than 0.6 without severe respiratory distress or apnea. The standard-care group was eligible for extubation at 6 hours of age and had prespecified criteria for surfactant redosing; however, subsequent ventilator management, including the decision to extubate to CPAP, was left to the discretion of the clinical team. This trial ended enrollment before reaching the goal sample size and was not able to differentiate the superior strategy. The RR of CLD or death was 0.78 (95% CI 0.59–1.03) for the INSURE group compared with the group receiving the standard traditional approach of intubation, surfactant administration, and continued mechanical ventilation.

The REVE (REduction of VEntilation) trial is a French RCT that is currently unpublished but has been presented in abstract form.[36] It compared early CPAP use after prophylactic surfactant administration (INSURE) with prophylactic surfactant followed by mechanical ventilation in 133 infants born at 25 to 27 weeks' gestation with mild respiratory distress. All infants received caffeine, and antenatal steroid use was very high. The full results are not available; however, the investigators concluded that the INSURE method of intubation with early surfactant administration followed by CPAP mostly benefits infants who are 25 to 26 weeks' gestational age.

LATE INSURE

The earliest studies of the INSURE method did not test INSURE as part of the initial stabilization of high-risk infants but rather as rescue treatment for spontaneously breathing infants managed on CPAP with already established RDS. Verder and colleagues'[31,32] studies demonstrated that infants who were rescued with the INSURE strategy were less likely to need continued mechanical ventilation and that this effect was more pronounced if the treatment was applied earlier in the course of the disease, before the oxygen requirement increases to approximately F_{IO_2} 0.4.[31,32] Several studies have followed comparing the INSURE procedure used later (>1 hours of life) as part of a rescue strategy for spontaneously breathing preterm infants with RDS on CPAP, to both the standard management of late rescue surfactant therapy and continued mechanical ventilation or to continued management on nasal CPAP without INSURE intervention. These studies are discussed later.

LATE INSURE VERSUS STANDARD CARE (RESCUE SURFACTANT AND MECHANICAL VENTILATION)

There are relatively few published reports comparing the use of the INSURE method later (>1 hour of life) in the course of established RDS to the standard approach of intubation, surfactant administration, and subsequent mechanical ventilation (**Table 4**). Each is discussed in detail next.

The VON has presented the results of a multicenter study randomizing 267 larger spontaneously breathing preterm infants (birth weight 1501–2500 g) with established RDS between 2 and 24 hours of life to either early intubation, surfactant treatment, and rapid extubation (INSURE) or standard respiratory management, including intubation and surfactant treatment based on predefined clinical indications.[37] This study has been presented in abstract form. A nonsignificant trend toward favoring the INSURE strategy for the primary outcome measure of the need for mechanical ventilation in the first week of life (RR 0.78 [95% CI 0.59–1.03]) was observed, a finding in keeping with Verder's work.

A report from a single center in Italy by Dani and colleagues[38] enrolled 27 infants born at less than 30 weeks' gestation with established RDS. Infants were eligible if they were on CPAP and were breathing spontaneously, displayed evidence of respiratory distress, and had an F_{IO_2} requirement of greater than 0.3. All enrolled patients were intubated for surfactant treatment, although infants in the INSURE arm received surfactant earlier than those randomized to standard management (mean 2.7 hours vs 3.5 hours, $P = .18$). Infants randomized to an INSURE strategy were extubated shortly after surfactant administration. At 7 days of life, none of the patients in the INSURE group were on a ventilator compared with 43% of those infants randomized to continued mechanical ventilation ($P = .026$). A second dose of surfactant was needed less frequently in the INSURE group compared with the infants randomized to surfactant followed by mechanical ventilation. Additionally, the duration on mechanical ventilation, on CPAP, and on any supplemental oxygen was statistically significantly shorter among infants treated with the INSURE early extubation strategy.

LATE INSURE VERSUS CONTINUED CPAP

As previously noted, the first RCT of the INSURE method was Verder and colleagues'[32] 1994 study performed in Scandinavia (**Table 5**). They enrolled 73 preterm infants (25–35 weeks' gestational age) with moderate to severe distress on CPAP to either INSURE or to continued CPAP. Eligible infants already on CPAP with established RDS had to be at least 2 hours of age. The median time of randomization was 12 hours. The INSURE treatment was considered to have failed if extubation was not possible within 1 hour of the surfactant instillation or if rescue reintubation was required within 5 days. Indications for rescue intubation, mechanical ventilation, and surfactant were available to both groups via standardized guidelines and based on an oxygen-tension ratio of less than 0.15 or severe apnea. As previously noted, the need for subsequent mechanical ventilation was reduced with the INSURE

Table 4
Late INSURE versus standard care (rescue surfactant and mechanical ventilation)

Author, Year	n	Population	Comparison	Status at Enrollment	Primary Outcome	Results of Primary Outcome	Notes
Soll et al,[37] 2003	267	Birth weight 1501–2500 g	Late INSURE vs STD care	2–24 h old with established RDS	Need for mechanical ventilation in first week of life	RR 0.78 (95% CI 0.59–1.03)	Larger infants Not published, presented in abstract form
Dani et al,[38] 2004	27	<30 wk gestation	Late INSURE vs STD care	Breathing spontaneously on CPAP, with evidence of RDS	Need for mechanical ventilation in first week of life	INSURE 0% Standard care 43% (P = .026)	INSURE infants received surfactant sooner (2.7 vs 3.5 h of life) Duration of mechanical ventilation, CPAP, O₂ use less among INSURE infants

Abbreviations: CI, confidence interval; CPAP, continuous positive airway pressure; INSURE, intubate, surfactant, and extubation; RDS, respiratory distress syndrome; RR, relative risk; STD, standard.

Table 5
Late INSURE versus continued CPAP

Author, Year	n	Gest Age	Comparison	Status at Enrollment	Primary Outcome	Results of Primary Outcome	Notes
Verder et al,[32] 1994	73	25–35	Late INSURE vs continued CPAP	At least 2 h old with a/A gradient <0.22	Need for mechanical ventilation	Late INSURE 43% Continued CPAP 85% ($P = .003$)	No difference in rate of CLD or mortality Median time of randomization ~12 h
Reininger et al,[39] 2005	105	29–35	Late INSURE vs continued CPAP	At least 30 min old on CPAP with O_2 requirement	Need for mechanical ventilation	Late INSURE 50% Continued CPAP 70% ($P = .04$)	Median enrollment at 6.5 h (range: 1.6–49 h) Larger, more mature infants Blinded study involving sham treatment No differences in CLD or mortality

Abbreviations: a/A, alveolar-arterial; CLD, chronic lung disease; CPAP, continuous positive airway pressure; Gest, gestational; INSURE, intubate, surfactant, and extubation.

treatment (85% vs 43%, $P = .003$). No significant differences in the rate of pneumo-thorax, mortality, or CLD were reported.

One additional study, reported by Reininger and colleagues,[39] examined the INSURE strategy used later (>1 hour of life) compared with continued CPAP in 105 larger infants (29 and 35 weeks' gestational age). Infants were eligible if they had established RDS, were stabilized on CPAP with an oxygen requirement, and were at least 30 minutes old. Infants were randomized typically at 6.5 hours; however, they ranged in age between 1.6 and 49.0 hours. Unlike many of the other studies of the INSURE method, this trial was blinded. Blinding was facilitated using privacy screens placed around the infants. A study team not involved in that infant's daily care administered surfactant to infants randomized to the INSURE strategy and these infants were extubated to CPAP while still behind the privacy screen. Infants random-ized to continued CPAP were not intubated nor received any placebo but were cared for in the interim behind the privacy screen for approximately 15 minutes. Uniform criteria for rescue mechanical ventilation and surfactant administration were used to manage both groups. Similar to Verder and colleagues' study, infants treated with the INSURE method were less likely to need subsequent mechanical ventilation (70% in CPAP-only group vs 50% in INSURE group), were less likely to need subse-quent surfactant, and had lower oxygen needs. There were no significant differences in the rate of pneumothorax, CLD, or mortality.

OTHER STUDIES FEATURING INSURE

The Texas Neonatal Research Group performed a multicenter trial that enrolled 132 larger (birth weight >1250 g) preterm (<36 weeks' gestation) infants with RDS between 4 and 24 hours of life.[40] Unlike the previously discussed studies, infants were not required to be routinely stabilized on CPAP before the intervention, although approx-imately two-thirds in each group were managed in this fashion. Infants randomized to the INSURE arm were intubated and extubated unless the F_{IO_2} was higher than before intubation. These infants were also not required to be extubated to CPAP following the INSURE treatment. Infants randomized to the standard arm had no prespecified treat-ment but could receive rescue surfactant and/or CPAP per the hospitals' routine guidelines. INSURE-treated infants were less likely to require subsequent mechanical ventilation for worsening respiratory disease (RR 0.60 [95% CI 0.37–0.99]) but actually had a higher median duration of mechanical ventilation (2.2 vs 0 hours) because only 29 out of 67 control infants required mechanical ventilation. There were no differences in any other outcome of interest (duration of CPAP, duration of supplemental oxygen, pneumothorax, or mortality). CLD was not reported, but discharge on home oxygen was not different between the groups. The investigators concluded that the INSURE method among these larger preterm infants (>1250 g) with mild to moderate RDS is not recommended. However, the omission of CPAP for functional residual capacity (FRC) stabilization before randomization or in the standard care arm makes this study difficult to interpret.

A Cochrane systematic review has been performed containing RCTs comparing early surfactant administration with less than 1 hour of mechanical ventilation followed by extubation (INSURE) versus selective surfactant administration, continued mechanical ventilation, and extubation from low respiratory support.[41] The investiga-tors included studies that gave surfactant either to spontaneously breathing infants with signs of RDS (who received surfactant for established RDS but before requiring intubation for frank respiratory failure) and infants at a high risk for RDS (who received prophylactic surfactant administration within 15–60 minutes after birth). Nine of the previously mentioned studies met selection criteria and were included in the review (6 as early treatment and 3 as prophylaxis). In the meta-analysis of the 6 studies that included early INSURE strategies, there were significant reductions in the need for oxygen use at 28 days of life (typical RR 0.43 [95% CI 0.20–0.92]), mechanical ventilation (typical RR 0.67 [95% CI 0.57–0.79]) and fewer air leak syndromes (typical RR 0.52 [95% CI 0.28–0.96]) but no differences in either CLD, mortality, or the combined outcome of CLD or mortality compared with the standard conventional strategy of selective surfactant administration and continued mechanical ventilation in infants with RDS. The protection against air-leak was more pronounced in a subanalysis using a low threshold for surfactant replacement of F_{IO_2} less than 0.45. The meta-analysis of the 3 studies featuring a prophylactic INSURE strategy with intubation of patients at a high risk for RDS immediately after birth for the purpose of surfactant administration followed by rapid extubation to nasal CPAP compared with initial stabilization on CPAP and selective surfactant administration demonstrated no significant advantage or difference between the two strategies.

Although the INSURE method seems to reliably reduce the burden of mechanical ventilation in preterm infants with RDS, some infants still fail, requiring reintubation and mechanical ventilation. Dani and colleagues[42] have identified independent risk factors for INSURE failure. Among preterm neonates born less than 30 weeks' gestation, having a birth weight less than 750 g or severe hypoxia (a/A gradient <0.44 on initial blood gas) has been demonstrated to be an independent risk factor for INSURE failure.

NASAL INTERMITTENT POSITIVE PRESSURE VENTILATION

Several studies have been performed examining the role of nasal intermittent positive pressure ventilation (NIPPV) as part of the initial stabilization of preterm infants. Although clinicians are increasingly trying to manage preterm infants without mechanical ventilation, the reality is that many preterm infants with RDS managed primarily on CPAP or extubated early to CPAP will fail, requiring intubation and stabilization on mechanical ventilation.[19,21,43] NIPPV use in preterm infants is an attempt to improve these failure rates. NIPPV is a method of noninvasive respiratory support in which intermittent ventilator-generated inflations via the nasal CPAP interface are used to augment CPAP.

Bhandari and colleagues[44] conducted an RCT that enrolled 41 infants less than 32 weeks' gestational age that were intubated and given surfactant for RDS. Infants were randomized to either continued management on conventional ventilation or extubation to NIPPV within 90 minutes of the surfactant administration. No differences in duration of endotracheal mechanical ventilation or oxygen use were observed; however, there was a significant reduction (from 52% to 25%, $P = .03$) in the combined outcome of CLD or death observed in the group that was extubated to NIPPV.

Two studies have been performed comparing NIPPV to CPAP as initial treatment of RDS to prevent intubation. Bisceglia and colleagues[45] randomized 88 preterm infants with RDS to either continued CPAP or NIPPV. The investigators reported improved P_{CO_2} levels and shorter duration of mechanical ventilation when it was indicated in the NIPPV group, but no difference was noted in the need for endotracheal ventilation. The investigators did not report mortality or CLD outcomes. A second study, reported by Kugelman and colleagues[46] randomized 84 infants born less than 35 weeks' gestation with clinical RDS to either NIPPV or CPAP. Infants from either arm were eligible for intubation, rescue surfactant administration, and mechanical ventilation using uniform criteria. In this trial, infants initially stabilized using NIPPV were less likely to be intubated (25% vs 49%, $P = .04$) and less likely to have CLD (2% vs 17%, $P = .03$).

One study has been performed comparing post-INSURE extubation to nCPAP versus NIPPV. Ramanathan and colleagues[47] performed an RCT enrolling 110 spontaneously breathing preterm infants born between $26 + 0$ and $29 + 6$ weeks' gestation that were administered surfactant at 60 minutes of life. In this report, infants intubated either in the DR or soon after admission as well as spontaneously breathing infants stabilized initially on CPAP were eligible for inclusion in the study. Infants randomized to extubation with CPAP remained on CPAP until at least 72 hours of life or until they no longer had an O_2 requirement. Infants randomized to extubation on NIPPV were weaned according to a standard guideline; however, infants were maintained on NIPPV for at least 24 hours following extubation. Both groups were reintubated for the same indications (severe apnea, FiO_2 >0.6, pH <7.25, PCO_2 >65 mm Hg). Days spent on endotracheal mechanical ventilation were shorter in the group randomized to NIPPV compared with CPAP (median 1 vs 7 days, $P = .006$). CLD was observed in 39% of the infants in the CPAP group compared with 21% in the NIPPV group (OR 2.4 [95% CI 1.02–5.6]). No differences were observed in mortality rates or in the combined outcome of mortality and CLD.

MIST AND OTHER METHODS OF SURFACTANT REPLACEMENT

The benefits seen with the INSURE method are likely secondary to surfactant replacement among infants who are surfactant deficient, thereby establishing an adequate FRC. However, to facilitate this treatment, intubation and some brief period of positive pressure endotracheal ventilation is required. As previously noted, both intubation and mechanical ventilation can be associated with adverse outcomes. An alternative to the INSURE procedure has been developed and has been referred to by some as minimally invasive surfactant therapy (MIST). The MIST procedure consists of instilling surfactant to the trachea via a thin catheter to spontaneously breathing infants stabilized on CPAP. Several observational studies have demonstrated that the technique is feasible and, in contrast to INSURE, seems well tolerated in the smallest infants.[48,49] One large multicenter RCT randomized 220 infants born between 26 to 28 weeks' gestation with a birthweight less than 1.5 kg to the MIST procedure if their FiO_2 was greater than 0.3 versus continuation on CPAP. This report is called the Avoidance of Mechanical Ventilation trial. Failure of either group was defined as the need for mechanical ventilation, PCO_2 greater than 65 mm Hg, or FiO_2 greater than 0.6. The study demonstrated that this approach is technically feasible; in 95% of the cases, surfactant replacement was performed on the first attempt. The group treated with MIST had less need for mechanical ventilation (absolute risk reduction -0.18 [95% CI -0.30 to -0.050]) and a decreased need for O_2 at 28 days of life (30% vs 45%, $P = .032$) compared with the CPAP-only group. There were no differences in mortality reported. No studies comparing the INSURE method versus the MIST method are available.

The MIST procedure, like the INSURE procedure, still requires the need for laryngoscopy. Other alternatives to direct laryngeal instillation of surfactant have been attempted and are under investigation. Several trials have been performed attempting to administer nebulized surfactant to spontaneously breathing preterm infants with RDS stabilized on CPAP as rescue or as prophylaxis; although some of these trials have demonstrated small clinical improvements, the earliest reports used less effective surfactant preparations and they have not demonstrated meaningful efficacy.[50–53] Other methods of surfactant deposition include directly into the nasopharynx immediately following delivery of the head[54] or via a laryngeal mask airway.[55] These approaches have great appeal but also have not been proven to be effective in large RCTs.

OPTIMIZATION OF THERAPY

Independent of the strategy to stabilize preterm infants with or at risk for RDS, several adjunctive therapies have been associated with improved outcome. Antenatal steroid administration has a well-documented diminution of the risk of RDS and is likely synergistic when used with surfactant replacement, such as the INSURE method.[31] This effect may also translate into a decreased risk in the development of CLD.[56] Caffeine prophylaxis has been proven to decrease apnea, decrease extubation failure, decrease time on mechanical ventilation, and decrease the risk of CLD development.[57] Opiate medications are recommended as part of premedication for elective intubation for the INSURE procedure. However, these medications are associated with unfavorable side effects in preterm infants struggling to breathe, such as respiratory depression and chest wall rigidity. Naloxone, an opiate antagonist, has been used to reverse the effects of opiates; however, shorter-acting opiates, such as remifenanil, are being evaluated for use in newborns.[58]

Accurate identification of infants at the highest risk for RDS or for the development of CLD would be helpful. One test being developed is based on sampling gastric aspirates from newborns for the quantity of lamellar bodies (a storage form of surfactant).[59] This technique has practical appeal because the size of the lamellar bodies is similar to the size of platelets, allowing for the use of readily available automated blood counters. Clinical studies are underway to further refine this method.

SUMMARY

Despite the lack of definitive evidence of a single superior strategy, a groundswell is taking place toward noninvasive respiratory support. Several well-designed trials suggest that strategies, including application of CPAP in the DR or early in the course of RDS in preterm infants, are as safe and at least as effective as the standard approach of intubation in the DR. Although prophylactic surfactant does not offer any definite benefit over selective treatment, it should be given as early as possible in the course of RDS, when it looks as if mechanical ventilation will be likely. Those probabilities will vary from nursery to nursery and will depend on the comfort level and experience of nurses with CPAP. Efforts to decrease the use of mechanical ventilation via the combination of maternal antenatal steroid administration and early INSURE strategies are associated with decreased morbidities associated with RDS and are likely an important part of a coordinated plan to reduce the risk of CLD. Newly developed techniques for administering exogenous surfactant and providing noninvasive respiratory support require further investigation. More trials comparing different techniques of respiratory support are justified and should include an evaluation of long-term respiratory and neurodevelopmental outcomes.

REFERENCES

1. Yost CC, Soll RF. Early versus delayed selective surfactant treatment for neonatal respiratory distress syndrome. Cochrane Database Syst Rev 2000;(2):CD001456.
2. National Quality Forum; [2012]. Available at: http://www.qualityforum.org/MeasureDetails.aspx?actid=0&SubmissionId=315#k=surfactant. Accessed July 19, 2012.

3. da Silva WJ, Abbasi S, Pereira G, et al. Role of positive end-expiratory pressure changes on functional residual capacity in surfactant treated preterm infants. Pediatr Pulmonol 1994;18(2):89–92.

4. O'Donnell CP, Kamlin CO, Davis PG, et al. Endotracheal intubation attempts during neonatal resuscitation: success rates, duration, and adverse effects. Pediatrics 2006;117(1):e16–21.

5. Kumar P, Denson SE, Mancuso TJ. Premedication for nonemergency endotracheal intubation in the neonate. Pediatrics 2010;125(3):608–15.

6. Cowan F, Whitelaw A, Wertheim D, et al. Cerebral blood flow velocity changes after rapid administration of surfactant. Arch Dis Child 1991;66(10 Spec No): 1105–9.

7. Avery ME, Tooley WH, Keller JB, et al. Is chronic lung disease in low birth weight infants preventable? A survey of eight centers. Pediatrics 1987;79(1):26–30.

8. Polin RA, Sahni R. Newer experience with CPAP. Semin Neonatol 2002;7(5): 379–89.

9. Jobe AH, Kramer BW, Moss TJ, et al. Decreased indicators of lung injury with continuous positive expiratory pressure in preterm lambs. Pediatr Res 2002; 52(3):387–92.

10. Ueda T, Ikegami M, Polk D, et al. Effects of fetal corticosteroid treatments on postnatal surfactant function in preterm lambs. J Appl Phys 1995;79(3):846–51.

11. Lindner W, Vossbeck S, Hummler H, et al. Delivery room management of extremely low birth weight infants: spontaneous breathing or intubation? Pediatrics 1999;103(5 Pt 1):961–7.

12. Gregory GA, Kitterman JA, Phibbs RH, et al. Treatment of the idiopathic respiratory-distress syndrome with continuous positive airway pressure. N Engl J Med 1971;284(24):1333–40.

13. Stefanescu BM, Murphy WP, Hansell BJ, et al. A randomized, controlled trial comparing two different continuous positive airway pressure systems for the successful extubation of extremely low birth weight infants. Pediatrics 2003; 112(5):1031–8.

14. Gupta S, Sinha SK, Tin W, et al. A randomized controlled trial of post-extubation bubble continuous positive airway pressure versus infant flow driver continuous positive airway pressure in preterm infants with respiratory distress syndrome. J Pediatr 2009;154(5):645–50.

15. Miller MJ, DiFiore JM, Strohl KP, et al. Effects of nasal CPAP on supraglottic and total pulmonary resistance in preterm infants. J Appl Phys 1990;68(1):141–6.

16. Zhang S, Garbutt V, McBride JT. Strain-induced growth of the immature lung. J Appl Phys 1996;81(4):1471–6.

17. Kamper J. Early nasal continuous positive airway pressure and minimal handling in the treatment of very-low-birth-weight infants. Biol Neonate 1999;76(Suppl 1): 22–8.

18. De Paoli AG, Lau R, Davis PG, et al. Pharyngeal pressure in preterm infants receiving nasal continuous positive airway pressure. Arch Dis Child Fetal Neonatal Ed 2005;90(1):F79–81.

19. Finer NN, Carlo WA, Duara S, et al. Delivery room continuous positive airway pressure/positive end-expiratory pressure in extremely low birth weight infants: a feasibility trial. Pediatrics 2004;114(3):651–7.

20. Ammari A, Suri M, Milisavljevic V, et al. Variables associated with the early failure of nasal CPAP in very low birth weight infants. J Pediatr 2005;147(3):341–7.

21. Morley CJ, Davis PG, Doyle LW, et al. Nasal CPAP or intubation at birth for very preterm infants. N Engl J Med 2008;358(7):700–8.

22. Soll RF, Morley CJ. Prophylactic versus selective use of surfactant in preventing morbidity and mortality in preterm infants. Cochrane Database Syst Rev 2001;(2):CD000510.

23. Finer NN, Carlo WA, Walsh MC, et al. Early CPAP versus surfactant in extremely preterm infants. N Engl J Med 2010;362(21):1970–9.

24. Rich W, Finer NN, Gantz MG, et al. Enrollment of extremely low birth weight infants in a clinical research study may not be representative. Pediatrics 2012; 129(3):480–4.

25. Dunn MS, Kaempf J, de Klerk A, et al. Randomized trial comparing 3 approaches to the initial respiratory management of preterm neonates. Pediatrics 2011; 128(5):e1069–76.

26. Rojas-Reyes MX, Morley CJ, Soll R. Prophylactic versus selective use of surfactant in preventing morbidity and mortality in preterm infants. Cochrane Database Syst Rev 2012;(3):CD000510.

27. Bjorklund LJ, Ingimarsson J, Curstedt T, et al. Manual ventilation with a few large breaths at birth compromises the therapeutic effect of subsequent surfactant replacement in immature lambs. Pediatr Res 1997;42(3):348–55.

28. Bohlin K, Bouhafs RK, Jarstrand C, et al. Spontaneous breathing or mechanical ventilation alters lung compliance and tissue association of exogenous surfactant in preterm newborn rabbits. Pediatr Res 2005;57(5 Pt 1):624–30.

29. Grossmann G, Nilsson R, Robertson B. Scanning electron microscopy of epithelial lesions induced by artificial ventilation of the immature neonatal lung; the prophylactic effect of surfactant replacement. Eur J Pediatr 1986; 145(5):361–7.

30. Verder H, Agertoft L, Albertsen P, et al. Surfactant treatment of newborn infants with respiratory distress syndrome primarily treated with nasal continuous positive air pressure. A pilot study. Ugeskr Laeger 1992;154(31): 2136–9 [in Danish].

31. Verder H, Albertsen P, Ebbesen F, et al. Nasal continuous positive airway pressure and early surfactant therapy for respiratory distress syndrome in newborns of less than 30 weeks' gestation. Pediatrics 1999;103(2):E24.

32. Verder H, Robertson B, Greisen G, et al. Surfactant therapy and nasal continuous positive airway pressure for newborns with respiratory distress syndrome. Danish-Swedish Multicenter Study Group. N Engl J Med 1994; 331(16):1051–5.

33. Sandri F, Plavka R, Ancora G, et al. Prophylactic or early selective surfactant combined with nCPAP in very preterm infants. Pediatrics 2010;125(6): e1402–9.

34. Rojas MA, Lozano JM, Rojas MX, et al. Very early surfactant without mandatory ventilation in premature infants treated with early continuous positive airway pressure: a randomized, controlled trial. Pediatrics 2009;123(1):137–42.

35. Tooley J, Dyke M. Randomized study of nasal continuous positive airway pressure in the preterm infant with respiratory distress syndrome. Acta Paediatr 2003;92(10):1170–4.

36. Truffert P, Storme L, Fily A. Randomised trial comparing nasal CPAP versus conventional ventilation in extremely preterm infants. In: Progrès en Neonatologie. 28eme Journees Nationales de Neonatologie. Paris: Societe Francaise de Neonatologie Ed; 2008. p. 377–83.

37. Soll RF, Conner JM, Howard D, the Investigators of the Early Surfactant Replacement Study. Early surfactant replacement in spontaneously breathing premature infants with RDS. Seattle, Washington: Pediatric Academic Society; 2003.

38. Dani C, Bertini G, Pezzati M, et al. Early extubation and nasal continuous positive airway pressure after surfactant treatment for respiratory distress syndrome among preterm infants <30 weeks' gestation. Pediatrics 2004;113(6):e560–3.

39. Reininger A, Khalak R, Kendig JW, et al. Surfactant administration by transient intubation in infants 29 to 35 weeks' gestation with respiratory distress syndrome decreases the likelihood of later mechanical ventilation: a randomized controlled trial. J Perinatol 2005;25(11):703–8.

40. Escobedo MB, Gunkel JH, Kennedy KA, et al. Early surfactant for neonates with mild to moderate respiratory distress syndrome: a multicenter, randomized trial. J Pediatr 2004;144(6):804–8.

41. Stevens TP, Harrington EW, Blennow M, et al. Early surfactant administration with brief ventilation vs. selective surfactant and continued mechanical ventilation for preterm infants with or at risk for respiratory distress syndrome. Cochrane Database Syst Rev 2007;(4):CD003063.

42. Dani C, Berti E, Barp J. Risk factors for INSURE failure in preterm infants. Minerva Pediatr 2010;62(3 Suppl 1):19–20.

43. Davis PG, Henderson-Smart DJ. Nasal continuous positive airways pressure immediately after extubation for preventing morbidity in preterm infants. Cochrane Database Syst Rev 2003;(2):CD000143.

44. Bhandari V, Gavino RG, Nedrelow JH, et al. A randomized controlled trial of synchronized nasal intermittent positive pressure ventilation in RDS. J Perinatol 2007;27(11):697–703.

45. Bisceglia M, Belcastro A, Poerio V, et al. A comparison of nasal intermittent versus continuous positive pressure delivery for the treatment of moderate respiratory syndrome in preterm infants. Minerva Pediatr 2007;59(2):91–5.

46. Kugelman A, Feferkorn I, Riskin A, et al. Nasal intermittent mandatory ventilation versus nasal continuous positive airway pressure for respiratory distress syndrome: a randomized, controlled, prospective study. J Pediatr 2007;150(5):521–6, 526.e1.

47. Ramanathan R, Sekar KC, Rasmussen M, et al. Nasal intermittent positive pressure ventilation after surfactant treatment for respiratory distress syndrome in preterm infants <30 weeks' gestation: a randomized, controlled trial. J Perinatol 2012;32(5):336–43.

48. Dargaville PA, Aiyappan A, Cornelius A, et al. Preliminary evaluation of a new technique of minimally invasive surfactant therapy. Arch Dis Child Fetal Neonatal Ed 2011;96(4):F243–8.

49. Kribs A, Vierzig A, Hunseler C, et al. Early surfactant in spontaneously breathing with nCPAP in ELBW infants–a single centre four year experience. Acta Paediatr 2008;97(3):293–8.

50. Berggren E, Liljedahl M, Winbladh B, et al. Pilot study of nebulized surfactant therapy for neonatal respiratory distress syndrome. Acta Paediatr 2000;89(4):460–4.

51. Jorch G, Hartl H, Roth B, et al. Surfactant aerosol treatment of respiratory distress syndrome in spontaneously breathing premature infants. Pediatrician 1997;24(3):222–4.

52. Mazela J, Merritt TA, Finer NN. Aerosolized surfactants. Curr Opin Pediatr 2007;19(2):155–62.

53. Finer NN, Merritt TA, Bernstein G, et al. An open label, pilot study of Aerosurf(R) combined with nCPAP to prevent RDS in preterm neonates. J Aerosol Med Pulm Drug Deliv 2010;23(5):303–9.

54. Kattwinkel J, Robinson M, Bloom BT, et al. Technique for intrapartum administration of surfactant without requirement for an endotracheal tube. J Perinatol 2004;24(6):360–5.

55. Trevisanuto D, Grazzina N, Ferrarese P, et al. Laryngeal mask airway used as a delivery conduit for the administration of surfactant to preterm infants with respiratory distress syndrome. Biol Neonate 2005;87(4):217–20.
56. Jobe AH. Antenatal factors and the development of bronchopulmonary dysplasia. Semin Neonatol 2003;8(1):9–17.
57. Schmidt B, Roberts RS, Davis P, et al. Caffeine therapy for apnea of prematurity. N Engl J Med 2006;354(20):2112–21.
58. Pereira e Silva Y, Gomez RS, Marcatto Jde O, et al. Morphine versus remifentanil for intubating preterm neonates. Arch Dis Child Fetal Neonatal Ed 2007;92(4): F293–4.
59. Verder H, Ebbesen F, Brandt J, et al. Lamellar body counts on gastric aspirates for prediction of respiratory distress syndrome. Acta Paediatr 2011;100(2): 175–80.

Which Continuous Positive Airway Pressure System is Best for the Preterm Infant with Respiratory Distress Syndrome?

J. Jane Pillow, BMedSci (Dist), MBBS, FRACP, PhD (Dist)[a,b,c,*]

KEYWORDS

- Continuous positive airway pressure • Noninvasive ventilation • Infant • Newborn
- Variable flow • Constant flow • Apnea • Respiratory distress syndrome

KEY POINTS

- Short binasal prongs are an effective and convenient patient-device interface for the delivery of CPAP to the newborn infant.
- Fluid-sealed (bubble) flow-opposition CPAP produces variable CPAP pressures that may promote enhance volume recruitment relative to other CPAP systems in patients with acute atelectatic disease.
- Fluidic (variable) flow-opposition CPAP systems provide effective CPAP with lower imposed extrinsic work of breathing compared to constant-pressure ventilator-derived flow opposition CPAP.
- Lower resistive work of breathing associated with fluidic flow devices may provide clinical advantage in the infant with chronic respiratory disease who has impaired respiratory muscle contractility and susceptibility to fatigue.
- Additional, adequately powered and appropriately designed clinically randomised trials that separately address the use of CPAP in specific clinical settings are necessary to determine which CPAP system is best for any given patient.

Commercial relationships: J Pillow has acted as a consultant for Fisher & Paykel Healthcare (Auckland, New Zealand) in the past and lectures in educational workshops organized by several ventilator companies including Drager Medical (Lubeck, Germany), Bunnel (Salt Lake City, UT), and SLE (Croydon, United Kingdom). She has received unrestricted research grants from Fisher & Paykel Healthcare and equipment loans from CareFusion (Yorba Linda, CA).

[a] The Centre for Neonatal Research and Education, The University of Western Australia, 35 Stirling Highway, Perth, Western Australia, Australia, 6009; [b] School of Women's and Infants' Health, The University of Western Australia, 35 Stirling Highway, Perth, Western Australia, Australia, 6009; [c] Neonatal Clinical Care Unit, King Edward Memorial Hospital, 374 Bagot Road, Subiaco, 6008, Western Australia, Australia
* c/- NCCU, King Edward Memorial Hospital, 374 Bagot Road, Subiaco, 6008, Western Australia, Australia.
E-mail address: jane.pillow@uwa.edu.au

INTRODUCTION

The resurgence of interest in noninvasive respiratory support over the last 2 decades has generated renewed interest in understanding the best way to deliver continuous positive airway pressure (CPAP). The development of the first CPAP device for adults can be traced back to Von Tiegel in 1914.[1] However, it was more than 60 years before the relevance of CPAP for the newborn infant with respiratory distress syndrome (RDS) was fully appreciated. In 1968, Harrison and colleagues[2] recognized that the increased intrapleural pressure associated with expiratory grunting arising from closure of the glottis and contraction of abdominal muscles effected a physiologic advantage for the infant; prevention of grunting through intubation of the trachea resulted in lower arterial oxygen tensions, which were restored when the tracheal tube was removed. Within a few years of this observation, Gregory and colleagues[3] realized that applying CPAP to the neonate with RDS (via a tracheal tube in 16 infants, and in another 2 infants via use of a pressure chamber positioned around the infant's head) abolished grunting and increased arterial oxygen levels. This study indicated that CPAP and grunting achieved similar physiologic effects, and that CPAP also reduced work of breathing. Gregory and colleagues achieved this effect using CPAP pressures up to 12 mm Hg (~ 16 cm H_2O), well in excess of current commonly applied CPAP pressures. The next few years marked a period of rapid innovation for noninvasive respiratory support, and the emergence of different methods and devices for application of this mechanical assistance. Such methods included negative thoracic pressure applied to infants placed in a hermetically sealed box,[4,5] application of CPAP using a mask that covered the mouth and nares,[6] development of nasal CPAP,[7] and the emergence of bubble nasal CPAP in 1975.[8]

Clinical interest in CPAP as a treatment modality for RDS also spurred studies to enhance our understanding of its physiologic benefits and potential adverse effects, both of which are important to understand the merits of different approaches to CPAP in the clinical setting: CPAP improves oxygenation as a consequence of lung volume recruitment and maintenance, avoidance of atelectasis,[9] and stabilization of the chest wall, with resultant enhanced compliance and reduced intrinsic work of breathing.[10] Improved matching of ventilation and perfusion results from reduced intrapulmonary shunting[11] and improved diffusion. CPAP reduces airway resistance, likely in part because of stenting and the resultant enhanced patency of the airways.[12] Other evidence of reduced work of breathing from CPAP includes a decrease in thoracoabdominal asynchrony,[13] tachypnea, nasal flaring, and rib recession.[14] Direct physical airway stimulation[12] as well as splinting of the upper airway[15] reduces obstructive and central apnea during CPAP therapy[16] and consequently also increases extubation success.[17]

Despite much of this physiologic understanding becoming evident in the early CPAP era, it is only in the last 15 to 20 years, with the reemergence of interest in CPAP, that we have seen further progress in the development of different CPAP support platforms. An understanding of the theoretic basis of these developments may assist the clinician in selecting the optimal form of CPAP for any given clinical setting. For the purposes of this review, discussion is limited to noninvasive CPAP except when discussion of CPAP delivered via a tracheal tube enhances understanding of physiologic principles, with a specific focus on nasal CPAP, the most commonly applied route in the newborn.

DESIRABLE FEATURES OF CPAP SYSTEMS

There are 3 important considerations when determining optimal CPAP therapy for any given clinical setting, including safety and the susceptibility of the patient to adverse effects, ease of care and application, and the desired physiologic outcomes (**Table 1**).

Safety and Minimization of Adverse Effects

Avoidance of harm is a fundamental concept of any clinical treatment. During CPAP, the most significant equipment features to consider include mechanisms to detect obstruction of flow, potential trauma or deformation of the nares, and adequate humidification. Consideration must be given to the potential for nasal trauma arising from incorrect sizing or placement of prongs, or deformation associated with abnormal nasal positioning over extended durations of CPAP support.

Pulmonary air leak and nasal mucosal trauma are most commonly reported as adverse events during neonatal CPAP. Pneumothorax and pulmonary interstitial emphysema likely result from shear trauma associated with repetitive cyclic expansion of atelectatic alveoli. However, obstruction of the expiratory tubing of the CPAP system, resulting in sustained increase of delivered pressures, may contribute to its development. Systems with free expiratory tubing positioned such that it may become obstructed by bedding material or occluded from other equipment represent a particular risk,[18] especially if an overpressure safety valve and alarm are not built into the system. Whereas a pressure-release valve on the inspiratory limb may limit transmission of excessive pressure transmitted to the infant in the event of an obstructed expiratory limb, additional monitoring is necessary to detect obstructed apnea, or impeded fresh gas flow arising from occlusion of the inspiratory circuit limb. Delivery of excessive pressure is a particular concern with heated humidified high-flow nasal cannula (HHHFNC) delivery systems: if the infant closes their mouth, and the cannulae are effectively sealed in the nares (because of secretions around the cannulae or inappropriate sizing), then because the gas flow is unidirectional (ie, there is no expiratory limb), the flow continues to increase the nasopharyngeal pressure until it finds an outlet: either through opening of the mouth, or in soft tissues, the lungs, or intestinal

Table 1
Considerations for selecting CPAP therapy

Consideration	Desirable Outcome
Safety and minimization of adverse effects	Detection of inspiratory limb obstruction and apnea
	Detection of expiratory limb obstruction and avoidance of air leak arising from overpressurization
	Minimization of nasal and mucosal trauma, septal necrosis
	Avoidance of nasal deformity (snubbing)
	Minimize risk of tube dislodgement and inhalation/ingestion
Nursing and care considerations	Ease and stability of fixation
	Ease of positioning
	Noninterference with developmental outcomes, including visual focus, ease of oral feeding, and kangaroo care
Clinical setting and desired physiologic outcomes	Recruitment of the atelectatic lung
	Minimization of obstructive apnea via stenting of airways
	Reducing extrinsic work of breathing in setting of impaired respiratory muscle function
	Bypass of nasal impedance to reduce intrinsic work of breathing
	Weaning of respiratory support and encouraging acquisition of developmental milestones

tract. The potential of this system to result in significant lung and gut overexpansion in this situation should be of concern to attending physicians. A recent report describes the development of subcutaneous scalp emphysema, pneumo-orbitis, and pneumo-cephalus, with concomitant use of the high-flow nasal cannula,[19] whereas others have acknowledged the potential for unpredictably high pressures to be delivered to the smallest infants.[20]

Attention to provision of adequate humidification to avoid nasal mucosal irritation and injury, and systems using circuits that avoid excessive condensation, is also vital. Nasal deformities include necrosis of the columella nasi, flaring of the nostrils (worsens with duration of nasal CPAP) and nasal snubbing that persists after cessation of pro-longed nasal CPAP therapy.[21] Snorkel-type fixation of the nasal prong interface may be more likely to produce nasal snubbing.

Rare complications reported during CPAP include dislodgement of a nasal prong from its metal connector with relocation of the tube to the stomach, requiring endo-scopic removal.[22] This complication is avoidable with the use of appropriately designed short binasal prongs, rather than adaptation of a tracheal tube for the delivery of nasopharyngeal CPAP. Nasal vestibular stenosis may complicate nasal CPAP, resulting in airway and feeding difficulties.[23] Auricular seroma caused by shearing forces associated with straps for attachment of the nasal CPAP application system can be prevented by careful positioning and padding of such straps when needed.[24] Vascular air embolism complicating bilateral tension pneumothoraces during nasal CPAP[25] and pneumopericardium in the absence of other air-leak syndrome[26] are also reported.

Ease of Care and CPAP Application

A system that is easy to apply and maintain is likely to reduce the risk of adverse effects. For example, tubing that lies across the side of the head requires careful head positioning and cushioning to avoid unnecessary pressure associated with prone positioning when the head is positioned to the side. Fixation of nasal prongs and facial masks that avoids dislodgement and ineffective pressure transmission is also vital. In older infants, ease of feeding and development of visual function and fixa-tion also warrants consideration in determining the most appropriate nasal interface.

Reason for CPAP Support and Desired Physiologic Outcomes

Choice of CPAP system should also give strong consideration to the underlying path-ophysiology necessitating CPAP support. Infants with acutely atelectatic lungs may derive particular benefit when CPAP strategies and systems that provide additional volume recruitment are used. In contrast, the infant with impaired respiratory muscle function may especially benefit from a system that minimizes extrinsic load imped-ance. The infant receiving CPAP to avert central apneic intervals may require only a stimulatory flow, or in the event of obstructive apnea, simply require provision of positive pressure sufficient to maintain upper airway patency. In the latter 2 cases, selection of a CPAP system may be weighted more heavily to selection of equipment that requires minimal maintenance and that facilitates acquisition of developmentally appropriate behaviors such as feeding and gaze fixation.

MAJOR COMPONENTS OF CPAP SYSTEMS

Major components requiring consideration when selecting the most appropriate CPAP system for any given patient are listed in **Table 2**.

Table 2 Components of a CPAP system	
Factor	**Relevance**
Pressure-generating device	Constant vs variable pressure influencing potential for gas exchange and airway recruitment Constant vs variable flow influencing work of breathing
Heated and humidified circuit	Delivery of appropriate gas energy and saturation content at high flow to avoid mucosal injury and avoidance of condensation
Blended gas source	Avoidance of hyperoxia/hypoxia
Patient interface	Influences ease of application, rebreathing, extrinsic work of breathing, and potential for local injury
Safety pressure release and alarm	Avoidance of overpressurization with obstruction of expiratory tubing Alert carer to potential deprivation of fresh gas associated with inspiratory limb obstruction

Patient Interfaces and Extrinsic Work of Breathing

Several different patient interfaces have been used for the delivery of CPAP to the nonintubated infant. Nonnasal interfaces have included masks, pressurized plastic bags, and head-box enclosures.[27] Assuming an adequate seal is achieved, these approaches have the benefit of avoiding mucosal damage, adverse consequences associated with tube obstruction, and absence of sudden pressure decreases. However, they restrict access to the head and face and have significant drawbacks with respect to integration of CPAP with oral feeding.

Nasal interfaces are most commonly selected and usually the most appropriate route for the delivery of CPAP to the newborn infant. Whereas nasopharyngeal CPAP was commonly used in the latter part of the twentieth century, this approach is associated with a high level of impedance during spontaneous breathing,[28] injury to and colonization of the nasopharyngeal space, and promotion of copious nasal secretions that increase the risk of airway occlusion.

In contrast, the short binasal prong, initially used by Wung and colleagues,[8] provides an easy-to-manage solution that also facilitates acquisition of developmentally timely oral feeding/sucking behaviors. Appropriate fixation of these devices also facilitates maintenance of CPAP support during spontaneous infant movements. Nasal deformities and mucosal injury are often associated with the prongs. Softer material of the nasal prongs may reduce the impact of local physical stress, provided the design incorporates a flare mechanism that reduces the risk of collapse of the prong walls, and occluded flow. Whereas small nasal masks can be similarly effective in delivering CPAP and reduce the risk of local trauma, difficulty achieving a seal to ensure consistent pressure delivery can limit their usefulness in some infants. High noise levels have also been reported with some systems: noise is flow dependent[29] and is higher in variable-flow devices with jet injectors than in constant-flow devices.[30]

Recently, humidified high-flow nasal cannulae have been popularized for noninvasive respiratory support. Although these small-diameter cannulae may seem to present a high extrinsic impedance load, the narrow diameter generates a jet flow that achieves more efficient penetration of the nasopharyngeal pathway, effectively reducing nasal dead space. Given that the nasal pathway contributes 50% to the intrinsic work of breathing in the nonintubated infant, the increased efficacy of this flow-delivery mechanism may provide mechanical advantage. The simple design of the cannulae, with adjustable length of the connecting tubing, which are secured behind the head, presents a minimally intrusive interface that does not interfere with developmental activities. A recently released nasal cannula system (RAM Cannula, Neotech, CA) combines the dead space clearing benefits of the small-diameter nasal prong (reducing the intrinsic work of breathing) and retains the benefits of a circuit that has inspiratory and expiratory limbs, including a 15-mm adapter to facilitate noninvasive ventilation. It represents a highly adaptable interface that may promote effective, noninvasive delivery not only of CPAP but also of conventional and high-frequency ventilatory modalities.

TYPES OF COMMERCIALLY AVAILABLE NASAL CPAP DEVICES

The range of commercially available, contemporary nasal CPAP devices was reviewed comprehensively in recent years.[31–33] A clear classification was provided by Black,[34] which defines each device as either using constant or variable flow, and subclassifies the devices according to method of CPAP generation. The categorization is shown in **Table 3** and detailed later.

Constant-Flow CPAP

Flow-opposition CPAP
Flow opposition, using a constant bias flow exiting through a fixed expiratory resistance, provides a simple solution for CPAP provision. Although the constant bias

Table 3
Categorization of CPAP modes

Flow Type	Subgroup	Example Systems	Mechanism of CPAP Generation
Constant flow	Flow opposition	Conventional CPAP	Patient's expiratory flow opposes a constant flow from the nasal prongs
	Electronic feedback control valve	SERVO-i Ventilator (Maquet, Fairfield, NJ) Air-Life nasal CPAP (Air-Life)	Variable resistance valve on the expiratory limb delivering constant flow and pressure to airway
	High-flow	Vapotherm (Vapotherm) Nasal High Flow (Fisher & Paykel Healthcare, NZ)	Unidirectional constant high flow and pressure delivered via narrow-diameter nasal cannula
	Liquid seal	Bubble (Fisher & Paykel Healthcare) Babi-Plus (A Plus Medical, CA) High-amplitude bubble	Expiratory limb is submerged in liquid (usually water/acetic acid) to the depth of desired CPAP. Variable (oscillatory) pressure is delivered
Variable flow	Fluidic flow opposition	Arabella (Hamilton Medical, UK), Infant Flow (CareFusion, San Diego, CA), SiPAP (CareFusion)	Gas is entrained during inspiration to maintain stable CPAP pressure. Expiratory flow is diverted via a separate expiratory limb

flow is usually applied to the device via a mechanical ventilator, it may also be delivered directly from the gas source. It thus represents a simple and uncomplicated approach to CPAP that does not require particularly specialized equipment.

HHHFNC treatment provides an alternative approach to flow-opposition CPAP. It was initially developed as an adjunctive therapy for use after weaning from CPAP that reduced the nasal mucosal complications associated with the delivery of cold dry air. However, there is increasing recognition that HHHFNC may generate pressures similar to those delivered during conventional CPAP treatment. HHHFNC differs from conventional flow-opposition CPAP in that the narrow diameter of the nasal cannula results in delivery of a high-velocity jet of gas into the nares that may clear the nasal dead space more effectively than other forms of nasal CPAP. Flows of up to 8 L/min during HHHFNC may reduce frequency and severity of apnea and bradycardia associated with prematurity and effect clinically significant amelioration of the severity of RDS.[35-38]

Electronic feedback control valve CPAP
Constant-flow CPAP may also be generated via inclusion of a variable expiratory resistance by incorporation of rapid servo-control between demand flow system and the expiratory valve that is regulated by software algorithms. The use of variable expiratory resistance provides potential for leak compensation, backup ventilation for apneic intervals, and monitoring of airway graphics. However, these features require retention of a flow sensor near the airway opening, which increases the extrinsic work of breathing and dead space and may diminish an infant's capacity to sustain spontaneous breathing over an extended interval. Furthermore, pressure monitoring within the ventilator rather than at the nasal airway opening reduces responsiveness to patient efforts.

Liquid-seal CPAP
Liquid-seal CPAP represents the simplest form of CPAP, requiring only provision of a constant bias flow, a patient interface (usually short binasal prongs or nasal mask) and creation of flow opposition and pressure by submerging the tip of the expiratory limb a set distance under the surface of the liquid (usually water). Flow escapes beneath the liquid surface via creation of bubbles. Pressure oscillation created by the bubbles is transmitted back to the nares, delivering a variable rather than constant pressure to the airway opening.

Variable Flow

Fluidic flow-opposition CPAP
The fluidic flow-opposition–coupled devices are modifications of the Benveniste valve, which has been used in Scandinavia since the early 1970s. The gas jet decelerates on entering the prongs, resulting in an increase in pressure, in accordance with the Bernoulli principle[33] If inspiratory flow exceeds available injector gas flow, additional gas is entrained from the expiratory tubing via jet mixing and the Coandä effect, to achieve required inspiratory flow demand. During expiration, gas jet flips and redirects inspiratory flow to the expiratory circuit. The fluidic flow-opposition devices offer potentially improved patient comfort (and hence patient-device interaction) because of separate flow pathways for inspiration and expiration. The promoted benefits include the provision of adequate inspiratory flow and maintain stable pressure at the airway opening[39] and rapid (4-millisecond) transition between inspiration and expiration. The overall effect is to lessen the imposed (extrinsic) work of breathing compared with other systems.[40] The systems allow for continuous flow of blended gas and airway pressure monitoring and use a thin soft silicone that flares during inspiratory flow to reduce potential leakage around the prongs. They differ from other nasal

CPAP systems by providing constant pressure with variable rather than constant flow. The 2 major commercially available devices differ with respect to the positioning of the gas injector jets. With the Infant Flow system (CareFusion, San Diego, CA), the gas injectors are positioned flush within the wall, whereas the Arabella device (Hamilton Medical, UK), has twin injector jets that extend partway into the chamber of the universal generator and exhaust into a larger cavity. The 2 devices also differ in the geometric angles that guide flow pathways.[33]

PHYSIOLOGIC CONSEQUENCES OF DEVICE SELECTION
Pressure Transmission

Constancy of the distending pressure waveform has been a focus of device development and refinement. However, in practice, the airway pressure waveform is rarely completely constant, because it varies in response to inspiratory/expiratory movements and the ability of the controller (ventilator) to servoadjust the gas delivery. The variable-flow (fluidic flow-opposition) devices achieve the most stable pressure throughout the respiratory cycle. In contrast, the liquid-seal (bubble CPAP) approach produces a highly variable noisy pressure waveform at the airway opening. The magnitude of the oscillatory pressure variations during bubble CPAP is influenced by the delivered flow.[41]

The use of HHHFNC is also associated with the delivery of positive pressure to the nasopharynx. However, the pressure delivered with a high-flow gas source is completely dependent on the level of leak present in the airway. There is currently limited information about the level of CPAP delivered to the individual baby using HHHFNC; however, some reports suggest that the pressures are unpredictable and can be excessive.[42] The positive distending pressure provided by HFNC varied with the patient's weight.[37] Infants with weights less than 2 kg and mean postmenstrual age of 30 weeks had similar esophageal pressures with HHHFNC using a flow of up to 2.5 L/min to those obtained with nasal CPAP. Using these flows, HHHFNC could match the esophageal pressures observed when babies received nasal CPAP of 6 cm H_2O. Whereas higher flows (up to 2.5 L/min) were required to achieve these pressures in bigger infants, calculations suggest that 6 cm H_2O nasal CPAP pressure can be achieved by flows of only 1.6 L/min in a 1-kg infant and as low as 1.3 L/min in a 500-g infant. Similar algorithms accounting for flow, cannula size, and body weight have been developed by Wilkinson and colleagues.[43] Whereas such algorithms now exist to guide flow selection, they depend on a predictable level of leak being present, and as Finer[44] points out, this does not necessarily reflect day-to-day clinical experience.

Although in the clinical setting, mean CPAP pressure level may be altered until the desired clinical effect of volume recruitment is achieved, the stochastic recruitment effect of the bubble CPAP system may effectively result in the need for a lower mean airway pressure to achieve the same level of volume recruitment, with potential reduced risk of air leak or adverse impact on pulmonary blood flow associated with higher CPAP pressures.

Lung Volume Recruitment

Recent studies suggest that lung volume recruitment and surfactant secretion may be enhanced by the incorporation of variability into the applied tidal volume delivery pattern. This stochastic resonance effect, achieved by superimposing a variable noise (eg, pressure oscillations associated with water-seal CPAP) on to the underlying subthreshold biological breathing pattern within the nonlinear respiratory system may promote enhanced oxygenation because of lung volume recruitment.[45] This concept has particular relevance to the use of constant-flow bubble CPAP, in clinical use since 1975.[8] In a preterm lamb model of RDS, bubble CPAP commenced immediately after birth had enhanced ventilation, oxygenation, lung mechanics, gas mixing efficiency, and lung volume compared with standard flow-opposition CPAP.[46] Di Blasi and colleagues[47] showed that changing the angulation of the tip of the submerged expiratory limb may amplify the oscillatory pressure amplitude and further enhance gas exchange efficiency. These features make bubble CPAP a particularly attractive option for noninvasive treatment of the infant with acute atelectasis.

Although variability of the applied pressure waveform may promote maintenance of lung volume during low tidal volume breathing (as may be expected in the preterm neonate with immature respiratory muscle pump capacity), evidence of a benefit of bubble CPAP in the clinically stable preterm infant after recovery from early respiratory distress is less clear. A clinical trial comparing fluidic flow-opposition nasal CPAP with bubble nasal CPAP showed superiority of bubble CPAP during the first 2 weeks of life (when atelectasis is most likely to be present), with no evidence of difference between the 2 treatments after that period.[48]

An alternative approach to the stochastic lung volume recruitment achieved with the oscillatory pressure waveform associated with bubble CPAP is the use of bilevel CPAP to enhance alveolar recruitment and promote sensory respiratory stimulation via additional air flow. The commercially available bilevel CPAP device (SiPAP, CareFusion, Yorba Linda, CA) combines the fluidic principles of the Infant Flow generator and permits spontaneous breathing at time-regulated alternating CPAP pressures as determined by device respiratory rate and time-high settings. This approach improves gas exchange compared with standard nasal CPAP in preterm infants.[49,50] The increase of the pressure to the secondary (high) pressure level is more gradual than that typically associated with constant-flow, noninvasive ventilation delivered by mechanical ventilators. In some countries, SiPAP breaths may be triggered from a Grasby capsule attached to the abdomen: the effectiveness of this triggering is highly dependent on correct capsule positioning.

Work of Breathing

A central concept in comparison of different CPAP devices relates to the imposed impedance and hence contribution of the device to work of breathing and resulting energy expenditure, oxygen consumption, and patient-device interaction. Minimization of work against the extrinsic system therefore enhances efficiency of respiration. Over the last decade, several in vitro and in vivo studies have attempted to identify differences between different nasal CPAP systems to identify the lowest imposed extrinsic impedance load. In vitro tests largely reflect extrinsic work of breathing (ie, the load impedance associated with the equipment). When nasal CPAP patient-device interfaces are compared, there is a clear reduction in resistance of short binasal prongs compared with longer single or binasal nasopharyngeal prongs,[28] which is translated clinically as reduced need for reintubation.[32] Although the lowest resistance was achieved with the Infant Flow interface (a fluidic flow-opposition device), there were marginal differences between this and other short binasal prongs, and the clinical differences are similarly less apparent.

Such in vitro studies do not examine the interaction between the device and the patient. Cook and colleagues[51] used a lung simulator to apply a standardized simulated-muscle-pressure waveform to identify the mechanical load effects on the breathing pattern. They observed marginally lower tidal volume and minute ventilation in bubble CPAP; however, this may have minimal relevance in the clinical setting because of the increased efficacy of the high-frequency oscillations in water-seal

CPAP compared with more constant-pressure modes. Cook and colleagues studied each system across a range of tidal volumes at a set compliance and resistance of the lung simulator to establish the flow dependence and concluded that there was no difference between the systems for neonates weighing less than 1 kg, but ventilator-derived nasal CPAP was potentially advantageous for larger infants. However, this conclusion is flawed because a constant compliance and resistance were maintained for the lung simulator throughout the tidal volume range, although these mechanical properties and respiratory muscle effort vary with body size.

However, assessments need to also consider patient–CPAP system interactions, and the potential of the equipment to reduce the intrinsic work of breathing through use of approaches that optimize airway patency and avoidance of atelectatic lung and, where relevant, promote lung volume recruitment. In acute situations in which intrinsic work of breathing is the predominant contributor to respiratory impedance, it may be reasonable to accept marginally higher extrinsic impedance during the period of acute lung volume recruitment when selection of an alternative CPAP device may achieve that recruitment more safely and effectively.

In contrast, infants with more chronic lung disease and particularly those who have received mechanical ventilation for extended periods may have accompanying respiratory muscle weakness because of apoptosis and atrophy of the respiratory muscles, increasing susceptibility to respiratory failure associated with increased extrinsic work of breathing. In this setting, minimizing extrinsic workload (eg, fluidic flow opposition), or significantly reducing intrinsic work of breathing by more effective flow penetration of the nasal dead space impedance through high-velocity jet streaming through small-diameter nasal prongs in HHHFNC, may provide effective clinical treatment solutions. Bypassing the nasal dead space may provide particular benefit, given that the nasal compartment contributes approximately 50% to the overall respiratory resistance.[52]

Gas Exchange and Clinical Outcomes

Data that compare efficacy of ventilation, oxygenation, and lung volume recruitment between different CPAP systems are limited. Lee and colleagues[53] compared bubble CPAP versus ventilator CPAP in intubated preterm infants before extubation. Each baby was alternated between the 2 delivery methods during short (30-minute) epochs. During bubble CPAP, infants had a lower minute volume and respiratory rate. Although some have suggested that the lower minute volume reflects increased work of breathing, there were no differences in arterial CO_2 levels, suggesting that bubble CPAP provides more efficient ventilation with less work of breathing than ventilator (constant-flow opposition) CPAP. Similarly, Morley and colleagues[54] found no difference in gas exchange between minimal bubbling and vigorous bubbling in extubated and clinically stable infants already treated with CPAP, and also no effect on breathing pattern. Differences in the constant flow used in the 2 groups (3 vs 6 L/min) may have influenced extrinsic work of breathing. Interpretation of the clinical implications for both of these cross-over trials is limited by the brevity (15–30 minutes) of each study epoch. In 3-hour studies comparing bubble with ventilator (constant-flow opposition) in newborn preterm lambs, we showed that reductions in CO_2 were not achieved until 30 minutes of age, and significant improvements in oxygenation required 2.5 hours to become evident.[46]

Several studies have compared bubble CPAP with fluidic flow-opposition CPAP. A randomized cross-over study using brief 5-minute to 10-minute epochs across a range of set pressures showed increased asynchrony and marginally higher resistive work of breathing in infants during bubble CPAP than when CPAP was delivered by the Infant Flow device.[14] CPAP pressures were determined as those set at the ventilator or by the depth of the submerged expiratory limb and did not account for the increased pressure delivered to the airway opening in this system, which may have influenced outcomes. The same investigators found that when they controlled for pressure measured at the airway opening, previously determined differences in work of breathing between bubble CPAP and ventilator-derived constant-flow opposition CPAP[55] were no longer present.[56] A randomized controlled trial of postextubation bubble CPAP (binasal prong not fully specified) versus the Infant Flow driver in 24-week to 29-week and 600-g to 1500-g infants showed no overall difference in 72 hours' or 7 days' successful extubation between the 2 groups.[48] However, bubble CPAP was associated with a lower duration of CPAP support before successful weaning to nasal cannula or unassisted breathing, and in the subgroup who were extubated before 14 days of invasive mechanical ventilatory support, there was a significant increase in the number of infants successfully extubated for 72 hours. Hence, over an extended interval and particularly when there may be a persisting tendency or presence of atelectatic lung disease, water-sealed CPAP may offer physiologic advantage over the fluidic flow-opposition systems, possibly because of increased pressure amplitude transmission and effective lung volume recruitment and efficient gas exchange in the presence of low compliance.

Several studies have compared the Infant Flow driver with ventilator-derived CPAP, with some evidence for the superiority of the Infant Flow driver (fluidic flow-opposition) device.[14,57,58] Compared with the constant-flow (ventilator-derived) flow-opposition device, fluidic (variable flow) flow-opposition reduced oxygen duration,[58] duration of respiratory support,[57] length of hospital stay,[58] and work of breathing[59] but failed to improve the extubation failure rate in extremely low-birth-weight infants.[58] A single study found no differences in lung volume recruitment or lung mechanics and work of breathing between the Infant Flow and Arabella CPAP systems in low-birth-weight infants.[60]

SUMMARY

Overall, the literature remains confusing because of differences in study design, including patient maturation and postnatal age, magnitude of leak, equivalence of testing conditions for different CPAP systems, and short study epochs, which may be insufficient to detect meaningful and relevant clinical outcomes. Nonetheless, it seems clear that short binasal prongs are an effective and convenient patient-device interface for the delivery of CPAP to the newborn infant. Compared with constant-pressure (ventilator-derived) flow-opposition CPAP, fluidic (variable) flow-opposition CPAP systems offer important and relevant clinical benefits. The distinction between fluid-sealed (bubble) CPAP and fluidic flow-opposition systems is less clear, although the stochastic recruitment benefits of bubble CPAP may offer advantage in acute atelectasis-prone patients with RDS. In contrast, the lower resistive work of breathing associated with fluidic flow devices may offer some clinical advantage in the infant with chronic respiratory disease, particularly in the presence of impaired respiratory muscle contractility and susceptibility to fatigue. Further investigation, with adequately powered and appropriately designed clinically randomized trials that separately address the use of CPAP in each of these clinical settings, is necessary to determine which CPAP is best.

REFERENCES

1. Von Reuss AR. The diseases of the newborn. London: John Bale, Sons and Danielsson; 1921. p. 286.

2. Harrison VC, Heese Hde V, Klein M. The significance of grunting in hyaline membrane disease. Pediatrics 1968;41:549–59.
3. Gregory GA, Kitterman JA, Phibbs RH, et al. Treatment of the idiopathic respiratory-distress syndrome with continuous positive airway pressure. N Engl J Med 1971;284:1333–40.
4. Bancalari E, Garcia OL, Jesse MJ. Effects of continuous negative pressure on lung mechanics in idiopathic respiratory distress syndrome. Pediatrics 1973;51:485–93.
5. Bancalari E, Gerhardt T, Monkus E. Simple device for producing continuous negative pressure in infants with IRDS. Pediatrics 1973;52:128–31.
6. Allen LP, Blake AM, Durbin GM, et al. Continuous positive airway pressure and mechanical ventilation by facemask in newborn infants. Br Med J 1975;4:137–9.
7. Kattwinkel J, Fleming D, Cha CC, et al. A device for administration of continuous positive airway pressure by the nasal route. Pediatrics 1973;52:131–4.
8. Wung JT, Driscoll JM Jr, Epstein RA, et al. A new device for CPAP by nasal route. Crit Care Med 1975;3:76–8.
9. Heldt GP, McIlroy MB. Dynamics of chest wall in preterm infants. J Appl Physiol 1987;62:170–4.
10. Gregory GA, Edmunds LH Jr, Kitterman JA, et al. Continuous positive airway pressure and pulmonary and circulatory function after cardiac surgery in infants less than three months of age. Anesthesiology 1975;43:426–31.
11. Saunders RA, Milner AD, Hopkin IE. The effects of continuous positive airway pressure on lung mechanics and lung volumes in the neonate. Biol Neonate 1976;29:178–86.
12. Richardson CP, Jung AL. Effects of continuous positive airway pressure on pulmonary function and blood gases of infants with respiratory distress syndrome. Pediatr Res 1978;12:771–4.
13. Locke R, Greenspan JS, Shaffer TH, et al. Effect of nasal CPAP on thoracoabdominal motion in neonates with respiratory insufficiency. Pediatr Pulmonol 1991;11:259–64.
14. Liptsen E, Aghai ZH, Pyon KH, et al. Work of breathing during nasal continuous positive airway pressure in preterm infants: a comparison of bubble vs variable-flow devices. J Perinatol 2005;25:453–8.
15. Miller MJ, Carlo WA, Martin RJ. Continuous positive airway pressure selectively reduces obstructive apnea in preterm infants. J Pediatr 1985;106:91–4.
16. Kurz H. Influence of nasopharyngeal CPAP on breathing pattern and incidence of apnoeas in preterm infants. Biol Neonate 1999;76:129–33.
17. Davis PG, Henderson-Smart DJ. Nasal continuous positive airways pressure immediately after extubation for preventing morbidity in preterm infants. Cochrane Database Syst Rev 2003;(2):CD000143.
18. Makhoul IR, Smolkin T, Sujov P. Pneumothorax and nasal continuous positive airway pressure ventilation in premature neonates: a note of caution. ASAIO J 2002;48:476–9.
19. Jasin LR, Kern S, Thompson S, et al. Subcutaneous scalp emphysema, pneumo-orbitis and pneumocephalus in a neonate on high humidity high flow nasal cannula. J Perinatol 2008;28:779–81.
20. Kubicka ZJ, Limauro J, Darnall RA. Heated, humidified high-flow nasal cannula therapy: yet another way to deliver continuous positive airway pressure? Pediatrics 2008;121:82–8.
21. Robertson NJ, McCarthy LS, Hamilton PA, et al. Nasal deformities resulting from flow driver continuous positive airway pressure. Arch Dis Child Fetal Neonatal Ed 1996;75:F209–12.
22. Peck DJ, Tulloh RM, Madden N, et al. A wandering nasal prong–a thing of risks and problems. Paediatr Anaesth 1999;9:77–9.

23. Smith LP, Roy S. Treatment strategy for iatrogenic nasal vestibular stenosis in young children. Int J Pediatr Otorhinolaryngol 2006;70:1369–73.
24. Eifinger F, Lang-Roth R, Woelfl M, et al. Auricular seroma in a preterm infant as a severe complication of nasal continuous positive airway pressure (nCPAP). Int J Pediatr Otorhinolaryngol 2005;69:407–10.
25. Wong W, Fok TF, Ng PC, et al. Vascular air embolism: a rare complication of nasal CPAP. J Paediatr Child Health 1997;33:444–5.
26. Alpan G, Goder K, Glick B, et al. Pneumopericardium during continuous positive airway pressure in respiratory distress syndrome. Crit Care Med 1984;12:1080–1.
27. Svenningsen NW, Jonson B, Lindroth M, et al. Consecutive study of early CPAP-application in hyaline membrane disease. Eur J Pediatr 1979;131:9–19.
28. De Paoli AG, Morley CJ, Davis PG, et al. In vitro comparison of nasal continuous positive airway pressure devices for neonates. Arch Dis Child Fetal Neonatal Ed 2002;87:F42–5.
29. Karam O, Donatiello C, Van Lancker E, et al. Noise levels during nCPAP are flow-dependent but not device-dependent. Arch Dis Child Fetal Neonatal Ed 2008;93:F132–4.
30. Kirchner L, Wald M, Jeitler V, et al. In vitro comparison of noise levels produced by different CPAP generators. Neonatology 2012;101:95–100.
31. Courtney SE, Barrington KJ. Continuous positive airway pressure and noninvasive ventilation. Clin Perinatol 2007;34:73–92, vi.
32. De Paoli AG, Davis PG, Faber B, et al. Devices and pressure sources for administration of nasal continuous positive airway pressure (NCPAP) in preterm neonates. Cochrane Database Syst Rev 2008;(1):CD002977.
33. Diblasi RM. Nasal continuous positive airway pressure (CPAP) for the respiratory care of the newborn infant. Respir care 2009;54:1209–35.
34. Black C. CPAP, yes! But how? Respir care 2010;55:638–9.
35. Holleman-Duray D, Kaupie D, Weiss MG. Heated humidified high-flow nasal cannula: use and a neonatal early extubation protocol. J Perinatol 2007;27:776–81.
36. Shoemaker MT, Pierce MR, Yoder BA, et al. High flow nasal cannula versus nasal CPAP for neonatal respiratory disease: a retrospective study. J Perinatol 2007;27:85–91.
37. Sreenan C, Lemke RP, Hudson-Mason A, et al. High-flow nasal cannulae in the management of apnea of prematurity: a comparison with conventional nasal continuous positive airway pressure. Pediatrics 2001;107:1081–3.
38. Woodhead DD, Lambert DK, Clark JM, et al. Comparing two methods of delivering high-flow gas therapy by nasal cannula following endotracheal extubation: a prospective, randomized, masked, crossover trial. J Perinatol 2006;26:481–5.
39. Huckstadt T, Foitzik B, Wauer RR, et al. Comparison of two different CPAP systems by tidal breathing parameters. Intensive Care Med 2003;29:1134–40.
40. Klausner JF, Lee AY, Hutchison AA. Decreased imposed work with a new nasal continuous positive airway pressure device. Pediatr Pulmonol 1996;22:188–94.
41. Pillow JJ, Travadi JN. Bubble CPAP: is the noise important? An in vitro study. Pediatr Res 2005;57:826–30.
42. Hasan RA, Habib RH. Effects of flow rate and airleak at the nares and mouth opening on positive distending pressure delivery using commercially available high-flow nasal cannula systems: a lung model study. Pediatr Crit Care Med 2011;12:e29–33.
43. Wilkinson DJ, Andersen CC, Smith K, et al. Pharyngeal pressure with high-flow nasal cannulae in premature infants. J Perinatol 2008;28:42–7.

44. Finer NN. Nasal cannula use in the preterm infant: oxygen or pressure? Pediatrics 2005;116:1216–7.
45. Suki B, Alencar AM, Sujeer MK, et al. Life-support system benefits from noise. Nature 1998;393:127–8.
46. Pillow JJ, Hillman N, Moss TJ, et al. Bubble continuous positive airway pressure enhances lung volume and gas exchange in preterm lambs. Am J Respir Crit Care Med 2007;176:63–9.
47. DiBlasi RM, Zignego JC, Smith CV, et al. Gas exchange with conventional ventilation and high-amplitude bubble CPAP (HAB-CPAP) during apnea in healthy and surfactant-deficient juvenile rabbits. PAS Annual Meeting. Baltimore, May 2–5, 2009. p. E-PAS20094735.8.
48. Gupta S, Sinha SK, Tin W, et al. A randomized controlled trial of post-extubation bubble continuous positive airway pressure versus Infant Flow Driver continuous positive airway pressure in preterm infants with respiratory distress syndrome. J Pediatr 2009;154:645–50.
49. Migliori C, Motta M, Angeli A, et al. Nasal bilevel vs. continuous positive airway pressure in preterm infants. Pediatr Pulmonol 2005;40:426–30.
50. Lista G, Castoldi F, Fontana P, et al. Nasal continuous positive airway pressure (CPAP) versus bi-level nasal CPAP in preterm babies with respiratory distress syndrome: a randomised control trial. Arch Dis Child Fetal Neonatal Ed 2010; 95:F85–9.
51. Cook SE, Fedor KL, Chatburn RL. Effects of imposed resistance on tidal volume with 5 neonatal nasal continuous positive airway pressure systems. Respir care 2010;55:544–8.
52. Hall GL, Hantos Z, Wildhaber JH, et al. Contribution of nasal pathways to low frequency respiratory impedance in infants. Thorax 2002;57:396–9.
53. Lee KS, Dunn MS, Fenwick M, et al. A comparison of underwater bubble continuous positive airway pressure with ventilator-derived continuous positive airway pressure in premature neonates ready for extubation. Biol Neonate 1998;73:69–75.
54. Morley CJ, Lau R, De Paoli A, et al. Nasal continuous positive airway pressure: does bubbling improve gas exchange? Arch Dis Child Fetal Neonatal Ed 2005; 90:F343–4.
55. Courtney SE, Pyon KH, Saslow JG, et al. Lung recruitment and breathing pattern during variable versus continuous flow nasal continuous positive airway pressure in premature infants: an evaluation of three devices. Pediatrics 2001;107:304–8.
56. Courtney SE, Kahn DJ, Singh R, et al. Bubble and ventilator-derived nasal continuous positive airway pressure in premature infants: work of breathing and gas exchange. J Perinatol 2011;31:44–50.
57. Buettiker V, Hug MI, Baenziger O, et al. Advantages and disadvantages of different nasal CPAP systems in newborns. Intensive Care Med 2004;30:926–30.
58. Stefanescu BM, Murphy WP, Hansell BJ, et al. A randomized, controlled trial comparing two different continuous positive airway pressure systems for the successful extubation of extremely low birth weight infants. Pediatrics 2003; 112:1031–8.
59. Pandit PB, Courtney SE, Pyon KH, et al. Work of breathing during constant- and variable-flow nasal continuous positive airway pressure in preterm neonates. Pediatrics 2001;108:682–5.
60. Courtney SE, Aghai ZH, Saslow JG, et al. Changes in lung volume and work of breathing: a comparison of two variable-flow nasal continuous positive airway pressure devices in very low birth weight infants. Pediatr Pulmonol 2003;36: 248–52.

Noninvasive Respiratory Support in the Preterm Infant

Vineet Bhandari, MD, DM

KEYWORDS

- SNIPPV • NIPPV • Nasal ventilation • Neonate • Respiratory distress syndrome
- Surfactant • Bronchopulmonary dysplasia

KEY POINTS

- Nasal intermittent positive pressure ventilation is a mode of noninvasive respiratory support that combines nasal continuous positive airway pressure and intermittent mandatory ventilation.
- Compared with nasal continuous positive airway pressure, synchronized or non-synchronized nasal intermittent positive pressure ventilation has been shown to be superior in keeping infants extubated.
- Pilot randomized controlled trials have suggested that use of synchronized nasal intermittent positive pressure ventilation or nasal intermittent positive pressure ventilation, with or without early surfactant (<2 hours of life), may decrease bronchopulmonary dysplasia.

INTRODUCTION

Noninvasive respiratory support in neonates can be achieved by a variety of interfaces using the mouth or nares and a positive pressure source. This article focuses on recent studies that have used nasal intermittent positive pressure ventilation (NIPPV) as a method of noninvasive ventilator assistance mostly in premature newborns. NIPPV is essentially a mode for providing intermittent mandatory ventilation using nasal prongs.[1]

A BRIEF HISTORY OF NIPPV

Early use of NIPPV was directed toward controlling apnea of prematurity,[2] but the report of increased risk of gastrointestinal perforations in sick neonates[3] put the technique into disfavor. Although a small randomized study of synchronized NIPPV (SNIPPV) using nasopharyngeal prongs showed promise,[4] only after two independently conducted randomized controlled trials (RCT) with adequate sample size[5,6]

Division of Perinatal Medicine, Department of Pediatrics, Yale University School of Medicine, Yale Child Health Research Center, Room 219, PO Box 208081, 464 Congress Avenue, New Haven, CT 06520, USA
E-mail address: vineet.bhandari@yale.edu

Clin Perinatol 39 (2012) 497–511
http://dx.doi.org/10.1016/j.clp.2012.06.008
0095-5108/12/$ – see front matter © 2012 Elsevier Inc. All rights reserved.

Table 1
SNIPPV studies in neonates

Author/Ref	Type	No. of Infants	SNIPPV Group[a]	Control Group[a]	Outcomes
Primary mode:					
Santin et al[27]	Prospective, Obs	59	SNIPPV: Rate: same as before extubation; PIP: increased by 2–4 over pre-extubation values; PEEP: ≤5; Flow: 8–10 L/min; Fio$_2$ adjusted for Spo$_2$: 90%–96%	Continued on CV, till ready to extubate to SNIPPV (secondary mode)	SNIPPV group had shorter duration of intubation, supplemental oxygen, parenteral nutrition, and hospitalization
Bhandari et al[29]	RCT	41	SNIPPV[b]: Rate: same as before extubation; PIP: increased by 2–4 over pre-extubation values; PEEP: ≤5; Flow: 8–10 L/min; Fio$_2$ adjusted for Spo$_2$: 90%–96%	Continued on CV, till ready to extubate to SNIPPV (secondary mode)	SNIPPV group had decreased BPD/death and BPD
Secondary mode:					
Friedlich et al[4]	RCT	41	SNIPPV[b]: Rate: 10; PIP: same as pre-extubation; PEEP: 4–6; Ti: 0.6 s; Fio$_2$ adjusted for Spo$_2$: 92%–95%	NP-CPAP: clinician discretion; Fio$_2$ adjusted for Spo$_2$: 92%–95%	Less failed extubation with SNIPPV at 48 h
Barrington et al[5]	RCT	54	SNIPPV: Rate: 12; PIP: 16 (to deliver at least 12); PEEP: 6;	NCPAP: 6	Less failed extubation with SNIPPV at 72 h
Khalaf et al[6]	RCT	64	SNIPPV: Rate: same as before extubation; PIP: increased by 2–4 over pre-extubation values; PEEP: ≤5; Flow: 8–10 L/min; Fio$_2$ adjusted for Spo$_2$: 90%–96%	NCPAP: 4–6; Flow: 8–10 L/min; Fio$_2$ adjusted for Spo$_2$: 90%–96%	Less failed extubation with SNIPPV at 72 h and 7 d

Study	Design	N	SNIPPV settings	Control settings	Outcomes
Kulkarni et al[28]	Retrospective, case-control	60	SNIPPV: Rate: same as before extubation; PIP: increased by 2–4 over pre-extubation values; PEEP: ≤5; Flow: 8–10 L/min; Fio$_2$ adjusted for Spo$_2$: 90%–96%	NCPAP: 4–6; Flow: 8–10 L/min; Fio$_2$ adjusted for Spo$_2$: 90%–96%	SNIPPV group had shorter duration of supplemental oxygen, and decreased BPD
Moretti et al[32]	RCT	63	SNIPPV: Rate: same as before extubation; PIP: 10–20; PEEP: 3–5; Flow: 6–10 L/min; Fio$_2$ adjusted for Spo$_2$: 90%–94%	NCPAP: 3–5; Flow: 6–10 L/min; Fio$_2$ adjusted for Spo$_2$: 90%–94%	Less failed extubation with SNIPPV at 72 h
Gao et al[45]	RCT	50	SNIPPV: Rate: 40; PIP: 20; PEEP: 5; Fio$_2$ adjusted for Spo$_2$: 88%–92%	NCPAP: 4–8; Flow: 8–10 L/min; Fio$_2$ adjusted for Spo$_2$: 88%–92%	Less failed extubation with SNIPPV
Bhandari et al[46]	Retrospective	469	SNIPPV: Rate: same as before extubation; PIP: increased by 2–4 over pre-extubation values; PEEP: ≤6; Flow: 8–10 L/min; Fio$_2$ adjusted for Spo$_2$: 85%–96%	NCPAP: 4–6; Flow: 8–10 L/min; Fio$_2$ adjusted for Spo$_2$: 85%–96%	SNIPPV group (BW 500–750 g) had decreased BPD, BPD/death, NDI and NDI/death

Rate: ventilator rate (breaths/minute).

Abbreviations: BPD, bronchopulmonary dysplasia; BW, birth weight; CV, conventional endotracheal tube ventilation; Fio$_2$, fraction of inspired oxygen; NCPAP, nasal continuous positive airway pressure (cm H$_2$O); NDI, neurodevelopmental impairment; NP-CPAP, nasopharyngeal continuous positive airway pressure (cm H$_2$O); Obs, observational study; PEEP, positive end-expiratory pressure (cm H$_2$O); PIP, peak inspiratory pressure (cm H$_2$O); RCT, randomized controlled trial; SNIPPV, synchronized nasal intermittent positive pressure ventilation; Spo$_2$, pulse oximeter oxygen saturation; Ti, inspiratory time (seconds).

^{a} Initial settings.
^{b} Nasopharyngeal.

Secondary Mode

A meta-analysis of the first three studies using the secondary mode[4–6] concluded that SNIPPV was more effective than NCPAP in preventing failure of extubation (relative risk, 0.21 [0.10–0.45]; risk difference, $-.32$ [$-.45$ to $-.20$]; number needed to treat, 3 [2–5]).[44] Successful extubation was defined as not requiring intubation within 72 hours. In a retrospective case-control study, the infants in the SNIPPV group had shorter duration of supplemental oxygen use and decreased BPD.[28] A subsequent RCT reported that successful extubation was accomplished in 90% in the SNIPPV (n = 32) versus 61% in the NCPAP group of infants (n = 31; $P = .005$).[32] In another RCT, infants randomized to SNIPPV (n = 25), compared with NCPAP group (n = 25), failed extubation less often with SNIPPV (24% vs 60%; $P<.05$).[45] In the largest retrospective analysis to date (n = 469), after controlling for confounding variables, use of SNIPPV in the birth weight category of 500 to 750 g was associated with decreased BPD and BPD/death.[46] These studies are summarized in **Table 1**. In a recent RCT comparing the use of SNIPPV (n = 40) with NCPAP (n = 40) in the management of apnea of prematurity,[47] ventilator duration was shorter in the SNIPPV group ($P<.01$), and arterial blood gases were better 2 hours after initiation of therapy, without any differences in other outcomes or complications.[47]

In a study by Kulkarni and colleagues,[28] introduction of SNIPPV in a NICU with no prior experience resulted in infants having significantly less need for supplemental oxygen and a decreased incidence of BPD, without affecting the incidence of other short-term morbidities. There were no differences between the two groups in nutritional intake or growth parameters.[28]

NIPPV STUDIES
Primary Mode

In a small study (n = 16), NIPPV was piloted to avoid intubation.[48] The success rate was 81%; however, the mean duration of NIPPV use was 23 hours, with no reported complications.[48] In an RCT, infants treated initially with NIPPV (n = 43) required less invasive mechanical ventilation than infants treated with NCPAP (n = 41; 25% vs 49%; $P<.05$). Infants in the NIPPV group had a significantly lower incidence of BPD compared with the NCPAP group (2% vs 17%, $P<.05$, and 5% vs 33%, $P<.05$, for infants with birth weight <1500 g).[38]

In another recent RCT, preterm infants with mild to moderate RDS (n = 88) were randomized to NIPPV versus NCPAP support.[49] Infants managed with NIPPV had lower P_{CO_2} values and decreased apnea (both $P<.05$), and exhibited a shorter duration respiratory support.[49] In a recent RCT by Sai Sunil Kishore and colleagues,[39] 76 neonates (28–34 weeks gestation) with respiratory distress within 6 hours of birth were randomized to receive NIPPV or NCPAP. The failure rate (defined as the need for intubation and mechanical ventilation) at 48 hours and 7 days was significantly less among infants randomized to NIPPV. The failure rate of NIPPV was significantly less in the subgroups of infants 28 to 30 weeks gestation and those who did not receive surfactant. In that combined subgroup of infants (28–30 weeks gestation who did not receive surfactant) the number needed to treat was 2.[39] There were no differences in other outcomes (including BPD), comparing NIPPV with NCPAP.[39]

In an RCT comparing NIPPV (n = 100) with bubble-NCPAP (n = 100), infants in the NIPPV group did not significantly differ in the need for mechanical ventilation at 72 hours of life.[40] However, significantly more infants in the NIPPV group remained extubated from 24 to 72 hours of life.[40] This also remained true for the infants who received surfactant therapy.[40] In another RCT of preterm infants less than 30 weeks gestational age requiring intubation and surfactant soon after delivery (n = 110), Ramanathan and colleagues found that extubation to NIPPV reduced the need for endotracheal tube ventilation, and BPD, using either the physiologic or clinical definition of BPD.[35] These two studies[29,35] suggest that early extubation to NIPPV may be an important modifier of the outcome of BPD, even if the total duration of mechanical ventilation is similar.

Secondary Mode

In the only such RCT, intubated premature infants (n = 48) were randomized to either NIPPV or NCPAP after extubation.[50] There were no differences in the primary outcome (reintubation within 7 days) or treatment-related complications.[50] This RCT had some important limitations. Despite randomization, there were significant differences in the demographics in the two groups. Specifically, infants randomized to NIPPV had lower birth weights and body weights at time of extubation. There were fewer males, more infants with RDS, and greater exposure to antenatal steroids. A critical technical issue in this study was that infants on NIPPV were kept on the same ventilator settings as pre-extubation, in contradiction to the increased settings (to compensate for the loss of distending pressure secondary to leak by the mouth or nose) done in most other studies.[5,6,29,38] These studies are summarized in **Table 2**.

Two studies compared NIPPV with NCPAP for the management of apnea of prematurity.[51,52] Although a meta-analysis was not possible, one trial showed a reduction in apnea frequency with NIPPV and the other a trend favoring NIPPV. Most recently, Pantalitschka and colleagues[53] conducted a randomized crossover trial of four nasal respiratory support systems. Each device was applied for 6 hours, with the total study duration of 24 hours. All infants were receiving caffeine. The median event rate was significantly higher at 6.7 per hour in infants receiving NIPPV by the conventional ventilator, compared with 4.4 per hour with NIPPV by the variable flow device, and 2.8 per hour with NCPAP by the variable flow device (P value <.03 for both).[53] There was no significant difference between NIPPV by the conventional ventilator and bubble-NCPAP modes.[53]

Finally, an evidence-based approach was used to introduce NIPPV in a nursery, as a routine for extremely low-birth-weight infants after extubation if apnea or respiratory insufficiency was evident.[18] It is noteworthy that there was a significant decrease in the number of extremely low-birth-weight infants discharged on supplemental oxygen (75% and 47%, after the introduction of NIPPV P = .01).[18]

SNIPPV VERSUS NIPPV

There is only one retrospective study comparing clinical outcomes in infants managed with SNIPPV versus NIPPV.[31] After adjusting for significant confounding variables, use of NIPPV versus SNIPPV (odds ratio, 0.74; 95% confidence interval, 0.42–1.30) was not associated with BPD/death or other common neonatal morbidities.[31]

NASAL HIGH-FREQUENCY VENTILATION STUDIES

Animal studies using the preterm lamb model have suggested that nasal high-frequency ventilation (NHFV) improves alveolarization,[54] with preservation of key homeostatic alveolar epithelial-mesenchymal markers.[55]

In human neonates, NHFV has been shown to be effective in CO_2 elimination.[56–58] In an RCT (n = 46), NHFV was found to decrease the duration and level of oxygen supplementation (both $P<.001$), compared with NCPAP, in infants with transient tachypnea of the newborn.[59]

Table 2
NIPPV studies in neonates

Author/Ref	Type	No. of Infants	NIPPV Group[a]	Control Group[a]	Outcomes
Primary mode:					
Manzar et al[48]	Prospective, Obs	16	Details not available.	N.A.	81% (n = 13) avoided intubation
Kugelman et al[38]	RCT	84	NIPPV: Rate: 12–30; PIP: 14–22; PEEP: 6–7; Ti: 0.3 s; Fio_2 adjusted for Spo_2: 88%–92%	NCPAP: 6–7; Fio_2 adjusted for Spo_2: 88%–92%	NIPPV group had decreased BPD
Bisceglia et al[49]	RCT	88	NIPPV: Rate: 40; PIP: 14–20; PEEP: 4–6	NCPAP: 4–6	NIPPV group had less apnea, shorter duration of respiratory support
Sai Sunil Kishore et al[39]	RCT	76	NIPPV: Rate: 50; PIP: 15–16; PEEP: 5; Ti: 0.3–0.35 s; Flow: 6–7 L/min; Fio_2 adjusted for Spo_2: 88%–93%	NCPAP: 5; Flow: 6–7 L/min; Fio_2 adjusted for Spo_2: 88%–93%	Less failed extubation with NIPPV at 48 h and 7 d
Meneses et al[40]	RCT	200	NIPPV: Rate: 20–30; PIP: 15–20; PEEP: 4–6; Ti: 0.4–0.35 s; Flow: 8–10 L/min; Fio_2 adjusted for Spo_2: 88%–92%	NCPAP: 5–6; Flow: 8–10 L/min; Fio_2 adjusted for Spo_2: 88%–92%	Less failed extubation with NIPPV at 24–72 h
Ramanathan et al[35]	RCT	110	NIPPV: Rate: 30–40; PIP: 10–15; PEEP: 5; Ti: 0.5 s; Flow: 8–10 L/min; Fio_2 adjusted for Spo_2: 84%–92%	NCPAP: 5–8; Fio_2 adjusted for Spo_2: 84%–92%	Less failed extubation with NIPPV and decreased clinical and physiologic BPD
Secondary mode:					
Khorana et al[50]	RCT	48	NIPPV: Same as pre-extubation ventilator settings	NCPAP: Same as pre-extubation PEEP	No differences in outcomes; however, there were significant differences in the demographics of the two groups

Rate: ventilator rate (breaths/minute).
Abbreviations: BPD, bronchopulmonary dysplasia; Fio_2, fraction of inspired oxygen; NCPAP, nasal continuous positive airway pressure (cm H_2O); NIPPV, nasal intermittent positive pressure ventilation; PEEP, positive end-expiratory pressure (cm H_2O); PIP, peak inspiratory pressure (cm H_2O); RCT, randomized controlled trial; Spo_2, pulse oximeter oxygen saturation; Ti, inspiratory time (seconds).
[a] Initial settings.

Although promising, RCTs with other neonatal respiratory disorders and larger sample sizes are needed to prove the safety and efficacy of this NHFV approach.[60]

COMPLICATIONS OF NASAL VENTILATION

Potential complications related to nasal ventilation are essentially the same as those for infants on NCPAP. These include obstruction of prongs because of secretions, hypoventilation, local trauma or bleeding, infection, skin irritation, and pressure necrosis.[1] One RCT noted a significant increase in the abdominal girth in the NIPPV group, but there were no issues with feeding tolerance or other complications.[39] Since the initial report of gastrointestinal perforations,[3] use of SNIPPV/NIPPV has not been associated with necrotizing enterocolitis or any gastrointestinal perforations.[1,20,31,46]

LONG-TERM OUTCOMES

Only two studies to date have reported on long-term neurodevelopmental outcomes in infants exposed to SNIPPV.[29,46] In a study by Bhandari and colleagues,[29] there were no differences in the Mental or Psychomotor Developmental Index scores between the infants managed with SNIPPV or continued on CV at a median corrected age of 22 months.

The second study revealed that after adjusting for significant covariates, infants who received SNIPPV (compared with those who received NCPAP) in the birth weight category 500 to 750 g were significantly less likely to have neurodevelopmental impairment (0.29 [0.09–0.94]; $P = .04$) and neurodevelopmental impairment/death (0.18 [0.05–0.62]; $P = .006$).[46]

STRATEGIZING NIPPV USE

If a specific NICU practices prophylactic surfactant administration, we suggest that the infant be extubated early to NIPPV, within 2 hours if possible. We do not recommend delaying surfactant administration by escalating therapy from NCPAP to NIPPV. For those NICUs initiating NIPPV at birth, we also recommend early surfactant be administered, if indicated,[61] followed by extubation to NIPPV. A recent approach of using a thin catheter to administer surfactant needs additional evaluation before it can be universally recommended.[62]

We suggest that extubation be attempted in the first week of life, specifically in the first 3 days.[30] We did not find pulmonary function parameters, measured just before extubation, very useful in predicting SNIPPV success[6]; hence, we attempt extubation in all infants if they meet certain criteria (**Table 3**).[1] The fear that an infant will require reintubation in the future should not be a reason to delay an extubation attempt[63] if the infant has been able to be weaned to appropriate settings.[1] We recommend the use of short binasal prongs. Once extubated, we adjust the ventilator to ensure bilateral good air entry and adequate chest rise. We also use the "decompression" orogastric tube[1] for bolus feeding. If the infant requires continuous feeds, an additional 5F catheter feeding tube is used. We usually check blood gas within an hour of extubation, and subsequently as clinically indicated. We adjust ventilator settings based on clinical judgment and blood gases, as would be done for an infant on invasive ventilation. Maximal NIPPV settings and indications for reintubation have been suggested.[1]

Table 3
(S)NIPPV use criteria:

1. (S)NIPPV (primary mode)
    1. Settings:
        - Frequency $\approx$ 40 per minute
        - PIP 4 cm H_2O > PIP required during manual ventilation (adjust PIP for effective aeration per auscultation)
        - PEEP 4–6 cm H_2O
        - Ti $\approx$ 0.45 s
        - FiO_2 adjusted to maintain SpO_2 of 85–93%
        - Flow 8–10 l m^{-1}
        - Caffeine 15–25 μgm ml or aminophylline level $\geq$8 μg ml^{-1}
        - Hematocrit $\geq$35%
    2. Monitor SpO_2, HR and respirations
    3. Obtain blood gas in 15–30 min
    4. Adjust ventilator settings to maintain blood gas parameters within normal limits
    5. Suction mouth and pharynx and insert clean airway Q4, as necessary
    6. Maximal support recommendations:
        $\leq$1000 g MAP 14 cm H_2O
        >1000 g MAP 16 cm H_2O
2. (S)NIPPV (secondary mode)
    1. Extubation criteria while on CV:
        - Frequency $\approx$ 15–25 per minute
        - PIP $\leq$16 cm H_2O
        - PEEP $\leq$5 cm H_2O
        - FiO_2 $\leq$0.35
        - Caffeine 15–25 μg ml^{-1} or aminophylline level $\geq$8 μg ml^{-1}
        - Hematocrit $\geq$35%
    2. Place on (S)NIPPV
        - Frequency $\approx$ 15–25 per minute
        - PIP 2–4 $\uparrow$> CV settings; adjust PIP for effective aeration per auscultation
        - PEEP $\leq$5 cm H_2O
        - FiO_2 adjusted to maintain SpO_2 of 85–93%
        - Flow 8–10 l m^{-1}
    3. Suction mouth and pharynx and insert clean airway Q4, as necessary
    4. Maximal support recommendations:
        $\leq$1000 g MAP 14 cm H_2O
        >1000 g MAP 16 cm H_2O
3. Considerations for re-intubation
    1. pH <7.25; $PaCO_2$ $\geq$60 mm Hg
    2. Episode of apnea requiring bag and mask ventilation
    3. Frequent (>2–3 episodes per hour) apnea/bradycardia (cessation of respiration for >20 s associated with a heart rate <100 per minute) not responding to theophylline/caffeine therapy
    4. Frequent desaturation (<85%) $\geq$3 episodes per hour not responding to increased ventilatory settings
4. (S)NIPPV weaning to oxyhood/nasal cannula
    1. Minimal (S)NIPPV settings
        - Frequency $\leq$20 per minute
        - PIP $\leq$14 cm H_2O
        - PEEP $\leq$4 cm H_2O
        - FiO_2 $\leq$0.3
        - Flow 8–10 l m^{-1}
        - Blood gases within normal limits
    2. Wean to:
        - Oxyhood adjust FiO_2 to keep SpO_2 85–93%
        - NC adjust flow (1–2 l m^{-1}) and FiO_2 to keep SpO_2 85–93%

From Bhandari V. Nasal intermittent positive pressure ventilation in the newborn: review of literature and evidence-based guidelines. J Perinatol 2010;30:505–12; with permission.

SUMMARY

Based on the studies discussed in this article, NIPPV should be the preferred mode for postextubation respiratory support in neonates. Although SNIPPV is preferable over NIPPV, there are limited options available with the phasing out of the Infant Star ventilator with StarSync. More adequately powered RCTs are required using the Comprehensive SiPaP (not approved for use in the United States) and the neurally adjusted ventilatory assist mode in the Servo-i ventilator, before the synchronized noninvasive modes can be recommended using these devices in neonates.

Although the data from the RCTs are promising, additional studies are required before the use of noninvasive respiratory support by NIPPV can be recommended as a therapeutic modality. It is important to have data on long-term pulmonary and neurodevelopmental outcomes.

As noted on the clinicaltrials.gov Web site, there are two active studies in China, one comparing Bi-PAP with NIPPV (NCT01318824) and another comparing NIPPV with NCPAP (using the VIP-Bird ventilator; NCT00780624). A large international multicenter trial comparing NIPPV with NCPAP (NCT00433212) has just been completed; results are awaited.

Caution must be exercised when comparing studies because different devices and ventilator settings could account for variability in the results. More studies are required to establish the efficacy of using early noninvasive respiratory support in the NIPPV mode, with or without surfactant administration, in the smallest infants with the highest risk for adverse pulmonary and neurodevelopmental outcomes.

REFERENCES

1. Bhandari V. Nasal intermittent positive pressure ventilation in the newborn: review of literature and evidence-based guidelines. J Perinatol 2010;30:505–12.
2. Moretti C, Marzetti G, Agostino R, et al. Prolonged intermittent positive pressure ventilation by nasal prongs in intractable apnea of prematurity. Acta Paediatr Scand 1981;70:211–6.
3. Garland JS, Nelson DB, Rice T, et al. Increased risk of gastrointestinal perforations in neonates mechanically ventilated with either face mask or nasal prongs. Pediatrics 1985;76:406–10.
4. Friedlich P, Lecart C, Posen R, et al. A randomized trial of nasopharyngeal-synchronized intermittent mandatory ventilation versus nasopharyngeal continuous positive airway pressure in very low birth weight infants after extubation. J Perinatol 1999;19:413–8.
5. Barrington KJ, Bull D, Finer NN. Randomized trial of nasal synchronized intermittent mandatory ventilation compared with continuous positive airway pressure after extubation of very low birth weight infants. Pediatrics 2001;107:638–41.
6. Khalaf MN, Brodsky N, Hurley J, et al. A prospective randomized, controlled trial comparing synchronized nasal intermittent positive pressure ventilation versus nasal continuous positive airway pressure as modes of extubation. Pediatrics 2001;108:13–7.
7. Moreau-Bussiere F, Samson N, St-Hilaire M, et al. Laryngeal response to nasal ventilation in nonsedated newborn lambs. J Appl Physiol 2007;102:2149–57.
8. Roy B, Samson N, Moreau-Bussiere F, et al. Mechanisms of active laryngeal closure during noninvasive intermittent positive pressure ventilation in nonsedated lambs. J Appl Physiol 2008;105:1406–12.

9. Lampland AL, Meyers PA, Worwa CT, et al. Gas exchange and lung inflammation using nasal intermittent positive-pressure ventilation versus synchronized intermittent mandatory ventilation in piglets with saline lavage-induced lung injury: an observational study. Crit Care Med 2008;36:183–7.

10. Andrade FH. Noninvasive ventilation in neonates: the lungs don't like it! J Appl Physiol 2008;105:1385–6.

11. Kugelman A, Bar A, Riskin A, et al. Nasal respiratory support in premature infants: short-term physiological effects and comfort assessment. Acta Paediatr 2008;97:557–61.

12. Owen LS, Morley CJ, Davis PG. Pressure variation during ventilator generated nasal intermittent positive pressure ventilation in preterm infants. Arch Dis Child Fetal Neonatal Ed 2010;95:F359–64.

13. Kiciman NM, Andreasson B, Bernstein G, et al. Thoracoabdominal motion in newborns during ventilation delivered by endotracheal tube or nasal prongs. Pediatr Pulmonol 1998;25:175–81.

14. Moretti C, Gizzi C, Papoff P, et al. Comparing the effects of nasal synchronized intermittent positive pressure ventilation (nSIPPV) and nasal continuous positive airway pressure (nCPAP) after extubation in very low birth weight infants. Early Hum Dev 1999;56:167–77.

15. Aghai ZH, Saslow JG, Nakhla T, et al. Synchronized nasal intermittent positive pressure ventilation (SNIPPV) decreases work of breathing (WOB) in premature infants with respiratory distress syndrome (RDS) compared to nasal continuous positive airway pressure (NCPAP). Pediatr Pulmonol 2006;41:875–81.

16. Ali N, Claure N, Alegria X, et al. Effects of non-invasive pressure support ventilation (NI-PSV) on ventilation and respiratory effort in very low birth weight infants. Pediatr Pulmonol 2007;42:704–10.

17. Chang HY, Claure N, D'Ugard C, et al. Effects of synchronization during nasal ventilation in clinically stable preterm infants. Pediatr Res 2011;69:84–9.

18. Jackson JK, Vellucci J, Johnson P, et al. Evidence-based approach to change in clinical practice: introduction of expanded nasal continuous positive airway pressure use in an intensive care nursery. Pediatrics 2003;111:e542–7.

19. Millar D, Kirpalani H. Benefits of non-invasive ventilation. Indian Pediatr 2004;41:1008–17.

20. Davis PG, Morley CJ, Owen LS. Non-invasive respiratory support of preterm neonates with respiratory distress: continuous positive airway pressure and nasal intermittent positive pressure ventilation. Semin Fetal Neonatal Med 2009;14:14–20.

21. Ramanathan R. Nasal respiratory support through the nares: its time has come. J Perinatol 2010;30(Suppl):S67–72.

22. de Winter JP, de Vries MA, Zimmermann LJ. Clinical practice: noninvasive respiratory support in newborns. Eur J Pediatr 2010;169:777–82.

23. Mahmoud RA, Roehr CC, Schmalisch G. Current methods of non-invasive ventilatory support for neonates. Paediatr Respir Rev 2011;12:196–205.

24. DiBlasi RM. Neonatal noninvasive ventilation techniques: do we really need to intubate? Respir Care 2011;56:1273–94 [discussion: 1295–7].

25. Kieran EA, Walsh H, O'Donnell CP. Survey of nasal continuous positive airways pressure (NCPAP) and nasal intermittent positive pressure ventilation (NIPPV) use in Irish newborn nurseries. Arch Dis Child Fetal Neonatal Ed 2011;96:F156.

26. de Medeiros SK, Carvalho WB, Soriano CF. Practices of use of nasal intermittent positive pressure ventilation (NIPPV) in neonatology in northeastern Brazil. J Pediatr (Rio J) 2012;88:48–53.

27. Santin R, Brodsky N, Bhandari V. A prospective observational pilot study of synchronized nasal intermittent positive pressure ventilation (SNIPPV) as

a primary mode of ventilation in infants > or = 28 weeks with respiratory distress syndrome (RDS). J Perinatol 2004;24:487–93.

28. Kulkarni A, Ehrenkranz RA, Bhandari V. Effect of introduction of synchronized nasal intermittent positive-pressure ventilation in a neonatal intensive care unit on bronchopulmonary dysplasia and growth in preterm infants. Am J Perinatol 2006;23:233–40.

29. Bhandari V, Gavino RG, Nedrelow JH, et al. A randomized controlled trial of synchronized nasal intermittent positive pressure ventilation in RDS. J Perinatol 2007;27:697–703.

30. Dumpa V, Northrup V, Bhandari V. Type and timing of ventilation in the first post-natal week is associated with bronchopulmonary dysplasia/death. Am J Perinatol 2011;28:321–30.

31. Dumpa V, Katz K, Northrup V, et al. SNIPPV vs NIPPV: does synchronization matter? J Perinatol 2012;32(6):438–42.

32. Moretti C, Giannini L, Fassi C, et al. Nasal flow-synchronized intermittent positive pressure ventilation to facilitate weaning in very low-birthweight infants: unmasked randomized controlled trial. Pediatr Int 2008;50:85–91.

33. Beck J, Reilly M, Grasselli G, et al. Patient-ventilator interaction during neurally adjusted ventilatory assist in low birth weight infants. Pediatr Res 2009;65:663–8.

34. Lista G, Castoldi F, Fontana P, et al. Nasal continuous positive airway pressure (CPAP) versus bi-level nasal CPAP in preterm babies with respiratory distress syndrome: a randomised control trial. Arch Dis Child Fetal Neonatal Ed 2010;95:F85–9.

35. Ramanathan R, Sekar KC, Rasmussen M, et al. Nasal intermittent positive pressure ventilation after surfactant treatment for respiratory distress syndrome in preterm infants <30 weeks' gestation: a randomized, controlled trial. J Perinatol 2012;32(5):336–43.

36. Ancora G, Maranella E, Grandi S, et al. Role of bilevel positive airway pressure in the management of preterm newborns who have received surfactant. Acta Paediatr 2010;99:1807–11.

37. O'Brien K, Campbell C, Havlin L, et al. Infant flow biphasic NCPAP versus infant flow NCPAP for the facilitation of successful extubation in infant's 1250 grams: a randomized controlled trial. EPAS 2009. 3450.3455.

38. Kugelman A, Feferkorn I, Riskin A, et al. Nasal intermittent mandatory ventilation versus nasal continuous positive airway pressure for respiratory distress syndrome: a randomized, controlled, prospective study. J Pediatr 2007;150:521–6.

39. Sai Sunil Kishore M, Dutta S, Kumar P. Early nasal intermittent positive pressure ventilation versus continuous positive airway pressure for respiratory distress syndrome. Acta Paediatr 2009;98:1412–5.

40. Meneses J, Bhandari V, Alves JG, et al. Noninvasive ventilation for respiratory distress syndrome: a randomized controlled trial. Pediatrics 2011;127:300–7.

41. De Paoli AG, Davis PG, Faber B, et al. Devices and pressure sources for administration of nasal continuous positive airway pressure (NCPAP) in preterm neonates. Cochrane Database Syst Rev 2008;(1):CD002977.

42. Bhandari V, Rogerson S, Barfield C, et al. Nasal versus nasopharyngeal continuous positive airway pressure use in preterm neonates. Pediatr Res 1996;39:196A (Abstract No. 1163).

43. Bhandari V. Non-invasive ventilation of the sick neonate: evidence-based recommendations. Journal of Neonatology 2006;20:214–21.

44. De Paoli AG, Davis PG, Lemyre B. Nasal continuous positive airway pressure versus nasal intermittent positive pressure ventilation for preterm neonates: a systematic review and meta-analysis. Acta Paediatr 2003;92:70–5.

45. Gao WW, Tan SZ, Chen YB, et al. Randomized trial of nasal synchronized intermittent mandatory ventilation compared with nasal continuous positive airway pressure in preterm infants with respiratory distress syndrome. Zhongguo Dang Dai Er Ke Za Zhi 2010;12:524–6 [in Chinese].

46. Bhandari V, Finer NN, Ehrenkranz RA, et al. Synchronized nasal intermittent positive-pressure ventilation and neonatal outcomes. Pediatrics 2009;124: 517–26.

47. Lin XZ, Zheng Z, Lin YY, et al. Nasal synchronized intermittent positive pressure ventilation for the treatment of apnea in preterm infants. Zhongguo Dang Dai Er Ke Za Zhi 2011;13:783–6 [in Chinese].

48. Manzar S, Nair AK, Pai MG, et al. Use of nasal intermittent positive pressure ventilation to avoid intubation in neonates. Saudi Med J 2004;25:1464–7.

49. Bisceglia M, Belcastro A, Poerio V, et al. A comparison of nasal intermittent versus continuous positive pressure delivery for the treatment of moderate respiratory syndrome in preterm infants. Minerva Pediatr 2007;59:91–5.

50. Khorana M, Paradeevisut H, Sangtawesin V, et al. A randomized trial of non-synchronized nasopharyngeal intermittent mandatory ventilation (nsNIMV) vs. nasal continuous positive airway pressure (NCPAP) in the prevention of extubation failure in pre-term <1,500 grams. J Med Assoc Thai 2008;91(Suppl 3):S136–42.

51. Ryan CA, Finer NN, Peters KL. Nasal intermittent positive-pressure ventilation offers no advantages over nasal continuous positive airway pressure in apnea of prematurity. Am J Dis Child 1989;143:1196–8.

52. Lin CH, Wang ST, Lin YJ, et al. Efficacy of nasal intermittent positive pressure ventilation in treating apnea of prematurity. Pediatr Pulmonol 1998;26:349–53.

53. Pantalitschka T, Sievers J, Urschitz MS, et al. Randomised crossover trial of four nasal respiratory support systems for apnoea of prematurity in very low birth-weight infants. Arch Dis Child Fetal Neonatal Ed 2009;94:F245–8.

54. Reyburn B, Li M, Metcalfe DB, et al. Nasal ventilation alters mesenchymal cell turnover and improves alveolarization in preterm lambs. Am J Respir Crit Care Med 2008;178:407–18.

55. Rehan VK, Fong J, Lee R, et al. Mechanism of reduced lung injury by high-frequency nasal ventilation in a preterm lamb model of neonatal chronic lung disease. Pediatr Res 2011;70:462–6.

56. van der Hoeven M, Brouwer E, Blanco CE. Nasal high frequency ventilation in neonates with moderate respiratory insufficiency. Arch Dis Child Fetal Neonatal Ed 1998;79:F61–3.

57. Hoehn T, Krause MF. Effective elimination of carbon dioxide by nasopharyngeal high-frequency ventilation. Respir Med 2000;94:1132–4.

58. Colaizy TT, Younis UM, Bell EF, et al. Nasal high-frequency ventilation for premature infants. Acta Paediatr 2008;97:1518–22.

59. Dumas De La Roque E, Bertrand C, Tandonnet O, et al. Nasal high frequency percussive ventilation versus nasal continuous positive airway pressure in transient tachypnea of the newborn: a pilot randomized controlled trial (NCT00556738). Pediatr Pulmonol 2010. [Epub ahead of print].

60. Carlo WA. Should nasal high-frequency ventilation be used in preterm infants? Acta Paediatr 2008;97:1484–5.

61. Stevens TP, Harrington EW, Blennow M, et al. Early surfactant administration with brief ventilation vs. selective surfactant and continued mechanical ventilation for

preterm infants with or at risk for respiratory distress syndrome. Cochrane Database Syst Rev 2007;(4):CD003063.

62. Gopel W, Kribs A, Ziegler A, et al. Avoidance of mechanical ventilation by surfactant treatment of spontaneously breathing preterm infants (AMV): an open-label, randomised, controlled trial. Lancet 2011;378:1627–34.

63. Robbins ME, Martin EM, Hitchner JC, et al. Early extubation attempts reduce length of stay in extremely premature infants even if re-intubation is necessary. EPAS 2011. 4532.4472.

Volume-Limited and Volume-Targeted Ventilation

Colin J. Morley, MD, FRCPCH, FRACP

KEYWORDS

- Infant • Newborn • Ventilation • Tidal volume • Respiratory distress

KEY POINTS

- Pressure limited ventilation was started because in the early days tidal volume targeted ventilators were not available.
- Neonates are ventilated because they have respiratory failure where they cannot breathe well enough to remove carbon dioxide.
- Arterial carbon dioxide levels are controlled by tidal volume and respiratory or ventilator rate.
- Pressure limited ventilation cannot carefully control tidal volume in breathing babies and changing lung pathology.
- Sophisticated ventilators are now available that cant target tidal volume and so are more physiological.
- Volume targeted ventilation is strongly associated with tighter tidal volume and carbon dioxide control, less death or BPD, fewer pneumothoraces and serious IVH, and less days of ventilation.

BACKGROUND

When pediatricians first started ventilating babies in the early 1970s there were no ventilators that were capable of delivering accurate tidal volumes to neonates, especially preterm neonates. Those that did deliver a tidal volume only delivered a set tidal volume into the entire ventilatory circuit, which included the baby. The volume of the ventilator circuit per se was several times greater than the volume of the baby's lungs, therefore much of the volume leaving the ventilator was lost by compression of the gas in the circuit. Furthermore, there were no pneumotachometers that could be used to accurately measure the volume of gas passing in and out of the endotracheal tube. Those that were available were inaccurate if any water condensed on the inside, and so were not suitable for long-term clinical use. A further problem was that cuffed

Disclosures: The author is Consultant to Fisher and Paykel Healthcare, Laerdal Global Health, and Dräger Medical.
Neonatal Research, The Royal Women's Hospital, Melbourne, Australia, 23 High Street, Great Shelford, Cambridge CB22 5EH, United Kingdom
E-mail address: colin@morleys.net

http://dx.doi.org/10.1016/j.clp.2012.06.016   **perinatology.theclinics.com** endotracheal tubes (ETT) were not available and so gas leaked around the ETT as pressure rose during inflation, reducing the volume of gas entering the alveoli.

This lack of appropriate technology meant that pediatricians could only apply pressure-limited ventilation (PLV), which was done by experience or from a protocol, watching chest movement, and adjusting the peak inflation pressure (PIP) until chest movement seemed appropriate. The effect of any pressure change was monitored by observing changes in blood gases. Neonatologists soon became experienced at using PLV; there was little thought about tidal volume because accurate measurement of tidal volumes in neonates was not possible.

Volutrauma (damage to the lungs caused by a large tidal volume overstretching the delicate alveoli and airways) has been associated with the development of lung injury.[1–5] PLV uses a fixed PIP. The delivered tidal volume varies from one inflation to the next as the baby breathes or lung physiology changes. Volume-targeted ventilation (VTV) aims to control the tidal volume with each inflation, thereby reducing the risk of volutrauma. Studies have reported reductions in tidal volume variation using VTV.[6–10] Hypocarbia has been associated with bronchopulmonary dysplasia and periventricular leukomalacia.[6,11–14] VTV reduces the incidence of both hypocapnia and hypercarbia.[6]

INDICATIONS FOR MECHANICAL VENTILATION OF A NEONATE

When considering whether VTV is the appropriate mode for ventilating neonates, it is important to consider the indications for mechanical ventilation in this population. The 3 main reasons to ventilate neonates are: (1) the infant is apneic and needs positive pressure ventilation; (2) the infant has developed respiratory failure, defined by a high and rising arterial CO_2 ($Paco_2$) level; and (3) the infant has inadequate oxygenation. However, improving oxygenation in a spontaneously breathing baby can often be achieved without mechanical ventilation.

The purpose of setting out the reasons for ventilation is to show that the indication for mechanical ventilation is largely to control CO_2.

PHYSIOLOGIC PRINCIPLES OF NEONATAL VENTILATION

Achievement of adequate oxygenation does not require gas to move regularly in and out of the lungs and so does not need rhythmic ventilation. Three factors control oxygenation.

1. Oxygenation is proportional to the exposed alveolar surface area. If the lung volume is abnormally low, oxygenation will also be low. Improving lung volume improves oxygenation. Applying a positive pressure to the lungs by altering the positive end-expiratory pressure (PEEP) if the infant is ventilated, or continuous positive airway pressure (CPAP) if the infant is spontaneously breathing, is an important way to improve oxygenation.[15–18]
2. Increase the inspired oxygen concentration (Fio_2).
3. Increase blood flowing through the lungs, particularly to the aerated areas. This flow can be improved by ensuring a reasonable blood pressure or by using pulmonary arterial dilating agents such as nitric oxide.

Therefore, oxygenation is improved by ensuring adequate lung aeration. It does not need gas to move in and out and is unrelated to the tidal volume.

To control $Paco_2$, gas containing CO_2 has to move out of the lungs. Mechanical ventilation is primarily about controlling $Paco_2$. Assuming there is sufficient blood passing the aerated alveoli and the dead space is not too large, the 2 functions that control the $Paco_2$ are the tidal volume and the rate of breathing or ventilation.[19] The tidal volume is the volume of gas that moves in and out of the lungs with each respiratory cycle.

Therefore, the primary function of mechanical ventilation is to control the $Paco_2$ by controlling the tidal volume and ventilator rate. It seems logical to control the $Paco_2$ by directly controlling the tidal volume rather than the PIP.

WHY USE VOLUME-TARGETED VENTILATION RATHER THAN PLV?

PLV was used for many years because it was the only mode of ventilation available. With PLV, a PIP is used to push a tidal volume into the lungs. However, a set PIP will not produce a specific tidal volume, because the size of the tidal volume will depend on how much the baby breathes and contributes to the tidal volume,[9] the amount of ETT leak, and the compliance and resistance of the lungs. The major problem with using PLV is that these can vary from breath to breath especially in an infant who is breathing spontaneously; therefore, using a set PIP will produce a variable tidal volume.[7,20]

Neonatal ventilators that can measure, target, and control tidal volume are currently available, and it is possible to ventilate babies by targeting tidal volume, a fact that should not be considered unusual. PLV has been used to control tidal volume indirectly by altering the PIP. Now tidal volume can be controlled more accurately by microprocessor control of the ventilator and in response to a baby's breathing pattern and tidal volume.

HOW DO VOLUME-TARGETED VENTILATORS CONTROL THE TIDAL VOLUME?

All of the author's experience with VTV has been gathered through using the Dräger Babylog 8000 (Dräger, Lübeck, Germany) in the volume guarantee mode.[9,21–26] The author does not have experience of using volume targeting with other neonatal ventilators, so what is written about them here has been gleaned from reading articles and manufacturers' literature and talking to neonatologists who use such ventilators. A problem is that the myriad of neonatal ventilators delivering VTV control the tidal volume in different ways. It can be very difficult to understand the jargon used to describe how the tidal volume is controlled, and this is compounded by failure of ventilator manufacturers to use the same terminology.

There are 2 main ways by which ventilators target tidal volume control. Each has its strengths and weaknesses.

Control of the Inflation Tidal Volume

With this technique, the ventilator controls the tidal volume entering the baby's lungs and when the set inflation tidal volume has been reached, inflation is stopped. The obvious advantage is that it controls the tidal volume as it is delivered. The disadvantage is that as it measures the tidal volume going into the ETT, it cannot accurately compensate for how much is lost through leak around the ETT. If the leak is 50% then the tidal volume delivered to the lung would be half that entering the ETT. Some ventilators may have a mechanism whereby the staff can adjust the ventilator setting for ETT leaks, but the technology cannot accurately respond to the ETT leak, as it varies inflation by inflation.

With some older volume-targeted ventilator modes, the set tidal volume is the inflation tidal volume leaving the ventilator and entering both the circuit and the baby. The main disadvantage is that the circuit has a relatively large compressible gas volume compared with a baby's tidal volume, so clinicians have to adjust the volume leaving the ventilator with each inflation to take this into account. If there is a flow sensor at the Wye connector measuring and displaying the tidal volume in and out of the baby, care providers have to adjust the tidal volume leaving the ventilator to control the delivered tidal volume. Although this is probably better than no volume control, it is not directly responding to the tidal volume delivered to the baby and cannot directly adjust the tidal volume for variable ETT leaks.

Control of the Expired Tidal Volume

With this technique, the tidal volume is regulated by the expired tidal volume, which makes intuitive sense, because the gas leaving the lung most closely represents the tidal volume that entered the lung when ETT leak was present. The problem is that the ventilator has to measure the expired tidal volume following an inflation and then use those data to determine the PIP needed to achieve the set expired tidal volume for the next inflation. Therefore, it is always working one inflation behind. An advantage is that the ETT leak in the previous breath has been calculated (inflation tidal volume minus expired tidal volume) so that the PIP is automatically adjusted by the ventilator to deliver a higher inflation tidal volume to compensate for the ETT leak. As ETT leak is almost always present and varies from inflation to inflation, this may be the better way to control the delivered tidal volume.

Some ventilators have 2 programs controlling the PIP used to deliver the tidal volume for each inflation, which depend on whether the inflation was or was not triggered by the baby. This aspect is important because if an inflation is triggered, the baby has created some of the tidal volume and so a lower PIP is needed to deliver the set tidal volume. If an inflation is not triggered, the baby is probably apneic and so a higher PIP is required to ensure an adequate tidal volume. If a ventilator uses one program to control triggered and untriggered inflations, it will be difficult to control the tidal volumes accurately.

HOW ACCURATE IS THE TIDAL VOLUME?

There are several reports about the accuracy of VTV.[6,7,9] McCallion and colleagues[9] studied the tidal volumes delivered to ventilated preterm babies with both triggered and untriggered inflations during volume guarantee ventilation with the Dräger Babylog. On average, both triggered and untriggered inflations were found to be almost identical to the set target expired tidal volume; however, there was a wide variation from 0% to 300% of the set volume. On careful examination of detailed recordings, the very high tidal volumes were found to be due to the baby taking a large breath such as crying,[9] and the very low tidal volumes were due to the infant having a forced expiration against an inflation.[27,28] Using the SLE5000 (SLE Ltd, South Croydon, UK), Patel and colleagues[29] demonstrated that the delivered tidal volumes were 10% to 20% higher than the set tidal volume with a wide range.

WHEN SHOULD VOLUME TARGETING BE USED?

VTV can be very useful as soon as mechanical ventilation is started, because all the clinician has to do is set the tidal volume to approximately 5 mL/kg and the ventilator will adjust its settings to try and ensure that the set volume is delivered. Using this method results in much better control of $Paco_2$ and tidal volume than using a set PIP, observing the chest-wall movement and intermittent blood gases.

VTV can also be useful when surfactant is given because surfactant has been shown to cause some obstruction to the airway.[23,25] With VTV the ventilator will adjust the PIP to ensure that the set tidal volume is delivered.

One of the major problems with PLV is that it delivers the set PIP even though the baby's breathing varies, meaning that if the baby is breathing hard the PIP is still delivered and will inappropriately augment the tidal volume. With VTV, the ventilator responds to the baby's breathing and adjusts the PIP to deliver the set tidal volume. If the baby is taking large breaths, the PIP may be lowered to almost zero. VTV is better at controlling the $Paco_2$; this is important, as hypocarbia is dangerous to the preterm infant's brain.

VTV is very useful for automatically weaning the ventilator. As the baby's respiratory condition improves, the ventilator automatically reduces the PIP.

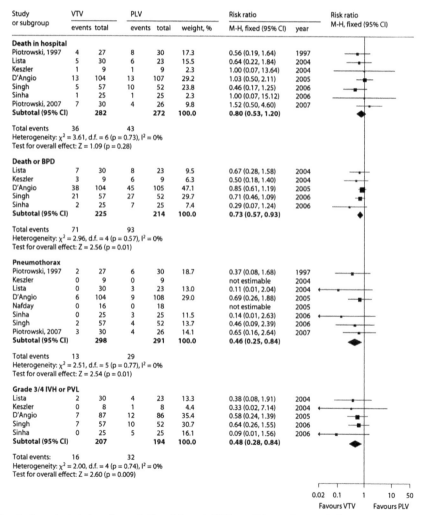

Fig. 1. Forest plot showing relative risk and 95% confidence intervals for meta-analysis of outcomes occurring during period of ventilation, before discharge, and after discharge. (From Wheeler KI, Klingenberg C, Morley CJ, et al. Volume-targeted versus pressure-limited ventilation for preterm infants: a systematic review and meta-analysis. Neonatology 2011;100(3):224; with permission.)

Table 1
Details of the trials included in the review

Authors,[Ref.] Year	No. of Subjects, Inclusion Criteria	VTV Ventilator Mode	PLV Ventilator Mode	Duration of Study	Hybrid Interventions	Comments	Outcomes Used in Meta-Analysis
Piotrowski et al,[31] 1997	N = 57, <2500 g	PRVC with Siemens Servo 300	Non-synch IMV (several ventilators)	Until extubation	Different triggers and ventilators in 2 groups	Controls inspired tidal volume entering circuit	Death in hospital, air leak, IVH, duration of ventilation
Sinha et al,[38] 1997	N = 50, >1200 g	AC+VC with Bird VIP	AC with Bird VIP	To ventilator weaning	Pressure trigger in VTV, flow trigger in PLV	Controls inspired volume entering circuit	Death in hospital, severe IVH or PVL, BPD, pneumothorax
Lista et al,[35] 2004	N = 53, 25–32 wk	PSV+VG with Dräger Babylog 8000+	PSV with Dräger Babylog 8000+	Until extubation		Controls expired tidal volume	Death in hospital, BPD, IVH, PVL, PIE, pneumothorax
Keszler[6] 2004	N = 18, <34 wk	AC+VG with Dräger Babylog 8000+	AC with Dräger Babylog 8000+	72 h or until extubation		Controls expired tidal volume	Death in hospital, low CO_2, pneumothorax, PIE, PVL, IVH
Nafday et al,[36] 2005	N = 34, <1500 g	PSV+VG with Dräger Babylog 8000+	SIMV with Dräger Babylog 8000+	24 h from enrollment	Different trigger modes in VTV and PLV groups	Controls expired tidal volume	Death in hospital, BPD, IVH, air leak

Study	N	(VTV mode)	(PLV/comparison mode)	Duration	Comments	Control mechanism	Outcomes
D'Angio et al,[34] 2005	N = 213, 500–1249 g	PRVC with Bird VIP	SIMV with Bird VIP	Extubation or mode failed	Different trigger modes in VTV and PLV groups	Controls inspired volume entering circuit	$Paco_2$, death in hospital, age at extubation, air leak, IVH, PVL, BPD, home O_2
Singh et al,[32] 2006 & 2009	N = 109, 600–1500 g	VC Bird VIP	PLV Bird VIP	To ventilator weaning		Controls inspired tidal volume entering circuit.	Duration of ventilation, death in hospital, BPD, IVH, home O_2
Cheema et al,[33] 2007	N = 40, <34 wk	AC+VG with Dräger Babylog 8000+	AC with Dräger Babylog 8000+	Until first blood gas		Controls expired tidal volume	Hypocarbia, Fio_2
Piotrowski et al,[37] 2007	N = 56, 24–34 wk	PRVC with Siemens Servo 300	SIMV with various ventilators	Until extubation	Different triggers and ventilators in 2 groups	Controls inspired tidal volume entering circuit	Time to extubation, air leak, IVH

Abbreviations: AC, assist control; BPD, bronchopulmonary dysplasia; IMV, intermittent mandatory ventilation; IVH, intraventricular hemorrhage; PC, pressure control; PIE, pulmonary interstitial emphysema; PLV, pressure-limited ventilation; PRVC, pressure-regulated volume control; PSV, pressure-support ventilation; PVL, periventricular leukomalacia; SIMV, synchronized intermittent mandatory ventilation; VC, volume control; VG, volume guarantee; VTV, volume-targeted ventilation.

Adapted from Wheeler KI, Klingenberg C, Morley CJ, et al. Volume-targeted versus pressure-limited ventilation for preterm infants: a systematic review and meta-analysis. Neonatology 2011;100(3):219–27; with permission.

Table 2
Summary of the meta-analysis results before hospital discharge

	Outcome	Studies	Patients	Meta-Analysis		95% CI	P Value	Favors	NNT
Ventilation	Hypocarbia	2	58	RR	0.56	(0.33–0.96)	.04	VTV	4
	Pneumothorax	8	589	RR	0.46	(0.25–0.84)	.01	VTV	17
	PIE	6	430	RR	1.21	(0.63–2.3)	.57		
	Any air leak	5	374	RR	0.79	(0.44–1.43)	.44		
	Duration of ventilation (raw data)	6	431	WMD	−2.36 d	(−3.9 to −0.83)	<.01	VTV	
Primary admission	BPD (36 wk)	5	413	RR	0.73	(0.53–1)	.05	VTV	
	Death before discharge	7	554	RR	0.8	(0.53–1.2)	.28		
	Death or BPD (36 wk)	5	439	RR	0.73	(0.57–0.93)	.01	VTV	8
	Severe IVH	6	494	RR	0.71	(0.45–1.11)	.13		
	PVL	4	351	RR	0.41	(0.15–1.16)	.09		
	PVL or severe IVH	5	401	RR	0.48	(0.28–0.84)	<.01	VTV	11
	Oxygen at discharge	2	270	RR	0.64	(0.3–1.36)	.24		
Follow-up	Severe neurodevelopmental impairment	2	213	RR	0.86	(0.47–1.59)	.63		
	Death or severe neurodevelopmental impairment	1	109	RR	0.54	(0.27–1.06)	.07		

Abbreviations: CI, confidence interval; NNT, number needed to treat; RR, relative risk; WMD, weighted mean difference.
From Wheeler KI, Klingenberg C, Morley CJ, et al. Volume-targeted versus pressure-limited ventilation for preterm infants: a systematic review and meta-analysis. Neonatology 2011;100(3):219–27; with permission.

COCHRANE REVIEW OF TIDAL VOLUME–TARGETED VENTILATION

A Cochrane systematic review of volume-targeted ventilation was published in 2010[21] and summarized in *Neonatology*.[30] It included all 9 randomized trials comparing VTV with PLV (**Fig. 1**) and excluded crossover studies, which only assessed short-term outcomes.[6,14,31–38] It included trials using several ventilators and modes. Three used the Siemens Servo 300 (Siemens, Erlangen, Germany) pressure-regulated volume control mode, which controls inflating tidal volume at the ventilator, not the Wye piece. The ventilator has a decelerating flow waveform and adjusts PIP in response to inspired tidal volume. Two trials used volume control with the Bird VIP ventilator (Viasys Healthcare, Palm Springs, CA, USA). This ventilator also controls tidal volume at the ventilator entering the inspiratory limb. Four trials used the Dräger Babylog 8000+ volume guarantee (VG) mode. This ventilator controls expiratory tidal volume measured at the Wye connector by altering the PIP. Five trials had further differences between the groups other than a "pure" comparison between PLV and VTV; these were called hybrid studies (**Tables 1** and **2**). The studies used different ventilators in the 2 groups, different modes, and different triggers for inspiration and/or expiration. In some, the weaning strategies differed between groups, and some infants crossed between groups. These differences have the potential to introduce bias.

The meta-analysis of the results during hospital admission showed that VTV significantly reduced the combined rates of death or bronchopulmonary dysplasia (BPD) (number needed to treat [NNT] = 8), and severe IVH (grade 3 or 4) or PVL (NNT = 11). There was a borderline reduction in BPD alone ($P = .05$). No statistically significant difference was observed in the risk of death before discharge, severe IVH, PVL, or oxygen treatment at discharge.

SUMMARY

Volume-targeted ventilation is physiologically more logical than pressure-limited ventilation and is associated with a reduced risk of pneumothorax, hypocarbia, duration of ventilation, death or bronchopulmonary dysplasia, and severe intraventricular hemorrhage. It should now be adopted as the main mode for mechanical ventilation of preterm neonates.

REFERENCES

1. Dreyfuss D, Saumon G. Role of tidal volume, FRC, and end-inspiratory volume in the development of pulmonary edema following mechanical ventilation. Rev Respir Dis 1993;148:1194–203.
2. Dreyfuss D, Saumon G. Ventilator-induced lung injury. Am J Respir Crit Care Med 1998;157:294–323.
3. Hernandez LA, Peevy KJ, Moise AA, et al. Chest wall restriction limits high airway pressure-induced lung injury in young rabbits. J Appl Physiol 1989;66(5):2364–8.
4. Bjorklund L, Ingimarsson J, Curstedt T, et al. Manual ventilation with a few large breaths at birth compromises the therapeutic effect of subsequent surfactant replacement in immature lambs. Pediatr Res 1997;42(No 3):348–55.
5. Clark RH, Gerstmann DR, Jobe AH, et al. Lung injury in neonates: causes, strategies for prevention, and long-term consequences. J Pediatr 2001;139(4): 478–86.
6. Keszler M, Abubakar K. Volume guarantee: stability of tidal volume and incidence of hypocarbia. Pediatr Pulmonol 2004;38(3):240–5.

7. Abubakar KM, Keszler M. Patient-ventilator interactions in new modes of patient-triggered ventilation. Pediatr Pulmonol 2001;32(1):71–5.

8. Herrera CM, Gerhardt T, Claure N, et al. Effects of volume-guaranteed synchronized intermittent mandatory ventilation in preterm infants recovering from respiratory failure. Pediatrics 2002;110(3):529–33.

9. McCallion N, Lau R, Morley CJ, et al. Neonatal volume guarantee ventilation: effects of spontaneous breathing, triggered and untriggered inflations. Arch Dis Child Fetal Neonatal Ed 2008;93(1):F36–9.

10. Scopesi F, Calevo MG, Rolfe P, et al. Volume targeted ventilation (volume guarantee) in the weaning phase of premature newborn infants. Pediatr Pulmonol 2007;42(10):864–70.

11. Erickson SJ, Grauaug A, Gurrin L, et al. Hypocarbia in the ventilated preterm infant and its effect on intraventricular haemorrhage and bronchopulmonary dysplasia. J Paediatr Child Health 2002;38(6):560–2.

12. Dammann O, Allred EN, Kuban KC, et al. Hypocarbia during the first 24 postnatal hours and white matter echolucencies in newborns < or = 28 weeks gestation. Pediatr Res 2001;49(3):388–93.

13. Greisen G, Munck H, Lou H. Severe hypocarbia in preterm infants and neurodevelopmental deficit. Acta Paediatr Scand 1987;76(3):401–4.

14. Cheema IU, Ahluwalia JS. Feasibility of tidal volume-guided ventilation in newborn infants: a randomized, crossover trial using the volume guarantee modality. Pediatrics 2001;107(6):1323–8.

15. Tusman G, Bohm SH, Vazquez de Anda GF, et al. 'Alveolar recruitment strategy' improves arterial oxygenation during general anaesthesia. Br J Anaesth 1999; 82(1):8–13.

16. Duncan AW, Oh TE, Hillman DR. PEEP and CPAP. Anaesth Intensive Care 1986; 14(3):236–50.

17. Suzuki H, Papazoglou K, Bryan AC. Relationship between PaO_2 and lung volume during high frequency oscillatory ventilation. Acta Paediatr Jpn 1992;34(5):494–500.

18. Naik S, Greenough A, Giffin FJ, et al. Manoeuvres to elevate mean airway pressure, effects on blood gases and lung function in children with and without pulmonary pathology. Eur J Pediatr 1998;157(4):309–12.

19. West JB. Chapter 2. Ventilation. Respiratory physiology—the essentials. London: Williams and Wilkins; 2004.

20. Abubakar K, Keszler M. Effect of volume guarantee combined with assist/control vs synchronized intermittent mandatory ventilation. J Perinatol 2005;25(10):638–42.

21. Wheeler K, Klingenberg C, McCallion N, et al. Volume-targeted versus pressure-limited ventilation in the neonate. Cochrane Database Syst Rev 2010;(11):CD003666.

22. McCallion N, Lau R, Dargaville PA, et al. Volume guarantee ventilation, interrupted expiration, and expiratory braking. Arch Dis Child 2005;90(8):865–70.

23. Klingenberg C, Wheeler KI, Davis PG, et al. A practical guide to neonatal volume guarantee ventilation. J Perinatol 2011;31(9):575–85.

24. Wheeler KI, Morley CJ, Hooper SB, et al. Lower back-up rates improve ventilator triggering during assist-control ventilation: a randomized crossover trial. J Perinatol 2012;32(2):111–6.

25. Wheeler KI, Morley CJ, Kamlin CO, et al. Volume-guarantee ventilation: pressure may decrease during obstructed flow. Arch Dis Child Fetal Neonatal Ed 2009; 94(2):F84–6.

26. Wheeler KI, Davis PG, Kamlin CO, et al. Assist control volume guarantee ventilation during surfactant administration. Arch Dis Child Fetal Neonatal Ed 2009; 94(5):F336–8.

27. Bolivar JM, Gerhardt T, Gonzalez A, et al. Mechanisms for episodes of hypoxemia in preterm infants undergoing mechanical ventilation. J Pediatr 1995;127:767–73.
28. Esquer C, Claure N, D'Ugard C, et al. Role of abdominal muscles activity on duration and severity of hypoxemia episodes in mechanically ventilated preterm infants. Neonatology 2007;92(3):182–6.
29. Patel DS, Rafferty GF, Lee S, et al. Work of breathing and volume targeted ventilation in respiratory distress. Arch Dis Child Fetal Neonatal Ed 2010;95(6):F443–6.
30. Wheeler KI, Klingenberg C, Morley CJ, et al. Volume-targeted versus pressure-limited ventilation for preterm infants: a systematic review and meta-analysis. Neonatology 2011;100(3):219–27.
31. Piotrowski A, Sobala W, Kawczynski P. Patient-initiated, pressure-regulated, volume controlled ventilation compared with intermittent mandatory ventilation in neonates: a prospective, randomised study. Intensive Care Med 1997;23: 975–81.
32. Singh J, Sinha SK, Alsop E, et al. Long term follow-up of very low birthweight infants from a neonatal volume versus pressure mechanical ventilation trial. Arch Dis Child Fetal Neonatal Ed 2009;94:360–2.
33. Cheema IU, Sinha AK, Kempley ST, et al. Impact of volume guarantee ventilation on arterial carbon dioxide tension in newborn infants: a randomised controlled trial. Early Hum Dev 2007;83(3):183–9.
34. D'Angio CT, Chess PR, Kovacs SJ, et al. Pressure-regulated volume control ventilation vs synchronized intermittent mandatory ventilation for very low-birth-weight infants: a randomized controlled trial. Arch Pediatr Adolesc Med 2005;159(9): 868–75.
35. Lista G, Colnaghi M, Castoldi F, et al. Impact of targeted-volume ventilation on lung inflammatory response in preterm infants with respiratory distress syndrome (RDS). Pediatr Pulmonol 2004;37(6):510–4.
36. Nafday SM, Green RS, Lin J, et al. Is there an advantage of using pressure support ventilation with volume guarantee in the initial management of premature infants with respiratory distress syndrome? A pilot study. J Perinatol 2005;25(3): 193–7.
37. Piotrowski A, Bernas S, Fendler W. A randomised trial comparing two synchronised ventilation modes in neonates with respiratory distress. Anaesth Intensive Ther 2007;39:74–9.
38. Sinha S, Donn S, Gavey J, et al. Randomised trial of volume controlled versus time cycled, pressure limited ventilation in preterm infants with respiratory distress syndrome. Arch Dis Child Fetal Neonatal Ed 1997;77:F202–5.

Synchronized Mechanical Ventilation Using Electrical Activity of the Diaphragm in Neonates

Howard Stein, MD[a],*, Kimberly Firestone, BS, RRT[b],
Peter C. Rimensberger, MD[c]

KEYWORDS

- Electrical activity of the diaphragm • Edi • Neuroventilatory cascade • Neural trigger
- Neurally adjusted ventilatory assist • NAVA • Synchrony
- Patient-ventilator interaction

KEY POINTS

- The electrical activity of the diaphragm (Edi) is measured by a specialized nasogastric/orogastric tube positioned in the esophagus at the level of the crural diaphragm.
- The peak of the Edi waveform represents neural respiratory effort on inspiration, and the Edi minimum represents the tonic activity of the diaphragm.
- Neurally adjusted ventilatory assist (NAVA) uses the Edi signal as a neural trigger and intrabreath controller to synchronize mechanical ventilatory breaths with the patient's respiratory drive and to proportionally support the patient's respiratory efforts on a breath-by-breath basis.
- NAVA improves patient-ventilator interaction and synchrony even in the presence of large air leaks, and might therefore be an optimal option for noninvasive ventilation in neonates.

Diaphragmatic electromyography (EMG) as a tool to study respiration was first described in 1959.[1] From 1983 to 1994 various investigators used the diaphragm EMG to study sleep state and response to CO_2 in infants.[2–5] In the 1990s work was done by Sinderby and Beck[6–8] to develop electrodes embedded in a nasogastric tube that permitted reliable diaphragm EMG signal acquisition, reflecting the patient's

Drs Stein and Rimensberger and Ms Firestone are all speakers for Maquet. There are no other relationships to disclose.

[a] Department of Neonatology, Toledo Children's Hospital, 2142 North Cove Boulevard, Toledo, OH 43606, USA; [b] Department of Neonatology, Akron Children's Hospital, One Perkins Square, Akron, OH 44308, USA; [c] Pediatric and Neonatal ICU, Department of Pediatrics, University Hospital of Geneva, Rue Gabrielle-Perret-Gentil 4, 1211 Genève 14, Geneva, Switzerland
* Corresponding author.
E-mail address: Howardstein@bex.net

Clin Perinatol 39 (2012) 525–542
http://dx.doi.org/10.1016/j.clp.2012.06.004
0095-5108/12/$ – see front matter © 2012 Elsevier Inc. All rights reserved.

neural respiratory drive in real time, and minimized artifacts and noise. Over the past decade diaphragmatic EMG measurements have been incorporated into a mechanical ventilator (Servo-I; Maquet, Solna, Sweden). The mode of ventilation that converts this electrical activity into a proportionally assisted and synchronized breath is known as neurally adjusted ventilatory assist (NAVA).[8–10]

MEASUREMENTS OF THE ELECTRICAL ACTIVITY OF THE DIAPHRAGM

The diaphragmatic EMG is also referred to as the electrical activity of the diaphragm (Edi). The magnitude of this diaphragmatic activation (and hence the Edi signal) is controlled by adjusting the stimulation frequency (rate coding) and the number of nerves that are sending the stimulus (nerve fiber recruitment). Edi is measured from an array of 8 bipolar electrodes inserted into the lower end of a specialized nasogastric tube, with sensors placed above the feeding holes, and positioned in the lower esophagus at the level of the crural diaphragm. Signals from each electrode pair are differentially amplified, digitized, and processed. The signal is filtered to remove electrical contamination from the heart, esophagus, and environment to give the highest possible signal-to-noise ratio.[9] The position of the diaphragm is determined along the electrode array[11] and the double-subtraction technique is then applied to the electrode pairs close to the diaphragm.[12] The signal amplitude of the signal segment is calculated, and the eventual residual signal disturbances are identified and replaced.[8] Measuring the Edi in the esophagus with the double-subtraction method removes potential contamination from postural and expiratory muscles, the subcutaneous layers, and changes in lung volume, body position, intra-abdominal pressure, and positive end-expiratory pressure (PEEP).[6,7,9,13–15] The signal integrity also does not seem to be influenced by milk going down the esophagus during oral feeding[16] or by bolus versus continuous feeds.[17] Failure to detect an Edi signal can be due to central failure to deliver a signal (apnea of prematurity, central hypoventilation syndrome, overassist, hyperventilation, brain injury, sedation), anatomic reasons (diaphragmatic hernia), or peripheral abnormalities (phrenic nerve conduction failure, disease or chemical paralysis of the neuromuscular junction or diaphragm).[9]

The specialized nasogastric tube (shown in **Fig. 1**) is placed like any other nasogastric tube by using the measurement of nose-ear-xiphoid distance for initial positioning. The position is then refined using a retrocardiac electrocardiography (ECG), obtained from electrodes on the catheter, the waveforms of which can be seen on a dedicated catheter-positioning screen on the Servo-I, as shown in **Fig. 2**. When the electrode array is in the correct position, the largest p-waves and QRS complexes should be in the upper lead and decrease in size to minimal or absent p waves and QRS complexes in the lower leads. The Edi signal is superimposed on the retrocardiac ECG as a blue color and should be on the second and third lead.

NEUROVENTILATORY COUPLING

During spontaneous breathing, the respiratory signal originates in the brainstem and is transmitted down the phrenic nerve to the diaphragm, causing electrical excitation. The diaphragm then contracts, expanding the chest wall muscles and causing negative pressure in the chest. This negative pressure results in air being drawn into the lung, producing lung expansion and changes in pulmonary pressures, flow, and volume (**Fig. 3**).[13,18] Neural feedback from various sensors regulates the respiratory drive during spontaneous breathing on a breath-by-breath basis. This complex

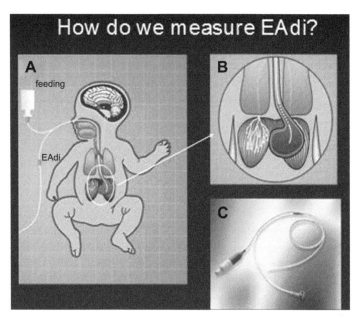

Fig. 1. Positioning of the specialized nasogastric tube with electrodes above and below the diaphragm. (*Courtesy of* J Beck and CA Sinderby, Toronto, ON.)

regulation system involves responses to stretch receptors in the lung, the Hering-Breuer reflex, and changes in lung compliance, upper airway receptors, peripheral chemoreceptors in the carotid body, and central chemoreceptors localized in the brainstem.[19,20]

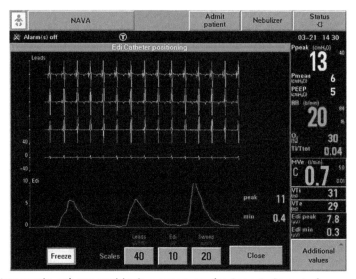

Fig. 2. Nasogastric catheter positioning screen on the Servo-I. Correct placement of the nasogastric tube shows the retrocardiac ECG signal progressing from large p and QRS complexes in the upper leads to small or absent complexes in the lower leads. The bottom tracing is the Edi signal, and the blue trace in the middle 2 leads is the Edi signal superimposed over the retrocardiac ECG tracing.

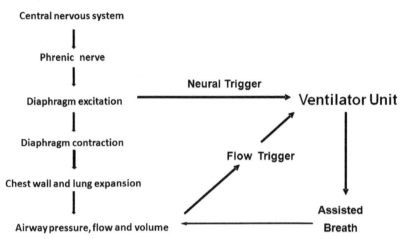

Fig. 3. Neuroventilatory cascade with the flow trigger and neural trigger. (*Adapted from* Sinderby C, Navalesi P, Beck J, et al. Neural control of mechanical ventilation in respiratory failure. Nat Med 1999;5:1434; with permission.)

PATIENT-VENTILATOR INTERACTION

The purpose of mechanical ventilation is to provide appropriate unloading of the respiratory muscles and to maintain adequate gas exchange until the respiratory disease that is responsible for the patient's respiratory failure has improved.[9,21] Short-term (less than 7 days) mechanical ventilation itself is known to be a cause of rapid diaphragmatic dysfunction and atrophy,[22–24] and long-term ventilation (more than 12 days) is also associated with failure of normal pulmonary growth and maturation.[24] Partial support modes that permit diaphragmatic effort or allow for periods of spontaneous breathing have been shown to alleviate some of the ventilator-induced diaphragmatic dysfunction (VIDD).[25] Strategies to promote synchronous ventilation, minimize mechanically delivered tidal volumes, and avoid both controlled mechanical ventilation and the use of paralytic agents are the best current approach to avoid VIDD and, possibly, ventilator-induced lung injury (VILI).[25,26]

The goal of synchronous ventilation is to provide a mechanical breath that is synchronous for timing of inspiratory effort and assists proportionally to the patient's needs.[9] Current neonatal ventilators offer 2 principal ventilator modes, assist-control/pressure-control ventilation (PCV) and pressure-support ventilation (PSV). The initiation of a breath can be triggered by the patient's respiratory effort in both modes; cycling is controlled either in time (for PCV) or by flow (for PSV), but the support level cannot be controlled proportionally to the patient's effort/demand breath by breath. Excessively high pressure-support levels may lead to ventilatory overassistance, resulting in suppression of the patient's respiratory drive, and may even lead to wasted respiratory efforts by the patient.[27]

Proportional-assist ventilation (PAV) offers, in addition to inspiratory triggering and cycling (controlled by either time or flow), an assist level (pressure or volume) proportional to patient-generated flow and volume.[21] However, all 3 types of ventilatory support (PSV, PCV, or PAV) are initiated only after the neuroventilatory cascade is complete (denoted as flow trigger in **Fig. 3**), and are in response to the patient's mechanical respiratory effort and not neural (central) respiratory need or drive. Asynchronous ventilation has the potential for adverse effects, which include the need for increased mean airway pressure and fraction of inspired oxygen (Fio$_2$), and fluctuations in blood pressure and intracranial pressure.[28] Sedation and/or muscle paralysis have been used to decrease the discomfort associated with asynchronous ventilation. These strategies have consequences including suppressing respiratory drive, prolonged duration of invasive mechanical ventilation, risk of developing edema, and unreliable assessments of neurologic status.[28]

Synchronization of neonatal ventilation is complicated because of unusually short inspiratory times, rapid respiratory rates, small tidal volumes, periodic breathing patterns, and often substantial and variable air leaks around the endotracheal tube.[29] These factors impose technological challenges especially with breath triggering, breath cycling, and termination. The ideal trigger device needs to (1) be sensitive enough to be activated by a small premature infant, without allowing for auto-triggering, (2) offer a rapid response time given the breathing characteristics of premature infants (short inspiratory times and rapid respiratory rates), (3) be able to compensate for variable air leaks, and (4) avoid the addition of additional dead space.[29] Previous triggering devices have included systems based on chest-wall impedance measurements, pneumatic capsule, and airway pressure or airway flow triggering.[28] All these triggering devices only detect initiation of the breath and synchronize a preset ventilator breath (for pressure control or time-cycled pressure-limited ventilation) or preset pressure (with PSV) with the patient. Further disadvantages of chest wall impedance triggering include susceptibility to chest-wall distortion and influences by cardiac and motion artifacts. The pneumatic capsule requires precise placement for accurate triggering, which is often impossible to achieve. This type of device is no longer available in the United States. Airway pressure triggering has limited efficacy in neonates.[28] Airway flow triggering is the triggering system most commonly used in neonates. Limitations include the addition of dead space by the flow sensor itself, auto-triggering secondary to endotracheal tube leaks, delays in response time, and failure to trigger.[28] The introduction of the Edi in the clinical setting has allowed further evaluation of the performance of the flow trigger, and **Fig. 4** shows examples of multiple types of ventilatory asynchrony seen with flow-triggered synchronized intermittent mandatory ventilation (SIMV) (pressure control) with pressure support.

PATIENT-VENTILATOR INTERACTION WITH EDI-CONTROLLED VENTILATION: HOW NAVA WORKS

During spontaneous breathing, electrical signals are generated in the respiratory center in the brainstem and travel via the phrenic nerves to activate the diaphragm. The electrical activity of the diaphragm is detected by electrodes embedded in the specialized nasogastric tube and is transmitted via wires in the nasogastric tube to the ventilator (see **Fig. 3**: neural trigger). The ventilator assists the spontaneous breath by delivering pressure directly and linearly proportional to the Edi. Therefore, the peak inspiratory pressure (PIP) delivered is proportional to the neural respiratory drive. Inspiration (pressure delivery) is maintained until the electrical activity decreases by 30% of the peak pressure generated, and then the breath is terminated. Using the Edi to control all aspects of the ventilator breath, the patient determines inspiratory pressure, inspiratory and expiratory time, and respiratory rate for each breath.[9,30] **Table 1** compares conventional ventilation with NAVA ventilation.

NAVA, like other modes of ventilation, has safety features available to protect the patient. The PIP limit can be set to prevent patients from taking excessively large breaths. When setting this limit, there needs to be consideration to allow the patient

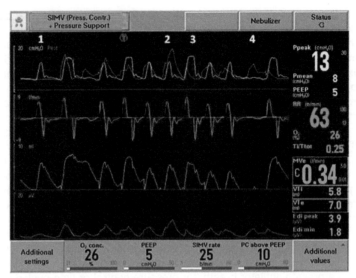

Fig. 4. Examples (1–4 in the top panel) of asynchronous ventilation in synchronized intermittent mandatory ventilation (SIMV) (pressure control). This panel shows the pressure (*first line*), flow (*second line*), and Edi (*fourth line*) tracings in a neonate on SIMV (pressure control). The Edi signal is converted to a pressure estimate (P.est), shown as a white line superimposed over the yellow pressure line in the upper tracing. The P.est represents what the pressure would be if the patient was in NAVA. (1) False (auto) triggering. There is no Edi signal but the ventilator delivers a flow-triggered pressure support breath shown in purple on the flow tracing. (2) Trigger delay, pressure and termination asynchrony. This flow-triggered, pressure support breath starts later than the start of the Edi signal; the breath is undersupported and terminated early compared with the neural respiratory drive. (3) Pressure and termination asynchrony. This flow-triggered, pressure control breath has accurate triggering but is significantly oversupported with excessive volume, and is terminated later than required by the neural respiratory drive. (4) Missed triggering. This Edi signal is completely missed by the flow trigger, and no breath is delivered.

the ability to generate sufficient inspiratory pressure to favor lung recruitment. NAVA ventilation depends on the Edi signal, which is detected by electrodes in the nasogastric tube. If a spontaneously breathing patient's nasogastric tube should become malpositioned, dislodged, or fail to detect the Edi, the ventilator switches into PSV. If the patient becomes apneic longer than a preset time, the ventilator switches to PCV. Once the Edi signal returns, NAVA ventilation resumes.

NAVA TERMINOLOGY

The development of NAVA ventilation has introduced several new terminologies not used in other ventilation modes.

Edi is the electrical activity of the diaphragm and is displayed for monitoring as a waveform. The Edi can be thought of as a respiratory vital sign. The Servo-I displays Edi not only as a waveform but also numerically on a breath-by-breath basis. For each breath, the highest Edi value of the waveform, the Edi_{peak}, represents neural inspiratory effort, and is responsible for the size and duration of the breath. The lowest Edi (Edi_{min}) represents the spontaneous tonic activity of the diaphragm, which prevents derecruitment of alveoli during expiration.[9]

Table 1 Comparison between conventional ventilation and NAVA	
Conventional Ventilation	**NAVA Ventilation**
Patient Controls Using Flow Trigger: Initiation of breath Rate (in some modes)	Patient Controls Using Neural Trigger: Initiation of breath Rate Inspiratory time Peak pressure Breath termination
Ventilator Controls: PEEP Fio_2 Peak pressure or tidal volume Inspiratory time Minimum rate Breath termination (expiratory time)	Ventilator Controls: PEEP Fio_2 NAVA level
Synchrony: Initiation of breath	Synchrony: Initiation of breath Size of breath Termination of breath

Reprinted from Stein HM, Firestone KS, Dunn D, et al. Bringing NAVA to the NICU. Advance for Respiratory Care and Sleep Medicine 2010;19:28–32; with permission.

Edi trigger is the minimum increase in electrical activity from the previous trough that triggers the ventilator to recognize the increase in electrical activity as a breath and not just as a baseline noise.[9]

The NAVA level is a conversion factor that converts the Edi signal into a proportional pressure. The unit of the NAVA level is cm H_2O per microvolt. The Edi is multiplied by this NAVA level to determine airway pressure delivered by the ventilator for each breath, as determined by the formula[9,31]:

$$Pressure\ above\ PEEP\ (cm\ H_2O) = NAVA\ level\ (cm\ H_2O/\mu V) \times Edi_{(peak-min)}\ (\mu V).$$

USING NAVA TO UNLOAD RESPIRATORY MUSCLES

In certain disease states whereby the respiratory muscles are unable to maintain adequate ventilation and oxygenation, partially or totally transferring workload from the respiratory muscles to the ventilator may be appropriate. As ventilatory assist increases, the inspiratory muscle workload is lessened and the respiratory drive is reduced. This process is reflected by a lower Edi. By increasing the NAVA level, the workload is shifted from the patient to the ventilator. However, even at the highest NAVA levels, when the ventilator assumes most of the work of breathing, the Edi continues to direct ventilation.[32–34] At these high NAVA levels transdiaphragmatic pressures are eliminated, indicating that the diaphragm is nearly completely unloaded.[34]

DETERMINING THE APPROPRIATE NAVA LEVEL

The Edi, in conjunction with the NAVA level, controls the NAVA ventilator support. However, in contrast to pressure-targeted or volume-targeted modes, the delivered pressure during NAVA is adjusted based on the neural feedback from the respiratory centers. As the NAVA level is increased the patient either maintains the Edi signal at

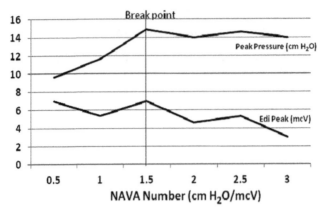

Fig. 5. Edi and peak pressure data from a 3-week-old 29-week infant, as the NAVA level is increased from 0.5 to 3 cm $H_2O/\mu V$. It appears that at a level of 1.5 cm $H_2O/\mu V$, the peak pressure no longer increases and the Edi$_{peak}$ starts to decrease, with further increases in NAVA level. The break point would then be determined to be a NAVA level of 1.5 cm $H_2O/\mu V$. (*Reprinted from* Stein HM, Firestone KS. NAVA ventilation in neonates: clinical guidelines and management strategies. Neonatology Today 2012;7:1–8; with permission.)

the current level, resulting in increased delivered inspiratory pressure from the ventilator, or the patient decreases the Edi signal to maintain the same inspiratory pressure. Adult and animal studies demonstrate that systematically increasing the NAVA level starts to unload the respiratory muscles and is followed by an initial increase in inspiratory pressure, airway pressure, and tidal volume while Edi remains constant; this is termed the first response, when respiratory muscles are insufficiently unloaded. When the NAVA level is further increased and reaches a "break point," respiratory muscle unloading becomes sufficient, at which time the Edi signal will start to decrease (ie, respiratory drive is decreasing) and the inspiratory pressure will reach a plateau, despite further increases in the NAVA level. The break point appears to be a unique value in each individual. In adults, this systematic approach to setting the NAVA levels offers a method to determine an appropriate assist level that results in sustained respiratory muscle unloading.[31–35] Above a certain support level, however, the Edi signal becomes erratic, indicating overassistance.[33,35] The NAVA level can be titrated daily as the respiratory disease evolves.[36] **Fig. 5** is an example from a premature neonate who underwent serial changes in NAVA levels to determine the adequate NAVA level needed to unload the respiratory muscles.[37] It is not known whether this break point is evident in all neonatal and pediatric patients or if it varies as neonatal respiratory disease and the need for ventilatory assist changes over time.

LITERATURE REVIEW OF STUDIES USING DIAPHRAGMATIC EMG
Studies in Animals

Studies in animals have shown that NAVA effectively unloaded respiratory muscles without increasing tidal volume.[27,38] Vagally mediated reflexes produce tonic Edi, which decreased with the addition of PEEP and functioned to prevent lung derecruitment.[38] Tonic activity disappeared with vagotomy, further supporting that vagally mediated reflexes were responsible for the increased tonic activity. Compared with PSV, some studies showed that NAVA reduced Edi and transdiaphragmatic pressure with little or no change in tidal volume and respiratory rate,[27,38] while other studies showed that NAVA decreased respiratory rate and increased inspiratory time while decreasing partial pressure of CO_2 (Pco_2) more rapidly than with PSV.[39] NAVA was as effective as low tidal volume strategies in reducing the incidence and severity of VILI, nonpulmonary organ dysfunction,[40] and VIDD.[41] Neurally triggered breaths reduced asynchrony, trigger delay, and pressure-time product, suggesting a reduction in the work of breathing as less effort was needed to trigger the ventilator and there was a faster response to respiratory effort.[42] Noninvasive ventilation with NAVA (NIV NAVA) was also able to provide synchronous ventilation with adequate blood gases, unloading of the respiratory muscles, and equivalent triggering on and cycling off via a noninvasive interface with significant (80%) and varying air leaks.[27,40] The NAVA level did, however, require augmentation up to 4-fold to achieve comparable diaphragmatic offloading as seen during invasive ventilation.

Studies in Healthy Adults

Increasing NAVA levels in healthy adults reduced inspiratory muscle workload and the respiratory drive during maximal inspiratory effort.[34] Even though the highest NAVA levels reduced the Edi by 60%, the Edi was never completely suppressed and the subject was always able to control the ventilator. As NAVA levels changed, lung-distending pressure (as represented by the difference between airway and esophageal pressure) remained constant.[43] In noninvasive ventilation (NIV) delivered via a helmet, the neural trigger had decreased delays between inspiratory effort and ventilator response in comparison with a pneumatic trigger.[44] Breathing comfort and subject-ventilator synchrony for triggering and cycling off was also improved with neural triggering.

Studies in Critically Ill Adults

PSV was compared with NAVA in patients with acute respiratory distress syndrome (ARDS) of varying etiology, those with exacerbation of chronic obstructive pulmonary disease, and postsurgical patients.[45–50] NAVA appeared to avert the risk of overassistance[45,46] by avoiding air trapping and cycling asynchrony,[48] improved patient-ventilator interaction,[45–48] reduced trigger delays and total asynchrony events,[45,46,49] and abolished ineffective efforts.[49] NAVA increased the variability of breathing pattern and complexity of flow delivered by the ventilator.[51] With NAVA, oxygenation improved despite reductions in tidal volume and respiratory drive (Edi) and there was no change in Pco_2.[50] When adequate NAVA levels (adequate unloading) were achieved, increasing the PEEP reduced ventilatory drive.[52] NAVA also improved the quality of sleep over PSV in terms of rapid-eye-movement sleep, fragmentation index, and ineffective efforts in a nonsedated adult population.[53] Using a helmet to deliver NIV, compared with PSV NAVA improved patient-ventilator interaction and synchrony, with no difference in gas exchange, respiratory rate, neural drive, and timing.[54] Critically ill patients who controlled their own tidal volume and respiratory rate on NAVA had a mean tidal volume of 6.8 mL/kg (range 5.9–9.9 mL/kg) with a mean respiratory rate of 25 breaths/min (range 18–30 breaths/min).[33,35,36,45,48–53]

Case studies suggest that the combination of extracorporeal membrane oxygenation (ECMO) lung support and NAVA deserve further study as a feasible treatment of severe ARDS.[55–57] NAVA has also been reported as a successful treatment in a patient with cystic fibrosis while waiting for a lung transplant.[58] The Edi and NAVA also function well in patients with polyneuromyopathy associated with critical illness.[59]

Edi monitoring can improve detection of patient-ventilator asynchrony in other ventilatory modes.[45–49,60–62] Edi, in relation to mechanical parameters such as tidal volume, may provide information about neuroventilatory efficiency, and may be useful to determine optimal PEEP and as a predictor for weaning.[52,63] Daily titration of the

NAVA level can also assist in ventilator weaning.[36] The Edi signal has been used to evaluate diaphragm function in a patient with advanced Duchenne muscular dystrophy,[64] as a possible marker for diaphragmatic fatigue,[65] and to evaluate recovery of diaphragmatic paralysis.[66]

Studies in Neonatal and Pediatric Patients

Studies have shown that NAVA improved patient-ventilator interaction and synchrony in neonates,[67–70] even in the presence of large air leaks.[71] When changing from conventional ventilation to NAVA, PIP decreased,[67,68,72–76] and respiratory rate increased in some studies[68,72] but remained the same or decreased in others.[67,73] Blood gases improved on NAVA in some studies[73,74,76] but remained the same in subjects studied on NAVA for less than 4 hours.[67,68,72] All studies showed no change in mean airway pressure, and no adverse events were noted while on NAVA. Specifically, in one retrospective review, there was no change in the rate of intraventricular hemorrhage, pneumothorax, or necrotizing enterocolitis.[73] Edi monitoring in neonatal and pediatric patients improved detection of patient-ventilator asynchrony in other ventilatory modes.[67–69,71,72,75] Studies in neonates on NAVA, who were ventilated for a variety of pulmonary problems, found a spontaneous mean tidal volume of 6.6 mL/kg (range 5.3–8.7 mL) and a mean respiratory rate of 46 breaths/min (range 35–59 breaths/min).[67,68,70–74]

Beck and colleagues[71] reported improved patient-ventilator interaction in 7 low-birth-weight neonates even in the presence of large air leaks. Neonates were ventilated with conventional ventilation (PSV or pressure-support volume guarantee) and then for 20 minutes with NAVA. The neonates were extubated and ventilated for another 20 minutes with NIV NAVA. Neonates on conventional ventilation initiated breaths comparable with NAVA but cycled off an average of 120 milliseconds before NAVA. Neural expiratory times and respiratory rates were lower during NAVA. There was no difference between NAVA and NIV NAVA.

Breatnach and colleagues[67] observed improved patient-ventilator synchrony during a 4-hour trial of NAVA in 16 children aged 2 days to 4 years. The patients were ventilated in a pneumatically triggered PSV mode for 30 minutes and then with NAVA for up to 4 hours. Improved synchrony for both triggering and breath termination with the neural trigger was noted when compared with the pneumatic trigger. In addition, there was a 28% reduction in peak airway pressure after 30 minutes on NAVA and a 32% reduction after 3 hours. There was no change in mean airway pressure, minute ventilation, expired tidal volume, respiratory rate, heart rate, partial pressure of oxygen in blood (Pao_2), and $Paco_2$. No adverse patient events or device effects were observed.

Bengtsson and Edberg[72] evaluated 30-minute study periods on NAVA in 21 children undergoing congenital heart surgery (4 were under 1 month of age and none were premature). Patients were alternated back and forth every 30 minutes between pneumatically triggered PSV and NAVA such that they were on each modality twice. The investigators found it was easy to insert the catheter and find the appropriate level of support during NAVA. Patients ventilated on NAVA had lower peak pressures and tidal volumes and higher respiratory rates than when on PSV. There was no change in mean airway pressure or blood gases. No serious adverse events occurred.

The 2 aforementioned studies compared PSV with NAVA inspiratory triggering based on pressure triggering. It must be questioned whether choosing flow triggering would have resulted in the same differences in asynchrony events between the 2 modes of ventilatory assist, or whether the pressure-support level chosen was adequate or eventually too high for the patients' needs. The latter scenario could explain the use of lower pressure levels during NAVA. However, Alander and colleagues,[68] who did a crossover trial in 18 neonatal and pediatric patients comparing flow, pressure, and NAVA-triggered ventilation for 10 minutes each, were unable to show a major difference between pressure and flow triggering during assist control. Neonates ventilated with NAVA were synchronous 91% of the time compared with 67% with pressure and 69% with flow-triggered ventilation. PIP decreased 13% on NAVA and respiratory rate increased. There was no change in mean airway pressure or blood gases. The investigators noted that in pressure and flow-triggered assist-control modes there was no spontaneous respiratory effort 8% to 12% of the time compared with 1.3% of the time on NAVA. No adverse events were noted during the study.

Emeriaud and colleagues[77] studied Edi signals in 16 infants, mechanically ventilated and ready to be weaned, on SIMV. Gestational age ranged from 28 to 40 weeks, age at study was 2.3 months (range 0.5–4 months), and weight at study was 4 kg (range 2.7–5.6 kg). These investigators showed that the diaphragm remained partially active during expiration of spontaneous breaths. Removal of PEEP increased the tonic activity, suggesting that infants had to compensate for the missing PEEP by tonic innervation of the diaphragm to maintain functional residual capacity. This finding indicates, as also suggested by experimental data by Beck and colleagues,[61] that the Edi signal might also be used to titrate PEEP levels in spontaneous-breathing patients with mild lung disease or on ventilatory assist for other reasons.

Beck and colleagues[78] characterized the neural breathing pattern in nonintubated preterm neonates. Ten neonates with a mean gestational age of 31 weeks (range 28–36 weeks) and birth weight of 1512 g (range 1158–1800 g) were studied for 1 hour daily for 4 days starting at a mean age of 7 days. Neonates were found to have a variable neural breathing pattern and elevated tonic Edi. Neural inspiratory times were found to average 0.28 seconds and decrease with increasing gestational age. Whether these average inspiratory times will be the same in neonates with restrictive lung disease (ie, hyaline membrane disease) is not yet known.

Zhu and colleagues[75] described 21 infants who underwent open heart surgery for congenital heart disease (mean age 2.9 months, mean weight 4.2 kg) who were ventilated with PSV and NAVA, each for 60 minutes, in a randomized order. Three cases were excluded because of postoperative bilateral diaphragmatic paralysis. The PIP and Edi on NAVA were significantly lower than on PSV. Postextubation Edi was higher in infants who needed reintubation or noninvasive mechanical ventilation than in those who extubated successfully (30.0 ± 8.4 vs 11.1 ± 3.6 µV). There were no differences in the heart rate, systolic blood pressure and central venous pressure, Pao_2/Fio_2 ratio, and Pco_2.

Stein and Howard[73] did a retrospective review on 52 neonates weighing less than 1500 g ventilated initially on SIMV (pressure control) and then changed to NAVA and followed up to 24 hours. The average gestational age was 26 weeks (range 22–32 weeks), age at study 2 weeks (range 0–56 days), and weight at study 958 g (range 465–1870 g). When on NAVA, these neonates had decreased peak inspiratory pressures (17%–20%) and Fio_2 requirements (15%) compared with those on SIMV (pressure control). Despite decreased pressures, in neonates ventilated with permissive hypercarbia, pH improved from 7.29 on SIMV to 7.34 on NAVA, and Pco_2 decreased from 54 on SIMV to 47 on NAVA. These changes were sustained over the study period. There was no change in mean airway pressure or respiratory rate. There was no change in the rate of intraventricular hemorrhage, pneumothorax, or necrotizing enterocolitis. Long-term respiratory outcomes were not evaluated.

Stein and colleagues[16] quantified Edi_{peak} and Edi_{min} values in 3 nonventilated spontaneously breathing term neonates. Two hundred forty data points were evaluated from each neonate. Edi_{peak} was 11 ± 5 and Edi_{min} was 3 ± 2 µV. Edi_{peak} was higher while awake than during sleep. Edi_{peak} was lower in the postprandial state than in the preprandial and feeding states. Edi_{min} was higher while awake than during sleep, but was not different among feeding states. There was no decrease or deterioration in the Edi signal during feeding, suggesting that there is no electrical interference from milk coating the esophagus or catheter. Although these are the first Edi values reported in healthy neonates, the study is limited by the small sample size.

Wolf and colleagues[79] evaluated extubation readiness in 20 mechanically ventilated patients (age 1 month to 18 years) using an Edi catheter. Patients who passed their extubation readiness test had a lower tidal volume to ΔEdi ratio than those who failed the test (pass: 24.8 ± 20.9 mL/µV vs fail: 67.2 ± 27 mL/µV). The investigators proposed that ventilated patients who generate a higher Edi in relation to tidal volume may have a better chance of successful extubation.

Bordessoule and colleagues[70] studied 10 infants ranging from 0.75 to 7 months old on mechanical ventilation for a variety of reasons. Mean age was 4.3 months and mean weight was 5.9 kg. The patients were successively ventilated with NAVA, pressure control (PCV), and PSV for 30 minutes each, and the last 5 minutes of each ventilator period were analyzed. In PCV and PSV, 4% and 6.5%, respectively, of neural efforts failed to trigger the ventilator versus none with NAVA, trigger delays were longer in PCV (193 milliseconds) and PSV (135 milliseconds) than with NAVA (93 milliseconds), and the ventilator cycled off before the end of neural inspiration sooner in PCV (in 12% of breaths) and PSV (in 21% of breaths) than with NAVA (0% of breaths). Asynchrony of the neural breath cycle with the ventilator was higher in PCV (24%) and PSV (25%) than with NAVA (11%). Variability of Edi was noted in all modes, but was only translated into ventilator breath variability during NAVA. Of interest, 5 patients received intermittent doses of fentanyl (1.3 µg/kg), morphine (0.08 µg/kg), or lorazepam (0.1 µg/kg) during the study period, and these medications, at these doses, did not appear to alter the respiratory drive, Edi signal, or respiratory variability.

Clement and colleagues[69] studied 23 infants ranging from 0 to 24 months in the weaning stage of mechanical ventilation for bronchiolitis. Mean age was 1.6 months and mean weight was 4.2 kg. The patients were randomized to start on either NAVA or volume-support ventilation in a prospective crossover study. The patient was on each mode for 120 seconds. When on NAVA there was less trigger delay (40 vs 98 milliseconds) and less response time (15 vs 36 milliseconds). There was also decreased work of breathing in NAVA as measured by the pressure-time product area.

Durrani and colleagues[80] described one term neonate with congenital diaphragmatic hernia post repair that met ECMO criteria despite management with high-frequency ventilation and nitric oxide. Because ECMO was logistically unavailable, a trial of NAVA was undertaken and the neonate was successfully extubated 3 weeks later. O'Reilly and colleagues[81] described in an abstract a series of 3 neonates (36–41 weeks' gestation) with congenital diaphragmatic hernia, of whom 2 were successfully managed using NAVA to facilitate extubation. One neonate resumed conventional ventilation after 24 hours on NAVA secondary to CO_2 retention. It is noteworthy that the neonate who had the diaphragm repaired with a patch (and did well on NAVA) had an Edi signal that was twice the value of the 2 neonates whose diaphragms were closed with suture only.

Vitale and colleagues[82] described a 15-year-old with cystic fibrosis who was managed on NAVA after a single lung transplant. The child had failed several attempts to wean off pressure-support mechanical ventilation because of infection, pneumothorax, and ventilator asynchrony causing gastric distention. After 22 days post transplant, the patient was placed on NAVA ventilation and was extubated within 3 days.

The investigators accredited improved patient-ventilator synchrony as the reason for extubation success with NAVA.

Stein[76] described a neonate with respiratory distress syndrome ventilated on NAVA before and after receiving surfactant. This neonate spontaneously increased PIP during, and for 40 minutes after, surfactant administration. The neonate then spontaneously decreased PIP (self-weaned their ventilator pressures), Edi_{peak} and Edi_{min}, and respiratory rate over the next few hours as lung compliance improved.

Liet and colleagues[74] described a series of 3 children (1 month, 3 years, and 28 days old) with severe respiratory syncytial virus–related bronchiolitis requiring mechanical ventilation with Fio_2 of at least 50%. Once on NAVA, respiratory rate and inspiratory pressure became extremely variable while breathing was easy and smooth. There were decreases in both oxygen requirements (57% ± 6% to 42% ± 18%) and peak airway pressure (28 ± 3 to 15 ± 5 cm H_2O).

Stein and Firestone provided clinical tips and management guidelines on the use of NAVA in neonates in 2010,[83] and updated their tips in 2012.[37] Because the clinical tips and management strategies are experience based and not evidence based, they have not been included in this review. However, given the limited clinical resources for the bedside caregiver on the application of NAVA ventilation in neonates, these references are included.

SUMMARY

The Edi signal represents the patient's neural respiratory drive and is used with NAVA ventilation to synchronize ventilatory support on a breath-by-breath basis. This technique may provide optimal ventilation based on the patient's ongoing needs, and uses all facets of physiologic respiratory control. Patients, even premature neonates, appear better than care providers at determining their ventilatory needs, and NAVA provides them the ability to use physiologic feedback to control ventilation and comfort for each breath. The Edi signal is becoming a valuable respiratory vital sign for both weaning and diagnostics. The patients can now "advise us" about what they want, directing their pattern of breathing with both timing and depth. NAVA also gives the caregiver access to previously inaccessible information about central respiratory desires.

Although the information available for neonatal use is still limited, research in this area has significantly increased in the last 3 years since NAVA received approval from the Food and Drug Administration. The challenge for health care practitioners remains the learning curve for the application of NAVA. Although the concept is straightforward, it is a new ventilation technique and process. Bedside caregivers need to be educated as to its nuances, which can be a time-consuming task. It appears that NAVA works well in neonates, but the question remains as to whether NAVA makes a difference in important clinical outcomes when applied both invasively and noninvasively in this population. Multicenter, randomized outcome trials to further investigate the promise of NAVA and NIV NAVA are awaited to determine whether this novel mode of ventilation will prevent intubation, facilitate extubation, decrease time on ventilators, reduce the incidence of chronic lung disease, decrease length of stay in hospital, and improve overall long-term outcomes.

REFERENCES

1. Petit JM, Milic-Emili G, Delhez L. New technique for the study of functions of the diaphragmatic muscle by means of electromyography in man. Boll Soc Ital Biol Sper 1959;35:2013–4 [in Italian].

2. Carlo WA, Martin RJ, Abboud EF, et al. Effect of sleep state and hypercapnia on alae nasi and diaphragm EMGs in preterm infants. J Appl Physiol 1983;54:1590–6.
3. Moriette G, Van Reempts P, Moore M, et al. The effect of rebreathing CO_2 on ventilation and diaphragmatic electromyography in newborn infants. Respir Physiol 1985;62:387–97.
4. Reis FJ, Cates DB, Landriault LV, et al. Diaphragmatic activity in preterm infants I. The effects of sleep state. Biol Neonate 1994;65:16–24.
5. Reis FJ, Cates DB, Landriault LV, et al. Diaphragmatic activity and ventilation in preterm infants II. The effects of inhalation of 3% CO_2 and abdominal loading. Biol Neonate 1994;65:69–76.
6. Beck J, Sinderby C, Lindstrom L, et al. Effects of lung volume on diaphragm EMG signal strength during voluntary contractions. J Appl Physiol 1998;85:1123–34.
7. Beck J, Sinderby C, Weinberg J, et al. Effects of muscle-to-electrode distance on the human diaphragm electromyogram. J Appl Physiol 1995;79:975–85.
8. Sinderby C. Neurally adjusted ventilatory assist (NAVA). Minerva Anestesiol 2002; 68:378–80.
9. Sinderby C, Beck J. Neurally adjusted ventilatory assist (NAVA): an update and summary of experiences. Sciences New York 2007;11:243–52.
10. Sinderby C, Spahija J, Beck J. Neurally-adjusted ventilatory assist. In: Vincent JL, Slutsky AS, Brochard L, editors. Mechanical ventilation. 1st edition. Heidelberg (Germany): Springer Berlin Heidelberg; 2005. p. 125–34.
11. Beck J, Sinderby C, Lindstrom L, et al. Influence of bipolar electrode positioning on measurements of human crural diaphragm EMG. J Appl Physiol 1996;81: 434–49.
12. Sinderby C, Beck J, Lindstrom L, et al. Enhancement of signal quality in esophageal recordings of diaphragm EMG. J Appl Physiol 1997;82:1370–7.
13. Sinderby C, Navalesi P, Beck J, et al. Neural control of mechanical ventilation in respiratory failure. Nat Med 1999;5:1433–6.
14. Barwing J, Pedroni C, Quintel M, et al. Influence of body position, PEEP and intra-abdominal pressure on the catheter positioning for neurally adjusted ventilatory assist. Intensive Care Med 2011;37:2041–5.
15. Barwing J, Ambold M, Linden N, et al. Evaluation of the catheter positioning for neurally adjusted ventilatory assist. Intensive Care Med 2009;35:1809–14.
16. Stein HM, Wilmoth J, Burton J. Electrical activity of the diaphragm in a small cohort of term neonates. Respir Care 2012;57:1–5.
17. Ng E, Schurr P, Reilly M, et al. Impact of feeding methods on breathing pattern in preterm infants. E-PAS 2010;4424.545.
18. Verbrugghe W, Jorens PG. Neurally adjusted ventilatory assist: a ventilation tool or a ventilation toy. Respir Care 2011;56:327–35.
19. Leiter JC, Manning HL. The Hering-Breuer reflex, feedback control, and mechanical ventilation: the promise of neurally adjusted ventilatory assist. Crit Care Med 2010;39:1915–6.
20. Sinderby C, Beck J. Proportional assist ventilation and neurally adjusted ventilatory assist—better approaches to patient ventilator synchrony? Clin Chest Med 2008;29:329–42.
21. Navalesi P, Colombo D, Della Corte F. NAVA ventilation. Minerva Anestesiol 2010; 76:346–52.
22. Levine S, Nguyen T, Taylor N, et al. Rapid disuse atrophy of diaphragmatic fibers in mechanically ventilated humans. N Engl J Med 2008;358:1327–35.
23. Froese AB, Bryan C. Effects of anesthesia and paralysis on diaphragmatic mechanics in man. Anesthesiology 1974;41:242–55.

24. Knisely AS, Leal SM, Singer DB. Abnormalities of diaphragmatic muscle in neonates with ventilated lungs. J Pediatr 1988;113:1074–7.
25. Petrof BJ, Jaber S, Matecki S. Ventilator-induced diaphragmatic dysfunction. Curr Opin Crit Care 2010;16:19–25.
26. Slutsky AS. Lung injury caused by mechanical ventilation. Chest 1999;116: 9S–15S.
27. Beck J, Campoccia F, Allo JC, et al. Improved synchrony and respiratory unloading by neurally adjusted ventilatory assist (NAVA) in lung-injured rabbits. Pediatr Res 2007;61:289–94.
28. Bhandari V. Synchronized ventilation in neonates: a brief review. Neonatology Today 2011;6:1–6.
29. Keszler M. State of the art in conventional mechanical ventilation. J Perinatol 2009;29:262–75.
30. Sinderby C, Spahija J, Beck J. Changes in respiratory effort sensation over time are linked to the frequency content of diaphragm electrical activity. Am J Respir Crit Care Med 2001;163:905–10.
31. Ververidis D, Van Gils M, Passath C, et al. Identification of adequate neurally adjusted ventilatory assist (NAVA) during systematic increases in the NAVA level. IEEE Trans Biomed Eng 2011;58:2598–606.
32. Lecomte F, Brander L, Jalde F, et al. Physiological response to increasing levels of neurally adjusted ventilatory assist (NAVA). Respir Physiol Neurobiol 2009;166: 117–24.
33. Brander L, Leong-Poi H, Beck J, et al. Titration and implementation of neurally adjusted ventilatory assist in critically ill patients. Chest 2009;135:695–703.
34. Sinderby C, Beck J, Spahija J, et al. Inspiratory muscle unloading by neurally adjusted ventilatory assist during maximal inspiratory efforts in healthy subjects. Chest 2007;131:711–7.
35. Patroniti N, Bellani G, Saccavino E, et al. Respiratory pattern during neurally adjusted ventilatory assist in acute respiratory failure patients. Intensive Care Med 2012;38(2):230–9.
36. Roze H, Lafrikh A, Perrier V, et al. Daily titration of neurally adjusted ventilatory assist using the diaphragm electrical activity. Intensive Care Med 2011;37: 1087–94.
37. Stein HM, Firestone KS. NAVA ventilation in neonates: clinical guidelines and management strategies. Neonatology Today 2012;7:1–8.
38. Allo JC, Beck JC, Brander L, et al. Influence of neurally adjusted ventilatory assist and positive end-expiratory pressure on breathing pattern in rabbits with acute lung injury. Crit Care Med 2006;34:2997–3004.
39. Campoccia Jalde F, Almadhoob AR, Beck J, et al. Neurally adjusted ventilatory assist and pressure support ventilation in small species and the impact of instrumental dead space. Neonatology 2009;97:279–85.
40. Brander L, Sinderby C, Lecomte F, et al. Neurally adjusted ventilatory assist decreases ventilator-induced lung injury and non-pulmonary organ dysfunction in rabbits with acute lung injury. Intensive Care Med 2009;35: 1979–89.
41. Huang D, Liu J, Wu X, et al. Effects of neurally adjusted ventilatory assist on prevention of ventilator-induced diaphragmatic dysfunction in acute respiratory distress syndrome in rabbits. Zhonghua Jie He He Hu Xi Za Zhi 2011;34: 288–93 [in Chinese].
42. Heulitt M, Clement K, Holt S, et al. Neurally triggered breaths have reduced response time, work of breathing, and asynchrony compared with pneumatically

triggered breaths in a recovering animal model of lung injury. Pediatr Crit Care Med 2012;13:e195–203.

43. Sarge T, Talmor D. Targeting transpulmonary pressure to prevent ventilator induced lung injury. Minerva Anestesiol 2009;75:293–9.

44. Moerer O, Beck J, Brander L, et al. Subject-ventilator synchrony during neural versus pneumatically triggered non-invasive helmet ventilation. Intensive Care Med 2008;34:1615–23.

45. Terzi N, Pelieu I, Guittet L, et al. Neurally adjusted ventilatory assist in patients recovering spontaneous breathing after acute respiratory distress syndrome: physiologic evaluation. Crit Care Med 2010;38:1830–7.

46. Colombo D, Cammarota G, Bergamaschi V, et al. Physiologic response to varying levels of pressure support and neurally adjusted ventilatory assist in patients with acute respiratory failure. Intensive Care Med 2008;34:2010–8.

47. Wu X, Huang Y, Yang Y, et al. Effects of neurally adjusted ventilatory assist on patient-ventilator synchrony in patients with acute respiratory distress syndrome. Zhonghua Jie He He Hu Xi Za Zhi 2009;32:508–12 [in Chinese].

48. Spahija J, De Marchie M, Albert M, et al. Patient-ventilator interaction during pressure support ventilation and neurally adjusted ventilatory assist. Crit Care Med 2010;38:518–26.

49. Piquilloud L, Vignaux L, Bialais E, et al. Neurally adjusted ventilatory assist improves patient-ventilator interaction. Intensive Care Med 2011;37:263–71.

50. Coisel Y, Chanques G, Jung B, et al. Neurally adjusted ventilatory assist in critically ill postoperative patients: a crossover randomized study. Anesthesiology 2010;113:925–35.

51. Schmidt M, Demoule A, Cracco C, et al. Neurally adjusted ventilatory assist increases respiratory variability and complexity in acute respiratory failure. Anesthesiology 2010;112:670–81.

52. Passath C, Takala J, Tuchscherer D, et al. Physiological response to changing positive end-expiratory pressure during neurally adjusted ventilatory assist in sedated critically ill adults. Chest 2010;138:578–87.

53. Delisle S, Ouellet P, Bellemare P, et al. Sleep quality in mechanically ventilated patients: comparison between NAVA and PSV modes. Ann Intensive Care 2011;1(1):42.

54. Cammarota G, Olivieri C, Costa R, et al. Noninvasive ventilation through a helmet in postextubation hypoxemic patients: physiologic comparison between neurally adjusted ventilatory assist and pressure support ventilation. Intensive Care Med 2011;37:1943–50.

55. Mauri T, Bellani G, Foti G, et al. Successful use of neurally adjusted ventilatory assist in a patient with extremely low respiratory system compliance undergoing ECMO. Intensive Care Med 2011;37:66–7.

56. Bein T, Osborn E, Hofman H, et al. Successful treatment of a severely injured soldier from Afghanistan with pumpless extracorporeal lung assist and neurally adjusted ventilatory support. Int J Emerg Med 2010;3:177–9.

57. Karagiannidis C, Lubnow M, Philipp A, et al. Autoregulation of ventilation with neurally adjusted ventilator assist on extracorporeal lung support. Intensive Care Med 2010;36:2038–44.

58. Roze H, Janvier G, Ouattara A. Cystic fibrosis patient awaiting lung transplantation ventilated with neurally adjusted ventilatory assist. Br J Anaesth 2010;105:97–8.

59. Tuchscherer D, Z'Graggen W, Passath C, et al. Neurally adjusted ventilatory assist in patients with critical illness-associated polyneuropathy. Intensive Care Med 2011;37:1951–61.

60. Colombo D, Cammarota G, Alemani M, et al. Efficacy of ventilator waveforms observation in detecting patient-ventilator asynchrony. Crit Care Med 2011;39: 2452–7.
61. Beck J, Gottfried SB, Navalesi P, et al. Electrical activity of the diaphragm during pressure support ventilation in acute respiratory failure. Am J Respir Crit Care Med 2001;164:419–24.
62. Rowley DD, Lowson SM, Caruso FJ. Diaphragmatic electrical activity signaling unmasks asynchrony and improves patient-ventilator interaction. Respir Ther 2009;4:51–3.
63. Liu H, Liu L, Tang R, et al. A pilot study of diaphragmatic function evaluated as predictors of weaning in chronic obstructive pulmonary disease patients. Zhonghua Nei Ke Za Zhi 2011;50:459–64 [in Chinese].
64. Beck J, Weinberg J, Hamnegard C, et al. Diaphragm function in advanced Duchenne muscular dystrophy. Neuromuscul Disord 2006;16:161–7.
65. Roze H, Richard J, Mercar A, et al. Recording of possible diaphragm fatigue under neurally adjusted ventilatory assist. Am J Respir Crit Care Med 2011; 184:1213–4.
66. Bordessoule A, Emeriaud G, Delnard N, et al. Recording diaphragm activity by an oesophageal probe: a new tool to evaluate the recovery of diaphragmatic paralysis. Intensive Care Med 2010;36:1978–9.
67. Breatnach C, Conlon NP, Stack M, et al. A prospective crossover comparison of neurally adjusted ventilatory assist and pressure-support ventilation in a pediatric and neonatal intensive care unit population. Pediatr Crit Care Med 2010;11:7–11.
68. Alander M, Peltoniemi O, Pokka T, et al. Comparison of pressure-, flow-, and NAVA-triggering in pediatric and neonatal ventilatory care. Pediatr Pulmonol 2012;47(1):76–83.
69. Clement K, Thurman T, Holt S, et al. Neurally triggered breaths reduce trigger delay and improve ventilator response times in ventilated infants with bronchiolitis. Intensive Care Med 2011;37:1826.
70. Bordessoule A, Emeriaud G, Morneau S, et al. Neurally adjusted ventilatory assist (NAVA) improves patient-ventilator interaction in infants compared to conventional ventilation. Pediatr Res 2012, doi: 10.1038/pr.2012.64 [Epub ahead of print].
71. Beck J, Reilly M, Grasselli G, et al. Patient-ventilator interaction during neurally adjusted ventilatory assist in low birth weight infants. Pediatr Res 2009;65:663–8.
72. Bengtsson JA, Edberg KE. Neurally adjusted ventilatory assist in children: an observational study. Pediatr Crit Care Med 2010;11:253–7.
73. Stein HM, Howard D. Neurally adjusted ventilatory assist (NAVA) in neonates less than 1500 grams: a retrospective analysis. J Pediatr 2012;160:786–9.
74. Liet J, Dejode J, Joram N, et al. Respiratory support by neurally adjusted ventilatory assist (NAVA) in severe RSV-related bronchiolitis: a case series report. BMC Pediatr 2011;11:92.
75. Zhu L, Shi Z, Ji G, et al. Application of neurally adjusted ventilatory assist in infants who underwent cardiac surgery for congenital heart disease. Zhongguo Dang Dai Er Ke Za Zhi 2009;11:433–6 [in Chinese].
76. Stein HM. NAVA ventilation allows for patient determination of peak pressures facilitating weaning in response to improving lung compliance during respiratory distress syndrome: a case report. Neonatology Today 2010;5:1–4.
77. Emeriaud G, Beck J, Tucci M, et al. Diaphragm electrical activity during expiration in mechanically ventilated infants. Pediatr Res 2006;59:705–10.
78. Beck J, Reilly M, Grasselli G, et al. Characterization of neural breathing pattern in spontaneously breathing preterm infants. Pediatr Res 2011;70:607–13.

79. Wolf G, Walsh B, Green M, et al. Electrical activity of the diaphragm during extubation readiness testing in critically ill children. Pediatr Crit Care Med 2010;12: e220–4.
80. Durrani N, Chedid F, Rahmani A. Neurally adjusted ventilatory assist mode used in congenital diaphragmatic hernia. J Coll Physicians Surg Pak 2011;21:637–9.
81. O'Reilly R, Freir N, Healy M, et al. A case series: NAVA and congenital diaphragmatic hernia. Am J Respir Crit Care Med 2009;179:A5820.
82. Vitale V, Ricci Z, Morelli S, et al. Neurally adjusted ventilatory assist and lung transplant in a child: a case report. Pediatr Crit Care Med 2010;11:e48–54.
83. Stein HM, Firestone KS, Dunn D, et al. Bringing NAVA to the NICU. Advancé for Respiratory Care and Sleep Medicine 2010;19:28–32.

Weaning Infants from Mechanical Ventilation

G.M. Sant'Anna, MD, PhD, FRCPC[a], Martin Keszler, MD[b,c],*

KEYWORDS

- Mechanical ventilation • Weaning • Extubation failure • Lung injury

KEY POINTS

- Weaning and extubation from mechanical ventilation (MV) remain an inexact science. Available evidence strongly suggests that early extubation is desirable, but our ability to predict the point at which this can be accomplished safely in extremely low-birth-weight infants remains limited.
- Volume-targeted ventilation may accelerate weaning from MV. There is a strong evidence base for using caffeine and distending airway pressure after extubation.
- Extubation failure remains frequent and may carry significant short and long-term consequences; achieving lower rates of extubation failure without unnecessarily increasing the duration of ventilation remains an elusive goal.
- Other adjuncts to weaning and extubation are less well established. Improved tools for predicting successful extubation in this vulnerable population are currently being explored with the hope of reducing extubation failure and the attendant risks of reintubation and prolonged MV.

INTRODUCTION

Mechanical ventilation (MV) is considered one of the major advances in neonatal medicine and is a widely used method of treatment, especially in the extremely preterm population. In a large cohort analysis of extremely low-birth-weight infants (ELBW) infants, 89% were treated with MV during the first day of life, and, almost 95% of survivors were invasively ventilated during their hospital stay.[1] Recently, a multicenter randomized controlled trial (RCT) compared the use of noninvasive and invasive respiratory support immediately after birth and showed that 83% of the ELBW infants initially assigned to noninvasive support required endotracheal (ET) intubation and MV during hospitalization.[2] In a large cohort of infants born at less than 28 weeks' gestational age

Disclosure: The authors have nothing to disclose.
[a] McGill University Health Center, 2300 Tupper Street, Montreal, Québec, Canada, H3Z1L2;
[b] Women and Infants Hospital of Rhode Island, Brown University, 101 Dudley Street, Providence, RI 02905, USA; [c] Warren Alpert Medical School, 222 Richmond Street, Providence, RI 02912, USA
* Corresponding author.
E-mail address: mkeszler@wihri.org

Clin Perinatol 39 (2012) 543–562
http://dx.doi.org/10.1016/j.clp.2012.06.003   **perinatology.theclinics.com**
0095-5108/12/$ – see front matter © 2012 Elsevier Inc. All rights reserved.

(GA), 74% were intubated and received surfactant therapy during their hospital stay.[3] The Continuous Positive Airway Pressure or Intubation (COIN) trial included only infants between 25 and 28 weeks of GA with adequate respiratory efforts at birth. Nevertheless, 46% of the infants initially assigned to noninvasive support required ET intubation and MV.[4] Thus, MV is a common therapy in neonatal intensive care units (NICUs), even in the current era of noninvasive respiratory support. Although MV offers essential support while the respiratory system recovers from acute failure and is necessary for survival, this therapy is associated with risks and complications, including mortality and neurodevelopmental impairments.[1,5] Therefore, when caring for extremely premature infants, clinicians should focus on weaning and removing MV as expeditiously as possible. Success of extubation is only 60% to 73% in ELBW infants.[6,7] Higher success rates (80%–86%) have been reported in some series that include all preterm infants.[8,9] Infants who fail and require reintubation, with its attendant risks, may experience deterioration of their respiratory status because of atelectasis. Episodes of hypoxemia or hypercapnia before reintubation may expose them to additional risks. Reintubation itself is unpleasant and may be traumatic and accompanied by bradycardia, hypercapnia, and alterations of cerebral blood flow and oxygenation.[10,11] On the other hand, many infants self-extubate and remain extubated subsequently.[12] Those infants may therefore have been exposed to MV and potential ventilator-induced lung injury for longer than necessary. Protracted MV is not benign; in preterm baboons, 5 days of elective MV resulted in a greater degree of brain injury when compared with only 1 day.[13] Using data from the National Institute of Child Health and Human Development Neonatal Research Network, Walsh and colleagues[1] showed that each week of additional MV was associated with a significant increase in the likelihood of neurodevelopmental impairment. In addition, the ET tube (ETT) acts as a foreign body, quickly becoming colonized and acting as a portal of entry for pathogens, increasing the risk of ventilator-associated pneumonia and late-onset sepsis.[14] Clearly, both premature extubation and unnecessarily prolonged MV are undesirable.

There is a striking paucity of good data to guide the clinician regarding optimal ways to wean respiratory support as well as to judge an infant's readiness for extubation. In this article, the available literature is summarized and reasonable evidence-based recommendations for expeditious weaning and extubation are formulated.

REDUCING VENTILATOR SUPPORT

Weaning from MV is usually achieved by the gradual reduction of ventilatory support until the settings are judged to be low enough to remove support. Considerable controversy persists regarding the best ways to accomplish this goal, but some general evidence-based guidelines can be formulated.

Pressure-Limited Ventilation

A Cochrane systematic review[15] comparing simple intermittent mandatory ventilation (IMV) with synchronized (sync) ventilation concluded that sync ventilation reduces the duration of MV. Which of the modes of sync ventilation is preferable remains a matter of debate, and there is no clear consensus regarding the relative merits of assist/control (AC) and sync IMV (SIMV). Available data do not clearly document superiority of 1 mode over another in terms of their effect on lung injury, but there is good evidence, as well as a sound physiologic rationale, for using modes that support every spontaneous breath in ELBW infants. Short-term studies have reported smaller and less variable tidal volume (V_T), less tachypnea, smaller fluctuations in blood pressure, and more rapid weaning from MV with AC, when compared with SIMV.[16,17] There are important physiologic considerations why SIMV does not provide optimal support in very premature infants. For example, with SIMV, the spontaneous breaths in excess of the set IMV rate are not supported, resulting in uneven tidal volumes and potentially a high work of breathing. This situation is especially true during weaning, when the number of unsupported breaths increases. This issue is most important in extremely small infants with correspondingly narrow ETT, because resistance to flow is inversely proportional to the fourth power of the radius (Poiseuille law: $R \propto L \times \acute{\eta}/r^4$, where $R =$ resistance, $L =$ length of the tube, $\acute{\eta} =$ viscosity and $r =$ radius). The impact on the ELBW infant may be substantial; 1 study showed a 4-fold increase in the work of breathing during SIMV, compared with AC.[17] The high airway resistance of the narrow ETT, limited muscle strength, and mechanical disadvantage conferred by the infant's excessively compliant chest wall typically result in small, ineffective V_T. Such small tidal volumes largely rebreathe dead space gas and contribute little to effective alveolar ventilation (alveolar ventilation = minute ventilation – dead space ventilation). Consequently, in order to achieve adequate alveolar minute ventilation, a relatively large V_T is required for the limited number of mechanical inflations provided by the ventilator.

Despite these considerations, many clinicians still prefer SIMV for weaning from MV, based largely on tradition and the belief that fewer mechanical breaths are inherently less damaging. However, it has now been unequivocally shown that excessive V_T directly causes lung injury, irrespective of the pressure required to generate that V_T. Thus, although the number of mechanical inflations with AC is larger, these inflations would be expected to be less injurious, because the V_T is about 33% smaller.[16] A rate of 60 inflations/min compared with 20 to 40 inflations/min resulted in less air leak with unsynchronized IMV,[15] lending further support to the presumed advantage of AC with its smaller V_T and higher ventilator rate over SIMV. Another misconception is that supporting every breath does not provide the infant with an opportunity for respiratory muscle training. This concern fails to account for the complex patient-ventilator interaction during sync ventilation. With sync ventilation, V_T is the result of the combined inspiratory effort of the patient (negative intrapleural pressure on inspiration) and the positive pressure generated by the ventilator. This combined effort (the baby pulling and the ventilator pushing) results in the transpulmonary pressure, which, along with compliance of the respiratory system, determines the V_T. During weaning, as ventilator peak inflation pressure is decreased, the infant gradually assumes a greater proportion of the work of breathing and in the process achieves training of the respiratory muscles. The ventilator pressure is decreased until it is only overcoming the added resistance of the ETT and circuit, at which point the infant is ready for extubation. The major disadvantage of SIMV can be mitigated by the use of pressure support (PS) for the spontaneous breaths. This combination is now available on all modern ventilators used in North American NICUs and should be used for small infants if the SIMV mode is chosen. The combination of SIMV + PS was shown to result in more rapid weaning from mechanical respiratory support than SIMV alone in ELBW infants[18] and to result in significantly lower work of breathing.[19] However, the combined mode results in added complexity and there is a paucity of information regarding how to optimally use this combination. The use of AC or PS alone is less complex and likely to be equally effective, provided sufficient positive end expiratory pressure (PEEP) is used during PS to maintain lung volume recruitment. Nonetheless, when used correctly, either approach avoids exhaustion of the ELBW infant's limited reserves and avoids setting up the baby for a failed extubation attempt. Ventilator settings at which extubation may be considered in infants 2 weeks of age or younger are provided in **Box 1**. Older infants may be able to be extubated from higher pressures.

Box 1
Ventilatory settings to consider extubation readiness in infants 2 weeks of age or younger. Older infants may be able to be extubated from higher pressures or tidal volumes

Conventional Ventilation (AC, SIMV/PS)

- SIMV: PIP $\leq$16 cm H_2O, PEEP $\leq$6 cm H_2O, rate $\leq$20, Fio_2 (fraction of inspired oxygen) <0.30
- AC/PSV, birth weight (BW) <1000 g: MAP $\leq$7 cm H_2O and Fio_2 <0.30
- AC/PSV, BW >1000 g: MAP $\leq$8 cm H_2O and Fio_2 <0.30

Volume ventilation

- Tidal volume $\leq$4.0 mL/kg (5 mL/kg if <700 g or >2 weeks of age) and Fio_2 <0.30

High-Frequency Oscillatory Ventilation

- BW <1000 g – MAP $\leq$8 cm H_2O and Fio_2 <0.30
- BW >1000 g – MAP $\leq$9 cm H_2O and Fio_2 <0.30

High-Frequency Jet Ventilation (HFJV)

- BW <1000 g: PIP $\leq$14 cm H_2O, MAP $\leq$7 cm H_2O and Fio_2 <0.30
- BW >1000 g: PIP $\leq$16 cm H_2O, MAP $\leq$8 cm H_2O and Fio_2 <0.30

Abbreviations: AC, assist control; MAM, mean airway pressure; PEEP, positive end-expiratory pressure; PIP, peak inflation pressure; PSV, pressure support ventilation, SIMV, synchronized intermittent positive pressure ventilation.

Volume-Targeted Ventilation

When tidal volume, rather than pressure, is the primary control variable, reduction in inflation pressure occurs automatically in response to improved lung compliance or increased respiratory effort of the infant. This reduction in support occurs continuously and in real time, rather than intermittently in response to blood gas measurements, and thus should accelerate the weaning process. A recent Cochrane meta-analysis,[20] which included both volume guarantee and volume-controlled ventilation, concluded that volume-targeted ventilation reduces significantly the duration of MV when compared with pressure-limited ventilation.

The specific V_T values that are optimal to accomplish weaning are not well established. However, the reduction in support is occurring automatically and the tidal volume/min ventilation requirements of the infant do not decrease substantially with improvement in lung disease; rather, the pressure needed to achieve the V_T is reduced. Therefore, reducing the target V_T below the normal physiologic value is counterproductive and inappropriately increases the work of breathing.[19] Infants who remain ventilator dependent for extended periods have increased V_T requirement over time,[21] as a result of (1) increasing anatomic dead space, referred to as acquired tracheomegaly,[22] and (2) increased physiologic dead space with the development of chronic lung disease and more heterogeneous lung aeration. In general, V_T should not be reduced below 4 mL/kg and in some infants not below 5 mL/kg during the weaning process to avoid excessive work of breathing (see **Box 1**). The goal is to have an infant who has adequate respiratory drive, with a pH less than 7.35, regardless of the $Paco_2$ (partial pressure of carbon dioxide, arterial). Drugs that might depress the respiratory drive should be avoided.

High-Frequency Ventilation

Although many clinicians are more comfortable changing from high-frequency ventilation to conventional modes, extubation directly from both jet and oscillatory ventilation is possible and may even be desirable. An early high-frequency oscillatory ventilation (HFOV) study compared 2 strategies of HFOV with conventional ventilation. The investigators found that only those infants who remained on HFOV until extubation had a lower incidence of bronchopulmonary dysplasia (BPD); infants who were changed to SIMV after 72 hours did not seem to benefit equally.[23] Similarly, the Neonatal Ventilation Study Group trial, which required infants to remain on HFOV during the first 2 weeks or until extubation, reported lower risk of BPD and shorter duration of ventilation, compared with conventional ventilation,[24] whereas the study by Johnson, which allowed early crossover to conventional ventilation did not show similar benefits.[25]

The way HFOV support is reduced is largely based on empiric, rather than experimental, data. In general, both pressure amplitude and mean airway pressure (Paw) are reduced progressively as tolerated. There is even less information about what constitutes extubatable settings during HFOV and HFJV than is available for conventional ventilation. In general, extubation is considered when mean Paw is around 8 cm H_2O (ie, slightly higher than with conventional ventilation) with Fio_2 less than 0.30. This situation is because with the usual 33% inspiratory time (1:2 ratio), the mean Paw measured in the ventilator circuit overestimates the tracheal pressure by 1 to 2 cm H_2O (see **Box 1**). Frequency is not reduced as a means of reducing support. With many HFOV devices, delivered V_T increases as frequency decreases, so that reducing ventilator frequency has the opposite effect from that on conventional ventilation. Some clinicians increase frequency on HFOV as a means of reducing pressure amplitude and V_T, but this approach of making ventilation more inefficient seems counterintuitive. Weaning from HFJV more closely parallels conventional ventilation, with stepwise reduction in peak and mean pressures. Frequency may be reduced slightly, because the V_T with HFJV is not affected by changes in frequency, but the primary means of reducing support is reduction in pressure amplitude. With both modalities, if support is reduced enough to allow mild respiratory acidosis, spontaneous breathing should become evident. As pressure amplitude continues to be reduced, the infant should take over progressively more of the respiratory effort, with visible spontaneous V_T, and when the settings are judged to be sufficiently low, extubation should be attempted. There are no studies of extubation readiness for infants on high-frequency ventilation. Ventilatory settings to consider extubation readiness in infants 2 weeks of age or younger receiving high-frequency ventilation are also provided in **Box 1**.

ADJUNCTIVE THERAPIES FOR WEANING
Permissive Hypercapnia

Accepting higher levels of $Paco_2$ during ventilation weaning to facilitate earlier extubation has been investigated extensively and is reviewed in detail elsewhere in this issue. Randomized clinical trials in preterm infants suggest that mild permissive hypercapnia is safe, but clinical benefits are modest.[26] The safe limits of hypercapnia both during the first few days when the risk of intraventricular hemorrhage is highest and later on during the chronic phase of BPD have not been definitively established.

Permissive Hypoxemia

Oxygen supplementation of preterm infants is a common intervention. The current knowledge of the optimal range of oxygen saturation (Spo_2) at various gestational and postnatal ages is still limited and target ranges used are wide, ranging as low as 70% for the low limit and as high as 98% for the high limit. Currently available information suggests that lower Spo_2 targets reduce the incidence and severity of retinopathy of prematurity (ROP) and lead to shorter requirements for ventilatory support and supplemental oxygen. However, there may be a small but significant increase in mortality with the lower Spo_2 targets. In the BOOST (Benefit Of Oxygen Saturation Targeting) trial, infants assigned to the high-saturation group (95%–98%) received oxygen for a longer duration (median, 40 days vs 18 days; $P<.001$), had higher rate of oxygen dependency at 36 weeks' postmenstrual age and a higher rate of home oxygen therapy, without any improvement in growth and neurodevelopment, when compared with infants assigned to a lower Spo_2 range of 91% to 94%.[27] The STOP-ROP (Supplemental Therapeutic Oxygen for Prethreshold Retinopathy of Prematurity) trial was prematurely interrupted and reported a trend toward a beneficial effect on ROP of a higher Spo_2 (96%–99%) target (odds ratio 0.72: 95% confidence interval [CI] 0.52, 1.01).[28] However, infants in the higher-oxygen target group had prolonged oxygen and ventilator dependence and prolonged hospitalization. This trial included only preterm infants with prethreshold ROP. The Neonatal Research Network SUPPORT (Surfactant, Positive Pressure, and Pulse Oximetry Randomized Trial) trial reported that a lower Spo_2 range (85%–89%) resulted in a substantial decrease in severe retinopathy among survivors, but increased mortality overall, raising serious concerns about the safety of this low target range, even though the mean Spo_2 in the low target group was close to the higher target range (see article elsewhere in this issue for more information about control of oxygenation). Similarly, the Benefits Of Oxygen Saturation Targeting (BOOST II) trials in Australia and New Zealand stopped recruitment after a safety analysis showed higher survival rates at 36 weeks' corrected GA in infants randomly assigned to Spo_2 targets of 91% to 95% rather than 85% to 89% while receiving supplemental oxygen.[29]

Other large RCTs are evaluating effects of higher (91%–95%) versus lower (85%–90%) Spo_2 targets from birth in extremely preterm infants. The Neonatal Oxygenation Prospective Meta-analysis (NeOProM) Collaboration has been formed and will conduct a prospective meta-analysis, using individual patient data, when all trials are complete.[30] The size of the combined data set will allow the effect of the interventions to be explored more reliably. The primary outcome to be assessed is a composite outcome of death or major disability at 18 to 24 months' postmenstrual age.[30] Meanwhile, the available evidence points toward avoidance of very low (83%–87%) and very high Spo_2 ranges (95%–98%); keeping Spo_2 between 88% and 93% may be the best approach until more data are available.

Caffeine

The use of caffeine in preterm infants has been investigated in several small studies and a large RCT for apnea of prematurity (CAP trial).[31] In this multinational trial, infants born with weights between 500 and 1250 g randomized to the caffeine arm were administered caffeine at the discretion of the responsible physician within the first 10 days of life. A little more than half of the patients in the caffeine group received the medication while on MV, 33% to facilitate the removal of the ETT and 20% to prevent postextubation apnea. A secondary analysis of the trial data showed that infants assigned to caffeine were ventilated for a shorter period, received less continuous positive airway pressure (CPAP) and oxygen supplementation, and had less BPD.[31] In a subsequent subanalysis, it was observed that earlier administration of caffeine was associated with faster weaning.[32] Although the administration of caffeine to preterm infants of less than 1250 g BW seems to be safe and effective for ventilator weaning, all these findings are secondary analyses and therefore should be interpreted with caution. In the large trial, caffeine was administered at a median age of

3 days, when infants were close to being disconnected from MV as per their physician's assessment.[31] Therefore, extrapolations for caffeine initiation immediately after birth or within a few hours of birth with the objective of improving any short-term or long-term outcome is not justified based on the available evidence.

Postnatal Corticosteroids

The use of postnatal steroids, either dexamethasone or hydrocortisone, has been the subject of several systematic reviews.[33–35] The use of systemic corticosteroids for the treatment of BPD has decreased sharply since the recognition of the dangers of liberal use of these drugs. However, corticosteroids can be effective and work well even at lower doses than previously used, presumably with less toxicity. As with all drugs, a careful risk-benefit assessment should be made and their use should be restricted to situations in which the risk of adverse outcome because of prolonged ventilator dependence is high. A policy statement from the American Academy of Pediatrics Committee on Fetus and Newborn was released in 2010 and included the following recommendations: (1) high daily doses of dexamethasone (approximately 0.5 mg/kg per day) have been shown to reduce the incidence of BPD but have been associated with numerous short-term and long-term adverse outcomes, including neurodevelopmental impairment, and there is no basis for postulating that high daily doses confer additional therapeutic benefit over lower-dose therapy; (2) low-dose dexamethasone therapy (<0.2 mg/kg per day) may facilitate extubation and may decrease the incidence of short-term and long-term adverse effects observed with higher doses of dexamethasone. Additional RCTs sufficiently powered to evaluate the effects of this therapy on rates of survival without BPD, as well as on other short-term and long-term outcomes, are warranted; (3) low-dose hydrocortisone therapy (1 mg/kg per day) given for the first 2 weeks of life may increase rates of survival without BPD, particularly for infants delivered in a setting of prenatal inflammation, without adversely affecting neurodevelopmental outcomes. Clinicians should be aware of a possible increased risk of isolated intestinal perforation associated with early concomitant treatment with inhibitors of prostaglandin; (4) existing data are insufficient to make a recommendation regarding treatment with high-dose hydrocortisone. Because available data are conflicting and inconclusive, clinicians must use their own clinical judgment to balance the adverse effects of BPD with the potential adverse effects of treatments for each individual patient.

A meta-regression analysis using published trial data indicated that the risk/benefit ratio is unfavorable in infants with mild disease but does favor the use of corticosteroids in the more immature and severely ill infants.[36] Very-low-birth-weight (VLBW) infants who remain on MV after 1 to 2 weeks of age are at high risk of developing BPD.[35] If corticosteroid therapy is used, it is preferable to administer a short course.[33,34] This decision should be made in conjunction with the infant's parents.

Diuretics

Diuretics have been shown to be ineffective in the treatment of acute respiratory distress syndrome (RDS).[37] However, furosemide, thiazides, and spironolactone are widely used in clinical practice for infants with BPD, largely based on short-term studies that reported improvement in lung mechanics and on anecdotal experience. The effects on duration of ventilatory support and oxygen administration, length of hospital stay, potential complications, survival, and long-term outcomes have not been investigated in appropriately designed and sufficiently large RCTs.[38–40] Some infants with BPD seem to be prone to interstitial pulmonary edema with fluid retention and show short-term benefits of diuresis. The apparent benefits of diuresis need to be balanced against the known adverse effects of these drugs, especially in view of the lack of convincing data in support of the chronic use of diuretics.

Chest Physiotherapy to Facilitate Weaning

Routine chest physiotherapy (CPT) in VLBW infants with RDS is not indicated and has been associated with increased risk of intraventricular hemorrhage (IVH).[41] There may be a role for CPT in prevention of postextubation atelectasis, but the data are inconclusive, as discussed later.

Optimal Nutritional Support

Insufficient attention has been paid to the importance of nutritional support in facilitating extubation. This concept is well established in the adult literature and is based on sound physiologic principles.[42,43] Maintaining infants on MV to facilitate weight gain is a practice that should be abandoned, but nutritional support should be aggressively pursued while the infant is intubated, as a means of optimizing strength and endurance after extubation.

Protocols for MV

More than 10 years ago, a collective task force facilitated by the American College of Chest Physicians developed a series of recommendations about ventilation weaning in adults and recommended that protocols designed for nonphysician health care providers should be developed and implemented.[44] This recommendation was based on the evidence from RCTs reporting improved outcomes in patients managed with ventilation protocols.[44] Although available evidence from the adult literature is compelling and justifies the use of health care provider-driven protocols in many settings, additional studies are needed to assess the efficacy of such an approach in the neonatal population. Only 3 RCTs in children have been published; these studies showed conflicting results and enrolled only a few term neonates.[45–47] Extrapolation of data from adults or children to prematurely born neonates is inappropriate, because of the unique aspects of the pulmonary physiology, respiratory mechanics, and epidemiology of lung injury. In 2009, an observational study from Canada showed that implementation of a weaning protocol for the management of infants with BW 1250 g or less, using objective criteria for weaning, extubation, and reintubation, resulted in significant improvement in short-term respiratory outcomes. After the protocol was implemented, infants were extubated earlier and an overall reduction of extubation failure and duration of MV was reported.[48] These studies support the adoption of ventilation protocols for neonatal intensive care, but well-designed clinical trials including the preterm population would benefit the practice of neonatology.

EXTUBATION READINESS

Failure of extubation is a common problem in extremely premature infants. Although neonatology has experienced major advances in MV and postextubation respiratory support, the science of determining if the patient is ready for extubation is still imprecise. Most preterm infants are easily extubated after a short period of MV but a few patients, for reasons such as respiratory muscle weakness, airway abnormalities, presence of a hemodynamically significant patent ductus arteriosus, immature respiratory control, residual lung injury, or nosocomial infection, become difficult to wean and require prolonged ventilation or fail 1 or multiple extubation attempts. The association between extubation failure and worse outcomes has been extensively investigated in adults and pediatric patients, in whom extubation failure was shown to prolong the overall duration of MV and length of hospital stay and increase the risks for nosocomial pneumonia and death.[49,50] In the preterm population, protracted MV is strongly associated with increased morbidity and mortality and is the major reason for neonatologists being proactive in weaning babies from the ventilator.[1,5,51] However, whether or not a premature disconnection followed by 1 or multiple episodes of extubation failure and reintubation directly contributes to worse short-term and long-term outcomes or is simply a marker for more immature, sicker infants is not clear. Nonetheless, an improved ability to predict when a preterm infant can be considered for extubation with the highest chance of success is highly desirable.

In the absence of strong evidence, the decision to extubate is most often based on the clinical judgment of the responsible physician. This process takes into account personal experience and bedside observation of the evolution of 1 or more parameters, usually blood gases, oxygen needs, and ventilator settings. Predictably, this strategy leads to substantial variation in practice and frequent failure of extubation. Ventilation studies involving preterm infants have described highly variable criteria for extubation for infants receiving different modes of ventilation, including SIMV, SIMV/PS, PSV, AC, volume guarantee, or HFOV. Thus, it becomes evident that there is no consensus on what constitutes the widely used expression minimal, or extubatable, ventilatory settings.

In preterm infants, the prevalence of extubation failure can range from 10% to 80% and is related to differences in the population studied, age at extubation, duration of MV before extubation, type of postextubation management, and time frame used for the definition. Failure occurs for several reasons, such as an inconsistent respiratory drive, weak respiratory pump, upper airway malacia, alveolar atelectasis, hemodynamic instability, glottic or subglottic edema, or residual lung injury (**Box 2**). The most common indications for reintubation are apnea and bradycardia (increased number or severity of episodes), respiratory acidosis, or severe hypoxemia, and increased work of breathing (intercostal and subcostal retractions, nasal flaring, grunting (**Box 3**). The criteria for reintubation are also variable. Typically, these infants are reintubated for any of the following conditions: $Paco_2$ greater than 60 or 65 with a pH less than 7.20 or 7.25, Fio_2 consistently greater than 0.5 or 0.6 to maintain Spo_2 between 88% and 92%, multiple episodes of apnea (>3–8 per hour), or severe apnea requiring positive pressure ventilation (**Box 4**).

Box 2
Risk factors for extubation failure

Lower GA (<26 weeks)

Prolonged ventilation (>10–14 days)

History of previous extubation failure

Use of sedatives (eg, morphine, fentanyl)

Multiple reintubations: upper airway problems

Evidence of residual lung injury: BPD, pulmonary interstitial emphysema

Extubation from high ventilatory settings

Extubation from high Fio_2

Hemodynamically significant PDA

Abbreviation: PDA, patent ductus arteriosus.

Box 3
Causes of extubation failure

Severe or multiple episodes of apnea

Hypoxemia

Hypercapnia

Upper airway obstruction

- Edema of the epiglottic area
- Subglottic edema/stenosis

Reintubation is not a benign procedure and may be associated with a variety of physiologic perturbations. Declining technical skills are also a problem, because fewer infants are being intubated. A recent study performed at a level III NICU in Canada reported that the ability of pediatric residents and neonatal fellows to perform a successful ET intubation did not meet the Neonatal Resuscitation Program (NRP) standards.[52] Although NRP states that a neonatal intubation attempt should last no longer than 20 seconds to avoid oxygen desaturation and bradycardia, the overall mean time for successful intubation was 51 ± 28 seconds, and attempts by pediatric residents and neonatal fellows were longer. Furthermore, 60% of ETTs were not optimally positioned within the airway on chest radiographs. Prospective trials performed to evaluate the use of premedication for elective and semielective ET intubations have reported even longer periods of time for a successful procedure and an average of almost 2 attempts per patient.[53,54] Therefore, reintubation of the extremely preterm infant carries a risk of prolonged and multiple unsuccessful attempts and complications associated with the procedure. Reintubation can cause tube malposition, traumatic injury to the nares or palate, glottis or trachea, lung or airway collapse, and infection.[52,55] These complications may cause or aggravate cardiorespiratory or neurologic disorders and, perhaps, result in long-term respiratory or neurologic disability. Severe bradycardia and large fluctuations in blood pressure, Spo_2, intracranial pressure, and oxygenation have been observed during intubation attempts, and these are only partially mitigated by premedication.[11] A recent study used 3-channel electroencephalographic monitoring during the ET intubation process and described significant changes in cerebral function.[56] All of these findings underscore the importance of achieving lower rates of extubation failure without unnecessarily increasing the duration of MV.

PREDICTORS OF EXTUBATION READINESS

Over the past decades, several studies have investigated prediction tools that could help neonatologists determine extubation readiness in neonates with the highest

---

Box 4
Criteria for reintubation

Severe apnea requiring positive pressure ventilation

Multiple episodes of apnea: >6 within 6 hours

Hypoxemia: Fio_2 >50% to maintain Spo_2 >88%

Hypercapnia: Pco_2 (partial pressure of carbon dioxide) >60 with pH <7.25

Excessive work of breathing with severe retractions

---

chances of success. Several of these studies were performed before routine or widespread use of antenatal steroids and surfactant. Also, postextubation management was different from current practice, with infants being extubated to a headbox with humidified oxygen or room air.[8,57–59] More recently, other predictors have been examined in infants exposed to antenatal steroids and surfactant treatments and provided with noninvasive ventilatory support during the immediate postextubation phase.

Physiologic Measurements

Szymankiewicz and colleagues investigated differences in pulmonary mechanics in ventilator-dependent preterm infants who were successfully or unsuccessfully extubated.[60] Just more than half of the babies were exposed to antenatal steroids, and surfactant was administered in ventilated patients only if Fio_2 was greater than 0.4 with an arterial/alveolar Po_2 (partial pressure of oxygen) ratio less than 0.22. Specific criteria for extubation and reintubation were applied, and 31% of the infants failed extubation. Significant differences were observed between success and failure patients in the values of dynamic compliance, respiratory system resistance, work of breathing, V_T, and minute ventilation measured on 10 quiet mechanical inflations with less than 10% leak. However, in this study, all infants received high doses of dexamethasone during the periextubation period (total dose = 1.5 mg/kg) and were treated with nasal CPAP of 10 cm H_2O only for the first 2 to 3 hours after extubation. Thereafter, infants were placed in oxygen hoods. Most failures were because of episodes of apnea; only 3 patients failed because of respiratory acidosis. No predictive values were calculated and validation of the findings was not performed. The application of a pressure-time index assessing respiratory muscle strength was able to predict successful extubation with high sensitivity and specificity, indicating a decreased diaphragmatic efficiency in neonates who failed extubation. However, this study was small and enrolled infants up to 36 weeks of GA and BW greater than 3 kg. Whether or not this index can be used in the smallest and most immature infants who are at the greatest risk of failure is unknown.

Spontaneous Breathing Trials

In adults, the use of a 30-minute to 120-minute spontaneous breathing trial (SBT) to assess extubation readiness is established evidence-based practice. In preterm infants, only a few studies have investigated a similar approach of a prolonged trial of ETT-CPAP and a meta-analysis concluded that preterm infants should be extubated directly from low ventilatory settings without a trial of ETT-CPAP.[61] The updated meta-analysis failed to identify recent investigations, and the 3 studies included in the analysis were performed more than 20 years ago, when the preterm population and ventilatory strategies were substantially different. Furthermore, the ETT-CPAP trials of those studies ranged from 6 hours to 24 hours in duration. For the last 2 decades, only 1 small single-center RCT investigated differences in weaning outcomes between clinical decision making alone and a minute ventilation test, which consisted of 10 minutes of ETT-CPAP at levels between 3 and 4 cm H_2O.[62] Infants with a median GA of 30 weeks were extubated if the ratio between spontaneous and mechanical minute ventilation was 50% and no adverse effects such as apnea, bradycardia, or an increase in oxygen requirement occurred. Although not significant, the percentage of patients requiring reintubation for 24 hours or longer was higher in the minute ventilation test group (24% vs 9%). The low level of CPAP likely caused some atelectasis and may have contributed to failure. Two small observational studies have investigated the use a trial of ETT-CPAP before extubation in neonates. Vento and colleagues[7] evaluated the percentage of time spent at a spontaneous expiratory minute ventilation less than 125 mL/min/kg during a 2-hour ETT-CPAP trial of 4 cm H_2O, performed after progressive weaning to an IMV rate of 6 inflations/min. Extubation failure was defined as need for reintubation within 72 hours after extubation. Forty-one infants were extubated to nasal CPAP of 4 to 5 cm H_2O; 11 patients required reintubation (26.8%). Using a cutoff value of more than 8.1% of the time spent less than spontaneous expiratory minute ventilation less than 125 mL/min/kg, these investigators obtained a sensitivity of 100% and specificity of 90%. The test was never validated in a prospective study and it is possible that infants at higher settings could have been successfully extubated. In 2006, Kamlin and colleagues[63] performed a 3-minute ETT-CPAP trial in preterm infants before extubation from ventilatory settings higher than used by Vento and colleagues. The test was simple and consisted of observing the clinical response by changes in Spo_2 and heart rate during the 3 minutes. The SBT showed a high positive predictive value, negative predictive value, sensitivity, and specificity and was adopted as standard of care at the investigators' institution. A prospective evaluation of this prediction tool at the same NICU found that infants were extubated earlier and from higher ventilator settings without any increase in the rate of extubation failure, compared with the period before the use of the SBT.[64]

Autonomic Nervous System Function

It is well known that in the healthy state, systems exhibit some degree of stochastic variability in physiologic functions, such as heart rate and respiration. This variability is produced by the dynamic behavior of the autonomic nervous system (ANS) and is a measure of complexity that is responsible for the greater adaptability and functionality of these systems. In preterm infants, loss of heart rate variability (HRV) has been shown to precede the onset of sepsis[65–68] and to be associated with worse clinical outcomes.[69–71]

The ventilation weaning process represents a period of transition from MV to spontaneous breathing and is associated with a change in autonomic activity.[72] Therefore, assessment of ANS function during ventilator weaning can provide information about physiopathologic imbalances.[73] In adults, reduced HRV and vagal withdrawal of the ANS activity were the primary changes in patients presenting with weaning failure.[74] Similarly, several studies have evaluated the ability of respiratory variability (RV) indexes to predict successful extubation; decreased RV been reported in patients who failed.[73,75,76] The combination of both indexes (HRV and RV) has been the subject of investigations during ventilator weaning in adults.[77,78] Only 1 study has evaluated RV in preterm infants before extubation. In this study, respiratory parameters obtained using a flow sensor during the 3-minute SBT were used for the calculation of RV. The combination of RV and clinical response to the SBT had a better accuracy in predicting successful extubation than either of the predictors alone.[79] Further investigations of variability indexes using more complex and sophisticated analysis over time are necessary and may provide important information for the clinician for the decision-making process during weaning and extubation.

POSTEXTUBATION MANAGEMENT
CPAP Versus Oxyhood or Nasal Cannula

The use of CPAP after extubation in preterm infants is superior to extubation to headbox or oxyhood.[80] The physiologic basis for this finding is the inability of the immature rib cage of the ELBW infant to maintain adequate functional residual capacity because of its excessive compliance/insufficient rigidity. In addition, after being intubated for some time, the infant's vocal cords are edematous, preventing effective grunting;

a mechanism the preterm infant normally uses to maintain internal distending pressure. Thus, some form of distending airway pressure should always be used for at least 24 hours after extubation.

There is insufficient evidence to clearly indicate if a heated humidified high-flow nasal cannula (HHHFNC) can be used to provide such distending airway pressure effectively.[81] Available evidence indicates that the pharyngeal pressure delivered via HHHFNC is inconsistent and low.[82,83] One study specifically addressing extubation success showed higher extubation failure with nasal cannula, compared with CPAP. Twelve of 20 infants randomized to HHHFNC were reintubated compared with 3 of 20 using Infant Flow CPAP ($P = .003$). The nasal cannula group had increased oxygen use and more apnea and bradycardia after extubation.[84] Two RCTs evaluating the use of HHHFNC in the prevention of extubation failure in preterm infants are actively enrolling patients (NCT 00609882 and ACTRN 12610000166077). Together, more than 700 patients will be evaluated. Results of these trials will help to elucidate the role of this therapy in this specific indication.

CPAP Versus Nasal Intermittent Positive Pressure Ventilation

Four small and single-center clinical trials have shown the beneficial effects of sync nasal intermittent positive pressure ventilation (NIPPV) to support the extremely preterm infant during the immediate postextubation phase.[85–87] Three of these studies were performed almost 20 years ago and used different interfaces and extubation failure definitions. Nevertheless, the use of nonsynchronized (nonsync) NIPPV became popular.[88–90] The exact mechanism by which NIPPV works is not understood and has been the subject of recent investigations performed in stable infants, several days after extubation. Chang and colleagues[91] reported no short-term benefits on ventilation and gas exchange of nasal ventilation when compared with nasal CPAP. Only sync NIPPV was associated with a decrease in the inspiratory work of breathing. However, active expiratory effort and expiratory duration increased during both modes of NIPPV. Owen and colleagues[92] confirmed these findings by reporting little effect on V_T during the use of nonsync NIPPV even when the positive pressure was delivered in synchrony with the patient's spontaneous breaths. These investigators also reported significant variations between the set and the delivered pressure (measured at the nose); in most of the patients, the achieved pressure was significantly less than the set pressure. During episodes of apnea, chest inflation was observed only 5% of the time, resulting in small tidal volumes (26.7% of spontaneous breath size), but nonetheless the number of oxygen desaturations was reduced. Many episodes of apnea are accompanied by airway obstruction,[93] and based on these findings, it seems that nasally delivered pressures may not be able to overcome this obstruction. Increased positive pressures may not be efficacious because of leaks but also because high levels of nasal positive pressure increase the electrical activity of glottal constrictor muscle (thyroarytenoid), as was shown in a series of experiments in newborn lambs.[94–96] This finding suggests that such airway closure can limit lung ventilation when increasing NIPPV levels. A large multinational RCT on the use of nonsync NIPPV in preterm infants (NCT00433212) has just been reported in abstract form and showed no difference in any of the major outcomes, including duration of ventilation or extubation failure. [Kirpalani, et al PAS 2012: E-PAS2012:1675.1].

Caffeine

A systematic Cochrane review of the literature[97] has indicated a relative risk of failed extubation of 0.48 for infants exposed to methylxanthines before extubation, and on that basis, caffeine is virtually always administered before extubation in ELBW infants, if it had not been initiated previously. The optimal dose to achieve extubation may be higher than that which has been traditionally used. A multicenter trial by Steer and colleagues[98] reported a significant reduction in failure to extubate for infants receiving a higher dose of 20 mg/kg/d (15.0% vs 29.8% in the infants receiving a dose of 5 mg/kg/d; relative risk [RR] = 0.51; 95% CI 0.31–0.85; number needed to treat = 7). A significant difference in duration of MV was seen in infants of less than 28 weeks' GA receiving the high dose of caffeine (14.4 ± 11.1 vs 22.1 ± 17.1 days; $P = .01$).

Postnatal Corticosteroids for the Prevention and Treatment of Postextubation Stridor

In neonates, 2 studies examined the use of steroids for the prevention of postextubation stridor. A meta-analysis revealed that the results were heterogeneous, with no overall statistically significant reduction in postextubation stridor (RR 0.42; 95% CI 0.07–2.32).[99] A study that was performed in high-risk neonates treated with multiple doses of steroids around the time of extubation showed a significant reduction in stridor.[100] Thus, this intervention does merit further investigation. Notwithstanding the equivocal data, the use of a short burst of low-dose corticosteroids has become widespread, largely based on favorable anecdotal experience. It may be prudent to reserve such therapy for infants who were intubated for prolonged periods, who have a history of traumatic or multiple endotracheal intubations, or who previously failed extubation because of subglottic edema.

Nebulized Racemic Epinephrine and Dexamethasone

Nebulization of racemic epinephrine is widely used to treat acute airway edema in pediatric croup and for postextubation stridor in newborn infants. Although anecdotal experience and short-term studies support its use,[101] a Cochrane meta-analysis[102] failed to identify any randomized studies that evaluated important clinical outcomes. There is similar paucity of clear evidence in support of nebulized dexamethasone.

CPT to Prevent Postextubation Atelectasis and Reintubation

CPT has been used around the world to improve removal of airway secretions and treat lung collapse, but the evidence to support its use in neonates is equivocal. In a meta-analysis,[41] active CPT performed every 1 to 2 hours was associated with a reduction in the need of reintubation within the first 24 hours after extubation. However, caution is required when interpreting any possible positive effects of this therapy because the studies are old and enrolled a small number of larger, more mature infants, and results were not consistent across the trials. Therefore, data on safety are insufficient and applicability to current practice may be limited.

SUMMARY

Weaning and extubation from MV remain an inexact science. Available evidence strongly suggests that early extubation is desirable, but our ability to predict the point at which this can be accomplished safely in ELBW infants remains limited. Volume-targeted ventilation may accelerate weaning from MV. There is a strong evidence base for using caffeine and distending airway pressure after extubation. Other adjuncts to weaning and extubation are less well established. Improved tools for predicting successful extubation in this vulnerable population are currently being explored, with the hope of reducing extubation failure and the attendant risks of reintubation and prolonged MV.

REFERENCES

1. Walsh MC, Morris BH, Wrage LA, et al. Extremely low birthweight neonates with protracted ventilation: mortality and 18-month neurodevelopmental outcomes. J Pediatr 2005;146(6):798–804.
2. Support Study Group of the Eunice Kennedy Shriver NICHD Neonatal Research Network, Finer NN, Carlo WA, et al. Early CPAP versus surfactant in extremely preterm infants. N Engl J Med 2010;362:1970–9.
3. Stoll BJ, Hansen NI, Bell EF, et al. Neonatal outcomes of extremely preterm infants from the NICHD neonatal research network. Pediatrics 2010;126(3): 443–56.
4. Morley CJ, Davis PG, Doyle LW, et al. Nasal CPAP or intubation at birth for very preterm infants. N Engl J Med 2008;358(7):700–8.
5. Miller JD, Carlo WA. Pulmonary complications of mechanical ventilation in neonates. Clin Perinatol 2008;35(1):273–81.
6. Stefanescu BM, Murphy WP, Hansell BJ, et al. A randomized, controlled trial comparing two different continuous positive airway pressure systems for the successful extubation of extremely low birth weight infants. Pediatrics 2003; 112(5):1031–8.
7. Vento G, Tortorolo L, Zecca E, et al. Spontaneous minute ventilation is a predictor of extubation failure in extremely-low-birth-weight infants. J Matern Fetal Neonatal Med 2004;15(3):147–54.
8. Dimitriou G, Greenough A, Endo A, et al. Prediction of extubation failure in preterm infants. Arch Dis Child Fetal Neonatal Ed 2002;86(1):F32–5.
9. Dimitriou G, Fouzas S, Vervenioti A, et al. Prediction of extubation outcome in preterm infants by composite extubation indices. Pediatr Crit Care Med 2011; 12(6):e242–9.
10. Marshall TA, Deeder R, Pai S, et al. Physiologic changes associated with endo-tracheal intubation in preterm infants. Crit Care Med 1984;12(6):501–3.
11. Venkatesh V, Ponnusamy V, Anandaraj J, et al. Endotracheal intubation in a neonatal population remains associated with a high risk of adverse events. Eur J Pediatr 2011;170(2):223–7.
12. Veldman A, Trautschold T, Weiss K, et al. Characteristics and outcome of unplanned extubation in ventilated preterm and term newborns on a neonatal intensive care unit. Paediatr Anaesth 2006;16(9):968–73.
13. Loeliger M, Inder T, Cain S, et al. Cerebral outcomes in a preterm baboon model of early versus delayed nasal continuous positive airway pressure. Pediatrics 2006;118(4):1640–53.
14. Garland JS. Strategies to prevent ventilator-associated pneumonia in neonates. Clin Perinatol 2010;37(3):629–43.
15. Greenough A, Dimitriou G, Prendergast M, et al. Synchronized mechanical ventilation for respiratory support in newborn infants. Cochrane Database Syst Rev 2008;(1):CD000456.
16. Hummler H, Gerhardt T, Gonzalez A, et al. Influence of different methods of synchronized mechanical ventilation on ventilation, gas exchange, patient effort, and blood pressure fluctuations in premature neonates. Pediatr Pulmonol 1996; 22(5):305–13.
17. Kapasi M, Fujino Y, Kirmse M, et al. Effort and work of breathing in neonates during assisted patient-triggered ventilation. Pediatr Crit Care Med 2001;2(1):9–16.
18. Reyes ZC, Claure N, Tauscher MK, et al. Randomized, controlled trial comparing synchronized intermittent mandatory ventilation and synchronized

intermittent mandatory ventilation plus pressure support in preterm infants. Pediatrics 2006;118(4):1409–17.

19. Patel DS, Sharma A, Prendergast M, et al. Work of breathing and different levels of volume-targeted ventilation. Pediatrics 2009;123(4):e679–84.

20. Wheeler K, Klingenberg C, McCallion N, et al. Volume-targeted versus pressure-limited ventilation in the neonate. Cochrane Database Syst Rev 2010;(11):CD003666.

21. Keszler M, Nassabeh-Montazami S, Abubakar K. Evolution of tidal volume requirement during the first 3 weeks of life in infants <800 g ventilated with volume guarantee. Arch Dis Child Fetal Neonatal Ed 2009;94(4):F279–82.

22. Bhutani VK, Ritchie WG, Shaffer TH. Acquired tracheomegaly in very preterm neonates. Am J Dis Child Fetal Neonatal Ed 1986;140(5):449–52.

23. Clark RH, Gerstmann DR, Null DM Jr, et al. Prospective randomized comparison of high-frequency oscillatory and conventional ventilation in respiratory distress syndrome. Pediatrics 1992;89(1):5–12.

24. Courtney SE, Durand DJ, Asselin JM, et al. High-frequency oscillatory ventilation versus conventional mechanical ventilation for very-low-birth-weight infants. N Engl J Med 2002;347(9):643–52.

25. Johnson AH, Peacock JL, Greenough A, et al. High-frequency oscillatory ventilation for the prevention of chronic lung disease of prematurity. N Engl J Med 2002;347(9):633–42.

26. Thome UH, Ambalavanan N. Permissive hypercapnia to decrease lung injury in ventilated preterm neonates. Semin Fetal Neonatal Med 2009;14(1):21–7.

27. Askie LM, Henderson-Smart DJ, Irwig L, et al. Oxygen-saturation targets and outcomes in extremely preterm infants. N Engl J Med 2003;349(10):959–67.

28. Supplemental Therapeutic Oxygen for Prethreshold Retinopathy of Prematurity (STOP-ROP), a randomized, controlled trial. I: Primary outcomes. Pediatrics 2000;105(2):295–310.

29. Stenson B, Brocklehurst P, Juszczak E, et al. Increased 36 week survival with high oxygen saturation target in extremely preterm infants. Arch Dis Child Fetal Neonatal Ed 2011;96(Suppl 1):Fa3–4.

30. Askie LM, Brocklehurst P, Darlow BA, et al. NeOProM: Neonatal Oxygenation Prospective Meta-analysis collaboration study protocol. BMC Pediatr 2011;11:6.

31. Schmidt B, Roberts RS, Davis P, et al. Caffeine therapy for apnea of prematurity. N Engl J Med 2006;354(20):2112–21.

32. Davis PG, Schmidt B, Roberts RS, et al. Caffeine for apnea of prematurity trial: benefits may vary in subgroups. J Pediatr 2010;156(3):382–7.

33. Doyle LW, Ehrenkranz RA, Halliday HL. Dexamethasone treatment in the first week of life for preventing bronchopulmonary dysplasia in preterm infants: a systematic review. Neonatology 2010;98(3):217–24.

34. Doyle LW, Ehrenkranz RA, Halliday HL. Postnatal hydrocortisone for preventing or treating bronchopulmonary dysplasia in preterm infants: a systematic review. Neonatology 2010;98(2):111–7.

35. Halliday HL, Ehrenkranz RA, Doyle LW. Late (>7 days) postnatal corticosteroids for chronic lung disease in preterm infants. Cochrane Database Syst Rev 2009;(1):CD001145.

36. Doyle LW, Halliday HL, Ehrenkranz RA, et al. Impact of postnatal systemic corticosteroids on mortality and cerebral palsy in preterm infants: effect modification by risk for chronic lung disease. Pediatrics 2005;115(3):655–61.

37. Stewart A, Brion LP, Soll R. Diuretics for respiratory distress syndrome in preterm infants. Cochrane Database Syst Rev 2011;(12):CD001454.

38. Brion LP, Primhak RA, Yong W. Aerosolized diuretics for preterm infants with (or developing) chronic lung disease. Cochrane Database Syst Rev 2006;(3):CD001694.

39. Stewart A, Brion LP, Ambrosio-Perez I. Diuretics acting on the distal renal tubule for preterm infants with (or developing) chronic lung disease. Cochrane Database Syst Rev 2011;(9):CD001817.

40. Brion LP, Primhak RA. Intravenous or enteral loop diuretics for preterm infants with (or developing) chronic lung disease. Cochrane Database Syst Rev 2000;(4):CD001453.

41. Hough JL, Flenady V, Johnston L, et al. Chest physiotherapy for reducing respiratory morbidity in infants requiring ventilatory support. Cochrane Database Syst Rev 2008;(3):CD006445.

42. Cresci G, Cué JI. Nutrition support for the long-term ventilator-dependent patient. Respir Care Clin North Am 2006;12(4):567–91.

43. Heyland DK, Dhaliwal R, Day A, et al. Validation of the Canadian clinical practice guidelines for nutrition support in mechanically ventilated, critically ill adult patients: results of a prospective observational study. Crit Care Med 2004; 32(11):2260–6.

44. MacIntyre NR, Cook DJ, Ely EW Jr, et al. Evidence-based guidelines for weaning and discontinuing ventilatory support: a collective task force facilitated by the American College of Chest Physicians; the American Association for Respiratory Care; and the American College of Critical Care Medicine. Chest 2001; 120(Suppl 6):375S–95S.

45. Randolph AG, Wypij D, Venkataraman ST, et al. Effect of mechanical ventilator weaning protocols on respiratory outcomes in infants and children: a randomized controlled trial. JAMA 2002;288(20):2561–8.

46. Restrepo RD, Fortenberry JD, Spainhour C, et al. Protocol-driven ventilator management in children: comparison to nonprotocol care. J Intensive Care Med 2004;19(5):274–84.

47. Schultz TF, Lin RJ, Watzman HM, et al. Weaning children from mechanical ventilation: a prospective randomized trial of protocol-directed versus physician-directed weaning. Respir Care 2001;46(8):772–82.

48. Hermeto F, Bottino MN, Vaillancourt K, et al. Implementation of a respiratory therapist-driven protocol for neonatal ventilation: impact on the premature population. Pediatrics 2009;123(5):e907–16.

49. Newth CJ, Venkataraman S, Willson DF, et al. Weaning and extubation readiness in pediatric patients. Pediatr Crit Care Med 2009;10(1):1–11.

50. Epstein SK. Extubation failure: an outcome to be avoided. Crit Care 2004;8(5): 310–2.

51. Natarajan G, Pappas A, Shankaran S, et al. Outcomes of extremely low birth weight infants with bronchopulmonary dysplasia: impact of the physiologic definition. Early Hum Dev 2012;88(7):509–15.

52. Bismilla Z, Finan E, McNamara PJ, et al. Failure of pediatric and neonatal trainees to meet Canadian Neonatal Resuscitation Program standards for neonatal intubation. J Perinatol 2010;30(3):182–7.

53. Dempsey EM, Al Hazzani F, Faucher D, et al. Facilitation of neonatal endotracheal intubation with mivacurium and fentanyl in the neonatal intensive care unit. Arch Dis Child Fetal Neonatal Ed 2006;91(4):F279–82.

54. Choong K, AlFaleh K, Doucette J, et al. Remifentanil for endotracheal intubation in neonates: a randomised controlled trial. Arch Dis Child Fetal Neonatal Ed 2010;95(2):F80–4.

55. Lee JJ, Ryu BY, Jang JS, et al. Two complications of tracheal intubation in a neonate: gastric perforation and lung collapse. Anesthesiology 2011; 115(4):858.

56. Shangle CE, Haas RH, Vaida F, et al. Effects of endotracheal intubation and surfactant on a 3-channel neonatal electroencephalogram. J Pediatr 2012; 161:252–7.

57. Balsan MJ, Jones JG, Watchko JF, et al. Measurements of pulmonary mechanics prior to the elective extubation of neonates. Pediatr Pulmonol 1990;9(4):238–43.

58. Kavvadia V, Greenough A, Dimitriou G. Prediction of extubation failure in preterm neonates. Eur J Pediatr 2000;159(4):227–31.

59. Dimitriou G, Greenough A. Computer assisted analysis of the chest radiograph lung area and prediction of failure of extubation from mechanical ventilation in preterm neonates. Br J Radiol 2000;73(866):156–9.

60. Szymankiewicz M, Vidyasagar D, Gadzinowski J. Predictors of successful extubation of preterm low-birth-weight infants with respiratory distress syndrome. Pediatr Crit Care Med 2005;6(1):44–9.

61. Davis PG, Henderson-Smart DJ. Extubation from low-rate intermittent positive airways pressure versus extubation after a trial of endotracheal continuous positive airways pressure in intubated preterm infants. Cochrane Database Syst Rev 2001;(4):CD001078.

62. Gillespie LM, White SD, Sinha SK, et al. Usefulness of the minute ventilation test in predicting successful extubation in newborn infants: a randomized controlled trial. J Perinatol 2003;23(3):205–7.

63. Kamlin CO, Davis PG, Morley CJ. Predicting successful extubation of very low birthweight infants. Arch Dis Child Fetal Neonatal Ed 2006;91(3):F180–3.

64. Kamlin CO, Davis PG, Argus B, et al. A trial of spontaneous breathing to determine the readiness for extubation in very low birth weight infants: a prospective evaluation. Arch Dis Child Fetal Neonatal Ed 2008;93(4):F305–6.

65. Fairchild KD, O'Shea TM. Heart rate characteristics: physiomarkers for detection of late-onset neonatal sepsis. Clin Perinatol 2010;37(3):581–98.

66. Griffin MP, Lake DE, O'Shea TM, et al. Heart rate characteristics and clinical signs in neonatal sepsis. Pediatr Res 2007;61(2):222–7.

67. Moorman JR, Delos JB, Flower AA, et al. Cardiovascular oscillations at the bedside: early diagnosis of neonatal sepsis using heart rate characteristics monitoring. Physiol Meas 2011;32(11):1821–32.

68. Saria S, Rajani AK, Gould J, et al. Integration of early physiological responses predicts later illness severity in preterm infants. Sci Transl Med 2010;2(48):48–65.

69. Moorman JR, Carlo WA, Kattwinkel J, et al. Mortality reduction by heart rate characteristic monitoring in very low birth weight neonates: a randomized trial. J Pediatr 2011;159(6):900–6.

70. Malarvili MB, Mesbah M. Newborn seizure detection based on heart rate variability. IEEE Trans Biomed Eng 2009;56(11):2594–603.

71. Griffin MP, Lake DE, Bissonette EA, et al. Heart rate characteristics: novel physiomarkers to predict neonatal infection and death. Pediatrics 2005;116(5): 1070–4.

72. Caminal P, Giraldo BF, Vallverdu M, et al. Symbolic dynamic analysis of relations between cardiac and breathing cycles in patients on weaning trials. Ann Biomed Eng 2010;38(8):2542–52.

73. Chaparro JA, Giraldo BF, Caminal P, et al. Analysis of the respiratory pattern variability of patients in weaning process using autoregressive modeling techniques. Conf Proc IEEE Eng Med Biol Soc 2011;2011:5690–3.

74. Shen HN, Lin LY, Chen KY, et al. Changes of heart rate variability during ventilator weaning. Chest 2003;123(4):1222–8.
75. Bien MY, Shui Lin Y, Shih CH, et al. Comparisons of predictive performance of breathing pattern variability measured during T-piece, automatic tube compensation, and pressure support ventilation for weaning intensive care unit patients from mechanical ventilation. Crit Care Med 2011;39(10):2253–62.
76. Papaioannou VE, Chouvarda IG, Maglaveras NK, et al. Study of multiparameter respiratory pattern complexity in surgical critically ill patients during weaning trials. BMC Physiol 2011;11:2.
77. Arcentales A, Giraldo BF, Caminal P, et al. Recurrence quantification analysis of heart rate variability and respiratory flow series in patients on weaning trials. Conf Proc IEEE Eng Med Biol Soc 2011;2011:2724–7.
78. Orini M, Giraldo BF, Bailon R, et al. Time-frequency analysis of cardiac and respiratory parameters for the prediction of ventilator weaning. Conf Proc IEEE Eng Med Biol Soc 2008;2008:2793–6.
79. Kaczmarek J, Kamlin COF, Morley CJ, et al. Variability of respiratory parameters and extubation readiness in ventilated neonates. Arch Dis Child Fetal Neonatal Ed 2012. [Epub ahead of print].
80. Davis PG, Henderson-Smart DJ. Nasal continuous positive airways pressure immediately after extubation for preventing morbidity in preterm infants. Cochrane Database Syst Rev 2003;(2):CD000143.
81. Wilkinson D, Andersen C, O'Donnell CP, et al. High flow nasal cannula for respiratory support in preterm infants. Cochrane Database Syst Rev 2011;(5):CD006405.
82. Spence KL, Murphy D, Kilian C, et al. High-flow nasal cannula as a device to provide continuous positive airway pressure in infants. J Perinatol 2007; 27(12):772–5.
83. Wilkinson DJ, Andersen CC, Smith K, et al. Pharyngeal pressure with high-flow nasal cannulae in premature infants. J Perinatol 2008;28(1):42–7.
84. Campbell DM, Shah PS, Shah V, et al. Nasal continuous positive airway pressure from high flow cannula versus Infant Flow for preterm infants. J Perinatol 2006; 26(9):546–9.
85. Barrington KJ, Bull D, Finer NN. Randomized trial of nasal synchronized intermittent mandatory ventilation compared with continuous positive airway pressure after extubation of very low birth weight infants. Pediatrics 2001;107(4):638–41.
86. Friedlich P, Lecart C, Posen R, et al. A randomized trial of nasopharyngeal-synchronized intermittent mandatory ventilation versus nasopharyngeal continuous positive airway pressure in very low birth weight infants after extubation. J Perinatol 1999;19(6 Pt 1):413–8.
87. Khalaf MN, Brodsky N, Hurley J, et al. A prospective randomized, controlled trial comparing synchronized nasal intermittent positive pressure ventilation versus nasal continuous positive airway pressure as modes of extubation. Pediatrics 2001;108(1):13–7.
88. Owen LS, Morley CJ, Davis PG. Neonatal nasal intermittent positive pressure ventilation: a survey of practice in England. Arch Dis Child Fetal Neonatal Ed 2008;93(2):F148–50.
89. Kieran EA, Walsh H, O'Donnell CP. Survey of nasal continuous positive airways pressure (NCPAP) and nasal intermittent positive pressure ventilation (NIPPV) use in Irish newborn nurseries. Arch Dis Child Fetal Neonatal Ed 2011;96(2): F156.
90. Morcillo SF, Gutierrez LA, Castillo SF, et al. Respiratory care in neonatal intensive care units. Situation in the year 2005. An Pediatr (Barc) 2009;70(2):137–42.

91. Chang HY, Claure N, D'Ugard C, et al. Effects of synchronization during nasal ventilation in clinically stable preterm infants. Pediatr Res 2011;69(1):84–9.

92. Owen LS, Morley CJ, Dawson JA, et al. Effects of non-synchronised nasal intermittent positive pressure ventilation on spontaneous breathing in preterm infants. Arch Dis Child Fetal Neonatal Ed 2011;96(6):F422–8.

93. Milner AD, Greenough A. The role of the upper airway in neonatal apnoea. Semin Neonatol 2004;9(3):213–9.

94. Roy B, Samson N, Moreau-Bussiere F, et al. Mechanisms of active laryngeal closure during noninvasive intermittent positive pressure ventilation in nonsedated lambs. J Appl Physiol 2008;105(5):1406–12.

95. Moreau-Bussiere F, Samson N, St-Hilaire M, et al. Laryngeal response to nasal ventilation in nonsedated newborn lambs. J Appl Physiol 2007;102(6):2149–57.

96. Praud JP, Samson N, Moreau-Bussiere F. Laryngeal function and nasal ventilatory support in the neonatal period. Paediatr Respir Rev 2006;7(Suppl 1): S180–2.

97. Henderson-Smart DJ, Davis PG. Prophylactic methylxanthines for endotracheal extubation in preterm infants. Cochrane Database Syst Rev 2010;(12):CD000139.

98. Steer P, Flenady V, Shearman A, et al. High dose caffeine citrate for extubation of preterm infants: a randomised controlled trial. Arch Dis Child Fetal Neonatal Ed 2004;89(6):F499–503.

99. Khemani RG, Randolph A, Markovitz B. Corticosteroids for the prevention and treatment of post-extubation stridor in neonates, children and adults. Cochrane Database Syst Rev 2009;(3):CD001000.

100. Couser RJ, Ferrara TB, Falde B, et al. Effectiveness of dexamethasone in preventing extubation failure in preterm infants at increased risk for airway edema. J Pediatr 1992;121(4):591–6.

101. Koren G, Butt W, Whyte H. Racemic epinephrine in very low birth weight infants with post-intubation upper airway obstruction: a controlled prospective study. J Perinatol 1986;6:24–6.

102. Davies MW, Davis PG. Nebulized racemic epinephrine for extubation of newborn infants. Cochrane Database Syst Rev 2002;(1):CD000506.

Control of Oxygenation During Mechanical Ventilation in the Premature Infant

Eduardo Bancalari, MD*, Nelson Claure, MSc, PhD

KEYWORDS

- Oxygen saturation targets • Hypoxemia • Hyperoxemia • Supplemental oxygen
- Premature infants

KEY POINTS

- Supplemental oxygen is a common therapy in premature infants, and can be associated with serious complications.
- In premature infants, hyperoxemia can only be the result of excessive supplemental oxygen.
- Targeting higher arterial oxygen saturation has been linked to lung and eye damage.
- Recent data suggest targeting lower saturation levels can reduce bronchopulmonary dysplasia and retinopathy of prematurity, but may increase the risk of death.
- In preterm infants receiving supplemental oxygen, arterial oxygen saturation is maintained within the intended range only about half of the time.
- Maintenance of arterial oxygen saturation within a target range in preterm infants is limited by frequent fluctuations owing to their respiratory instability, limited staff availability, and tolerance of high saturation levels.
- Stricter policies accompanied by education and establishment of clear guidelines are effective in improving the maintenance of oxygen saturation targets.
- Automatic control of supplemental oxygen can improve the maintenance of oxygen saturation targets, but the long-term benefits of this method are yet to be determined.

Extremely premature infants frequently spend long periods of time on supplemental oxygen. While this therapy is essential for their survival, it is also associated with many complications such as retinopathy of prematurity (ROP), bronchopulmonary dysplasia (BPD), and systemic oxidative damage. Hyperoxia may also contribute to central nervous system (CNS) damage in the immature infant.[1]

Conflict of interest statement: The system for closed-loop inspired oxygen discussed herein was developed and patented by Drs Claure and Bancalari, who are Faculty of the University of Miami. The University of Miami, the assignee for this patent, has a licensing agreement with CareFusion. CareFusion provided research support for the studies with this system.

Division of Neonatology, Department of Pediatrics, University of Miami Miller School of Medicine, University of Miami, Miami, Florida

* Corresponding author. PO Box 016960 R-131, Miami, FL 33101.

E-mail address: EBancalari@miami.edu

The association between prolonged oxygen exposure and high arterial oxygen tensions and an increased risk of ROP in the premature has been shown in many experimental and clinical studies. The authors demonstrated that maintenance of transcutaneous oxygen tensions of more than 80 mm Hg for extended periods of time was associated with a significant increase in the incidence and severity of ROP.[2] Furthermore, there have been 2 prospective randomized trials that evaluated different oxygen targets in premature infants, the STOP-ROP study and the BOOST trial.[3,4] Both showed that exposure to higher oxygen saturation targets was associated with an increased risk of chronic pulmonary damage, reflected by a greater need for respiratory medications or a higher proportion of infants requiring oxygen at 36 weeks postmenstrual age. These results were confirmed recently by the SUPPORT trial wherein preterm infants, 24 to 28 weeks gestational age, were randomly assigned to a low saturation target range (85%–89%) or a higher range of 91% to 95%.[5] The incidence of severe ROP was more than double in infants randomized to the high saturation group, and the incidence of BPD, defined as supplemental oxygen at 36 weeks, was also significantly higher in the high saturation group. An unexpected and disturbing finding of this trial was an increased mortality in infants randomized to the lower saturation group (adjusted relative risk 1.27, 95% confidence interval 1.01–1.60). There is also increasing evidence suggesting that exposure to high oxygen may be associated with CNS damage characterized by increased apoptosis of neural cells in experimental animals and by white matter lesions in premature infants.[1,6]

Therefore, neonatologists face a difficult task in balancing the risks of too little oxygen with those associated with excessive oxygen use in premature infants. Insufficient oxygen can increase the risk of neurologic damage, induce changes in the pulmonary vasculature, and impair growth, and may also increase mortality. On the other hand, too much oxygen increases the risk of lung injury and BPD, retinal damage and ROP, and may also cause CNS injury. It is very difficult to find the right balance between these 2 extremes, and it is not clear as to what the most appropriate oxygenation target for premature infants at different stages of maturity should be. Because of this, there is wide variation in oxygenation targets in neonatal units around the world. This situation was illustrated by Tin and Wariyar,[7] who did a survey of 100 centers in the United Kingdom and showed large variability in the pulse oximeter high and low saturation alarm settings used in the different institutions. High saturation alarm values ranged from 92% to 100% while the lower alarms ranged from 75% to 95%. There is also a large variation between centers regarding the saturation thresholds used for oxygen supplementation in infants with BPD, as reported in a survey of almost 200 neonatal centers. The saturation thresholds ranged from 85% to 96%.[8]

During routine care clinicians are usually more concerned with the effects of hypoxia than with hyperoxia, and for this reason premature infants frequently receive more oxygen than is required to maintain adequate oxygenation. This becomes evident when comparing the incidence of BPD in the different centers of the National Institute of Child Health and Human Development Network, as defined by clinical use of oxygen at 36 weeks' gestation versus that defined by a physiologic test intended to determine the actual inspired oxygen concentration required to maintain oxygen saturations above 90%. In almost every institution, infants received more oxygen than needed to maintain acceptable oxygen saturations.[9] The difference in the level of concern regarding hypoxemia and hyperoxemia was observed in a study that was primarily aimed at assessing a computerized system for ventilator management. These investigators observed that clinical staff was more likely to respond to correct conditions leading to hypoxemia than those leading to hyperoxemia.[10]

CONTINUOUS OXYGENATION MONITORING

Measurements of arterial oxygen tension (Pa_{O_2}) are considered the gold standard to determine the adequacy of oxygenation. This technique requires invasive catheters that are commonly used during the acute phase of respiratory failure but rarely beyond that period. Subsequently, intermittent sampling can be used to determine the oxygenation status, but this is only a snapshot view and provides limited information on oxygenation stability. Pulse oximetry (Sp_{O_2}) provides continuous information on oxygenation noninvasively, and is now part of the standard of care for infants receiving supplemental oxygen.

Before pulse oximetry was introduced in neonatal intensive care, adjustments of inspired oxygen concentration and ventilator settings were carried out, attempting to maintain Pa_{O_2} between 50 and 80 mm Hg. With the introduction of pulse oximetry, the adjustments of inspired oxygen and ventilator settings were guided by saturation values obtained with this simple noninvasive monitoring method. Most of the initial studies showed a relatively tight relationship between Sp_{O_2} and Pa_{O_2}, suggesting that if babies were kept with Sp_{O_2} between 85% and 95%, the likelihood of having Pa_{O_2}s less than 40 or greater than 80 mm Hg was small. However, recent clinical data[11,12] showed that although most Sp_{O_2} values between 85% and 95% are associated with Pa_{O_2} values between 40 and 80 mm Hg, there are a significant number of Pa_{O_2} values that fall outside this range. More concerning are data published recently whereby pulse oximetry Sp_{O_2} values were compared with actual saturation measured by cooximetry in arterial blood samples, which showed a significant overestimation of saturation by pulse oximetry.[13] This discrepancy was more striking, as the saturation values decreased to below 90%. This finding is of concern because if, in fact, pulse oximetry overestimates low saturation values, a significant risk of hypoxemia could be introduced unless one periodically correlates Sp_{O_2} with actual measurements of Pa_{O_2} or saturation. Because of the serious potential implications of this limitation of pulse oximetry, these observations need to be confirmed in larger, well-controlled prospective studies.

LIMITATIONS FOR KEEPING PREESTABLISHED OXYGEN TARGETS

In the clinical setting it is extremely difficult to maintain infants within a predefined oxygenation target. A prospective multicenter study that included 14 centers using different clinically defined saturation targets demonstrated that on average, infants in these centers spent less than 50% of the time within the predefined oxygenation target.[14] An average of 16% of the time was spent below target and 36% of the time above target. The variation between institutions for the time above target was striking and ranged between 5% and 90%, while time within target varied from 6% to 75% and time below target ranged from 0% to 47%. The effectiveness in keeping babies within a target is very much unit dependent and, among many factors, it may be in part related to the short-term physiologic responses that can be induced by different oxygenation targets. Infants with chronic lung disease have substantially more hypoxemic episodes when their saturations are targeted between 87% and 91% than when the target is 94% to 96%.[15] Similar findings were described recently in a subgroup of infants from the SUPPORT trial, showing that infants randomized to the saturation target of 85% to 89% had a significantly higher number of hypoxemia episodes than those targeted to the higher range, between 91% and 95%. The number of hypoxemic events after 80 days was more than double in infants who were maintained on the lower saturation target ranges.[16]

As mentioned earlier, one of the major problems in keeping the infants within a desired range is the continuous fluctuations in oxygenation that require constant attendance and tight alarm settings. These fluctuations can lead to desensitization of the staff to the frequent alarms. It is also difficult to convey a strong message to the staff regarding the importance of strictly keeping the targets, because the evidence for the harmful effects of short-term fluctuations in oxygenation is not strong.

For preterm infants on respiratory support with fluctuations in oxygenation that are caused by changes in ventilation, the ability to stay within a predetermined oxygenation target is difficult. During routine clinical care, the most common response from the staff to episodes of hypoxemia is an increase in inspired oxygen concentration. Although this may help reverse these hypoxemic episodes, it is not the most effective response if the hypoxemia is due to hypoventilation secondary to agitation or any other condition that impairs ventilation, such as airway obstruction.[17–19] Hence, increasing the inspired oxygen concentration alone may not be the most appropriate intervention to treat episodes of hypoxemia. The correct intervention may require the clinical staff to evaluate these patients and take the most effective action based on the disturbance in physiology. Such intervention may include changes in ventilator settings, suctioning the airway, repositioning the infant, and so forth.

Keeping these infants at a higher oxygen saturation level reduces the number of hypoxemia episodes, which is why nurses or respiratory therapy staff usually tolerate higher saturation levels than are needed. This scenario was clearly evident in the SUPPORT trial, where the median oxygen saturation level for the low and the higher oxygen groups were well above the intended targets. In fact, the median value of the saturation distribution for the low target group was closer to the high range than to the intended lower target.[5]

WHAT CAN BE DONE TO IMPROVE THE MAINTENANCE OF OXYGENATION TARGETS?

The challenge in maintaining oxygen targets depends on the instability of each infant and on the mechanisms of the hypoxemia episodes. Its success is closely dependent on the availability, education, and attitude of the medical and nursing staff. An interesting observation was published recently showing that a higher nurse to patient ratio produced a much better control and higher proportion of time within oxygenation target ranges than in units where the nurse to patient ratio was lower.[20] It is interesting that this improvement in maintaining oxygen targets was mainly due to a reduction in hyperoxemia. Furthermore, patients cared for in neonatal intensive care units (NICUs) where there was a low nurse to patient ratio (1:3) spent significantly more time in hyperoxemia, but less time in hypoxemia. This finding illustrates what happens in most NICUs when the bedside nurse does not have enough time to continuously monitor oxygenation; babies are placed on higher inspired oxygen concentration than is needed, which leads to more hyperoxemia but, at the same time, less exposure to hypoxemia.

The proper use of alarms available in pulse oximeters is another effective step toward improving maintenance of oxygenation targets. In most centers the alarms have been traditionally set at a wider range than the actual oxygen targets in an attempt to reduce the number of alarms and minimize the desensitization of the staff to too-frequent alarms. However, there is clear evidence that in centers where tighter alarm settings are used, the proportion of time within target is higher than in units with wider alarm settings[14]; this is mainly attributable to less hyperoxemia when tighter settings are used. Therefore, to better achieve oxygenation targets the alarms should be set as close as possible to the targeted range, because the clinical staff is likely to be more responsive to the alarms than to actual saturation values. This holds especially true when there is a low nurse to patient ratio and the nurse cannot be continuously at bedside.

As mentioned earlier, training, motivation, and attentiveness of the clinical staff play a crucial role in maintaining adequate oxygenation. Considerable improvements on the maintenance of oxygenation targets have been reported after specific educational interventions along with protocol development.[21] Maintenance of adequate oxygenation targets may be hindered by insufficient communication of unit policies as well as personal biases that infants do better at certain targets. A recent survey of NICU nurses in the United States showed that 36% of them were not aware or were unsure about their center's policies on oxygen saturation alarms while only 42% of them were aware of their center's policy and were able to identify the alarm ranges.[22]

Another issue that may also limit the efficacy of the staff in maintaining the targeted oxygen saturation ranges is the lack of specific oxygen titration guidelines. While on one hand the staff is asked to keep saturations in a certain range, on the other there are seldom guidelines on how to respond in terms of timing and magnitude of the changes in inspired oxygen to episodes of hypoxemia or hyperoxemia.

The response to hypoxemia varies widely between centers and caregivers. Acute changes in oxygenation are often related to changes in ventilation. Hence, adjustments in inspired oxygen should be accompanied by verification of the adequacy of ventilation. Although most neonatal ventilators allow clinicians to determine changes in ventilation, these functions are rarely used by the clinical staff.

Because most of the hypoxemia episodes are related to agitation, reduced functional residual capacity and hypoventilation, the authors evaluated the effect of tidal volume targeting in infants with frequent hypoxemia episodes. A volume-targeting strategy significantly reduced the duration of the hypoxemia episodes and the time spent at low saturation values when compared with pressure-regulated ventilation. However, this required targeting a tidal volume slightly higher than the infants required routinely.[23]

Aware of the intense effort required to maintain oxygen saturations in these infants and limitations in staffing during routine neonatal care, several groups of investigators have developed automated systems that can perform this repetitive task without the constant presence of a bedside nurse or respiratory therapist. All these systems have achieved a significant improvement in time within target when compared with manual control.[24–32] As expected, this advantage was more striking when the automated systems were compared with routine care rather than those studies that had a dedicated nurse at the bedside.

One of these systems has been developed at the University of Miami, and was evaluated in a prospective, randomized, multicenter crossover trial in infants who experienced frequent episodes of hypoxemia.[33] These infants had a mean gestational age of 25 weeks and were approximately 4 weeks old. The automated system was compared with standard clinical care during study periods of 24 hours. In both periods, manual or automated, the saturation target was 87% to 93%. **Fig. 1** shows a recording of the fraction of Fio_2 and Spo_2 in an infant during automated control followed by routine manual adjustment of Fio_2. During the manual control, it is apparent that the staff responded with an increase in Fio_2 mainly to the most severe episodes, but the infant was frequently left with an excessive Fio_2 resulting in saturations close to 100%. By contrast, during automated control the basal Fio_2 was continuously adjusted to avoid hyperoxemia. However, this was accompanied by more episodes of hypoxemia. These episodes were generally less severe and of shorter duration than those observed during the period of manual control.

Table 1 shows the proportion of time spent in the different saturation ranges during the manual and automated control periods. There was a significant increase in the time spent within target during the automated period, and this was mainly due to

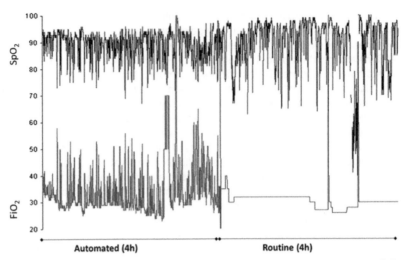

Fig. 1. Recording of Fio_2 and Spo_2 from an infant undergoing automated control followed by manual adjustment of Fio_2 illustrates the staff responses mainly to the most severe episodes of hypoxemia. The infant is frequently left with excessive Fio_2, resulting in high Spo_2. This recording shows more fluctuations in Spo_2 and Fio_2 during automated control, reflecting the fact that the system responds to every fluctuation. During automated control there are fewer episodes of hyperoxemia and severe hypoxemia.

a reduction in time with saturations above 93% and especially above 98%. On the other hand, there was a larger proportion of time spent between Spo_2 80% and 86%, which occurred because during the automated period there was a reduction in Fio_2 and a shift in Spo_2 toward the center of the target range. This shift, which did not occur during manual control, increased the likelihood of saturations below the target range. This situation was limited to oscillations just below the target range, while the times with Spo_2 below 80% or 75% were similar between the automated and manual periods. As mentioned earlier, the automated system reduces the Fio_2 to a point where the Spo_2 remains close to the mid target range, whereas the clinical staff usually keeps saturation closer to the upper limit of the target Spo_2 range. The automatic increase in Fio_2, although of limited efficacy in aborting the episodes of hypoxemia, attenuates their severity and duration, as shown by a decrease in the number of long episodes of hypoxemia with saturation below 75% for more than a minute or below 85% for more than 2 minutes.

Based on these results, it is possible to conclude that automation of inspired oxygen control can improve the maintenance of the target Spo_2 and reduce hyperoxemia, accompanied by a reduction in Fio_2 (and baseline saturations) and an increase in the number of fluctuations slightly below the target. As expected, automation results in a very significant reduction in the workload of the nursing staff, allowing them to dedicate this time to other tasks of patient care.

The advantage of the automated systems over manual control depends on the effectiveness of standard care. In units where there is favorable patient/nurse ratio and the nurse can stay at the bedside most of the time, the advantage of the automated systems is likely to be less than if used in units where there is a lower nurse/patient ratio with less nursing time to do the frequent adjustments required to maintain oxygen saturation within range.

Table 1
Proportion of time within different ranges of Spo$_2$, episodes of hypoxemia, inspired oxygen concentration, and workload during manual and automatic Fio$_2$ adjustments in infants with frequent fluctuations in oxygenation

	Manual	Automatic	P value
Target Spo$_2$ 87%–93% (% time)	32 ± 13	40 ± 14	<.001
Spo$_2$ >93% while on >21% O$_2$ (% time)	37 ± 12	21 ± 20	<.001
Spo$_2$ >98% while on >21% O$_2$ (% time)	5.6 (2.7–11.4)	0.7 (0.1–7.5)	.003
Spo$_2$ <87% (% time)	23 ± 9	32 ± 12	<.001
Spo$_2$ <80% (% time)	9.5 ± 6.1	9.8 ± 6.3	.693
Episodes with Spo$_2$ <87% (per hour)	11 ± 8	19 ± 16	<.001
Prolonged episodes with Spo$_2$ <85% for >120 s (per 24 h)	35 ± 17	22 ± 16	<.001
24-h median Fio$_2$	0.37 (0.24–0.49)	0.32 (0.24–0.39)	<.001
Manual Fio$_2$ adjustments (no. per 24 h)	112 ± 59	10 ± 9	<.001

Adapted from Claure N, Gerhardt T, Everett R, et al. Closed-loop controlled inspired oxygen concentration for mechanically ventilated very low birth weight infants with frequent episodes of hypoxemia. Pediatrics 2001;107:1120–24.

It is important that some of the potential limitations of automated systems are mentioned. Perhaps the most important is that similar to manual control, the reliability of any of these systems depends on the accuracy of the pulse oximeter signal. Automation can produce more fluctuation in oxygenation because the Fio$_2$ is adjusted every time the saturation value fluctuates out of range, whereas nurses tend to accept periods of hyperoxemia or hypoxemia in the hope that they will reverse spontaneously.

It is also very important that the response of the clinician be in accordance with the specific mechanism that is producing the hypoxemia. A nurse at the bedside is more likely to identify the mechanism and determine the most effective response than is an automated system, which will only change the inspired oxygen concentration. Identification of the mechanism leading to hypoxemia by the clinician should be standard of care independently of the use of this type of automatic system. The earlier automatic response should only prevent worsening of the hypoxemia until the proper corrective action takes place and the exposure to higher supplemental oxygen is reduced after the episode of hypoxemia resolves.

An important limitation of any automated system is that it may give a false sense of confidence to the clinical staff, which may reduce their attentiveness to the patient and cause them to rely excessively on the automated system. Although this remains speculative, careful application of any automatic system is warranted. Such care may be particularly important in situations when an automated increase in Fio$_2$ may mask a significant deterioration in the patient's clinical condition. Any persistent increase in Fio$_2$ during automatic control should be promptly reported by the automatic system and investigated by the caregiver.

SUMMARY

Maintenance of oxygen saturation targets is a very demanding and tedious task because of the frequency with which oxygenation changes, especially in small infants receiving prolonged respiratory support. Whereas hypoxemia episodes are usually related to changes in lung physiology, hyperoxemia is always induced by excessive inspired oxygen concentration. Infants will seldom be hyperoxemic as long as they are breathing room air. It is clear that the achievement of oxygenation targets can be improved by a higher nurse to patient ratio and by intense staff training. Automated control systems can also improve target maintenance, and this is achieved mainly by reducing exposure to hyperoxemia. The long-term benefits and safety of this strategy are yet to be determined in clinical trials.

At present the ideal oxygen saturation targets for premature infants are unclear, but based on the results of the SUPPORT trial and preliminary reports of the BOOST II trial,[34] it is important to avoid low saturation values because of the reported increase in mortality. Based on this evidence, most clinicians today are recommending saturations between 90% and 95% to assure proper oxygenation while simultaneously avoiding hypoxemia and hyperoxemia. These results, along with upcoming data from the Canadian Oxygen Trial, should be carefully considered when deciding on oxygen target goals in extremely premature infants. It will also be critical to evaluate the long-term effects of these different oxygen management strategies and define whether infants of different gestational or postnatal ages require different targets.

ACKNOWLEDGMENTS

The authors are grateful to the University of Miami Project New Born for their long-standing support.

REFERENCES

1. Collins MP, Lorenz JM, Jetton JR, et al. Hypocapnia and other ventilation-related risk factors for cerebral palsy in low birth weight infants. Pediatr Res 2001;50:712–9.
2. Flynn JT, Bancalari E, Snyder ES, et al. A cohort study of transcutaneous oxygen tension and the incidence and severity of retinopathy of prematurity. N Engl J Med 1992;326:1050–4.
3. Anonymous. Supplemental therapeutic oxygen for prethreshold retinopathy of prematurity (STOP-ROP), a randomized, controlled trial. I: primary outcomes. Pediatrics 2000;105:295–310.
4. Askie LM, Henderson-Smart DJ, Irwig L, et al. Oxygen-saturation targets and outcomes in extremely preterm infants. N Engl J Med 2003;349:959–67.
5. SUPPORT Study Group of the Eunice Kennedy Shriver NICHD Neonatal Research Network, Carlo WA, Finer NN, et al. Target ranges of oxygen saturation in extremely preterm infants. N Engl J Med 2010;362:1959–69.
6. Felderhoff-Mueser U, Bittigau P, Sifringer M, et al. Oxygen causes cell death in the developing brain. Neurobiol Dis 2004;17:273–82.
7. Tin W, Wariyar U. Giving small babies oxygen: 50 years of uncertainty. Semin Neonatol 2002;7:361–7.
8. Ellsbury DL, Acarregui MJ, McGuinness GA, et al. Variability in the use of supplemental oxygen for bronchopulmonary dysplasia. J Pediatr 2002;140:247–9.
9. Walsh MC, Yao Q, Gettner P, et al. National Institute of Child Health and Human Development Neonatal Research Network. Impact of a physiologic definition on bronchopulmonary dysplasia rates. Pediatrics 2004;114:1305–11.
10. Carlo WA, Pacifico L, Chatburn RL, et al. Efficacy of computer-assisted management of respiratory failure in neonates. Pediatrics 1986;78:139–43.
11. Castillo A, Sola A, Baquero H, et al. Pulse oxygen saturation levels and arterial oxygen tension values in newborns receiving oxygen therapy in the neonatal intensive care unit: is 85% to 93% an acceptable range? Pediatrics 2008;121:882–9.

12. Quine D, Stenson BJ. Arterial oxygen tension (Pao_2) values in infants <29 weeks of gestation at currently targeted saturations. Arch Dis Child Fetal Neonatal Ed 2009;94:F51–3.

13. Rosychuk RJ, Hudson-Mason A, Eklund D, et al. Discrepancies between arterial oxygen saturation and functional oxygen saturation measured with pulse oximetry in very preterm infants. Neonatology 2012;101:14–9.

14. Hagadorn JI, Furey AM, Nghiem TH, et al. AVIOx Study Group. Achieved versus intended pulse oximeter saturation in infants born less than 28 weeks' gestation: the AVIOx study. Pediatrics 2006;118:1574–82.

15. McEvoy C, Durand M, Hewlett V. Episodes of spontaneous desaturations in infants with chronic lung disease at two different levels of oxygenation. Pediatr Pulmonol 1993;15:140–4.

16. Di Fiore JM, Walsh M, Finer N, et al. Low oxygen saturation target range is associated with increased incidence of intermittent hypoxemia [abstract: E-PAS2011: 3305.7]. J Pediatr 2012, http://dx.doi.org/10.1016/j.jpeds.2012.05.046.

17. Bolivar JM, Gerhardt T, Gonzalez A, et al. Mechanisms for episodes of hypoxemia in preterm infants undergoing mechanical ventilation. J Pediatr 1995; 127:767–73.

18. Dimaguila MA, Di Fiore JM, Martin RJ, et al. Characteristics of hypoxemic episodes in very low birth weight infants on ventilatory support. J Pediatr 1997; 130:577–83.

19. Esquer C, Claure N, D'Ugard C, et al. Role of abdominal muscles activity on duration and severity of hypoxemia episodes in mechanically ventilated preterm infants. Neonatology 2007;92:182–6.

20. Sink DW, Hope SA, Hagadorn JI. Nurse:patient ratio and achievement of oxygen saturation goals in premature infants. Arch Dis Child Fetal Neonatal Ed 2011;96: F93–8.

21. Ford SP, Leick-Rude MK, Meinert KA, et al. Overcoming barriers to oxygen saturation targeting. Pediatrics 2006;118:S177–86.

22. Nghiem TH, Hagadorn JI, Terrin N, et al. Nurse opinions and pulse oximeter saturation target limits for preterm infants. Pediatrics 2008;121:e1039–46.

23. Polimeni V, Claure N, D'Ugard C, et al. Effects of volume-targeted synchronized intermittent mandatory ventilation on spontaneous episodes of hypoxemia in preterm infants. Biol Neonate 2006;89:50–5.

24. Beddis JR, Collins P, Levy NM, et al. New technique for servo-control of arterial oxygen tension in preterm infants. Arch Dis Child 1979;54:278–80.

25. Dugdale RE, Cameron RG, Lealman GT. Closed-loop control of the partial pressure of arterial oxygen in neonates. Clin Phys Physiol Meas 1988;9:291–305.

26. Bhutani VK, Taube JC, Antunes MJ, et al. Adaptive control of the inspired oxygen delivery to the neonate. Pediatr Pulmonol 1992;14:110–7.

27. Morozoff PE, Evans RW. Closed-loop control of SaO_2 in the neonate. Biomed Instrum Technol 1992;26:117–23.

28. Sun Y, Kohane IS, Stark AR. Computer-assisted adjustment of inspired oxygen concentration improves control of oxygen saturation in newborn infants requiring mechanical ventilation. J Pediatr 1997;131:754–6.

29. Morozoff EP, Smyth JA. Evaluation of three automatic oxygen therapy control algorithms on ventilated low birth weight neonates. Conf Proc IEEE Eng Med Biol Soc 2009;2009:3079–82.

30. Claure N, Gerhardt T, Everett R, et al. Closed-loop controlled inspired oxygen concentration for mechanically ventilated very low birth weight infants with frequent episodes of hypoxemia. Pediatrics 2001;107:1120–4.

31. Urschitz MS, Horn W, Seyfang A, et al. Automatic control of the inspired oxygen fraction in preterm infants: a randomized crossover trial. Am J Respir Crit Care Med 2004;170:1095–100.
32. Claure N, D'Ugard C, Bancalari E. Automated adjustment of inspired oxygen in preterm infants with frequent fluctuations in oxygenation: a pilot clinical trial. J Pediatr 2009;155:640–5.
33. Claure N, Bancalari E, D'Ugard C, et al. Multicenter crossover study of automated adjustment of inspired oxygen in mechanically ventilated preterm infants. Pediatrics 2011;127:e76–83.
34. Stenson B, Brocklehurst P, Tarnow-Mordi W, et al. Increased 36-week survival with high oxygen saturation target in extremely preterm infants. N Engl J Med 2011; 364:1680–2.

Noninvasive Monitoring by Photoplethysmography

Rakesh Sahni, MD

KEYWORDS

- Perfusion index • Photoplethysmogram • Pleth variability index • Pulse oximetry
- Oxygen saturation

KEY POINTS

- Pulse oximeters use the photoplethysmogram (PPG) to compute blood oxygen saturation and pulse rate.
- The PPG contains an abundance of information related to cardiac hemodynamics.
- With recent advances in signal processing, indices such as perfusion index (PI) and pleth variability index (PVI) have been developed to assess circulatory information from the PPG.
- The PPG waveform can be used to assess microcirculation (ie, PI) and intravascular fluid volume (ie, PVI).

INTRODUCTION

The development of pulse oximetry is unarguably the most important advance in clinical monitoring in the past 3 decades. Pulse oximeters, which compute blood oxygen saturations (Sp_{O_2}) using photoplethysmography with at least 2 different light wavelengths, often display a photoplethysmogram (PPG) to help clinicians distinguish between reliable Sp_{O_2} measurements (associated with clean, physiologic waveforms) and unreliable measurements (associated with noisy waveforms). Because of the success of pulse oximetry and recent advances in digital signal processing, there is growing research interest in seeking circulatory information from the PPG and developing techniques for a wide variety of novel applications. This article reviews the basic physics of photoplethysmography, physiologic principles behind pulse oximetry operation, and recent technological advances in the usefulness of the PPG waveform to assess and monitor the microcirculation and intravascular fluid volume during intensive care.

PHOTOPLETHYSMOGRAPHY AND PULSE OXIMETRY
Photoplethysmography

Photoplethysmography is a noninvasive optical technique widely used in the monitoring of the pulsations associated with changes in blood volume in a peripheral

Division of Neonatal-Perinatal Medicine, Department of Pediatrics, College of Physicians and Surgeons, Columbia University, 3959 Broadway MSCHN 1201, New York, NY 10032-3702, USA
E-mail address: rs62@columbia.edu

Clin Perinatol 39 (2012) 573–583
http://dx.doi.org/10.1016/j.clp.2012.06.012
0095-5108/12/$ – see front matter © 2012 Elsevier Inc. All rights reserved.

vascular bed.[1–4] In photoplethysmography, the emitted light, which is made to transverse the skin, is reflected, absorbed, and scattered by the tissue and blood. The intensity of the modulated transmitted or reflected light that reaches the photodetector is measured and the variations in the photodetector current are assumed to be related to blood volume changes underneath the probe.[1,5] These variations are electronically amplified and recorded as a voltage signal called the photoplethysmograph.

The photoplethysmographic signal is divided into 2 components (**Fig. 1**):

1. A pulsatile or alternating current (AC) component synchronous with the heart rate that is assumed to be related to the arterial blood volume pulse. The AC component pulse shapes indicate vessel compliance and cardiac performance.
2. A nonpulsatile direct current (DC) component, a constant voltage offset, the magnitude of which is determined by the nature of the material through which the light passes (skin, subcutaneous fat, muscles, cartilage, bones, and capillary and venous blood).

Physiologic Principles of Pulse Oximetry Operation

Theoretic descriptions of pulse oximetry often begin with a discussion of the Beer-Lambert law of light absorption, which describes the elements that contribute to the pulse oximeter waveform.[6]

$$A_{total} = E_1 C_1 L_1 + E_2 C_2 L_2 + \cdots + E_n C_n L_n$$

where A_{total} is the absorption at a given wavelength, E_n is the extinction coefficient (absorbency), C_n is the concentration, and L_n is the path length.

It is conceptually most useful to view the pulse oximeter waveform as measuring the change in blood volume (more specifically path length), during a cardiac cycle, in the region being studied. The general consensus is that the PPG waveform comes from the site of maximum pulsation within the arteriolar vessels where pulsatile energy is converted to smooth flow just before the level of the capillaries.[7,8]

Pulse oximeters are currently equipped with a light source comprising 2 light-emitting diodes (LEDs), 1 emitting at the red spectrum and the other at the infrared spectrum, most commonly at wavelengths of 660 and 940 nm respectively, and a light detector (photodiode). The probe of the device must be positioned in such a manner that the emitter and the detector are exactly opposite each other with 5 to 10 mm of tissue between them.[9,10] Emission of these 2 wavelengths alternates at frequencies of

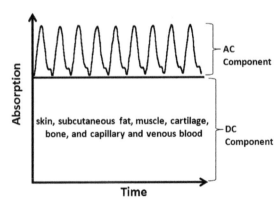

Fig. 1. Light absorption at the measurement site showing the variable alternating current (AC) and the constant direct current (DC) components by distinct tissue characteristics.

0.6 to 1.0 kHz[9,11,12] and the nonabsorbed energy is detected by a semiconductor detector. A microprocessor subtracts the absorption by skin, subcutaneous fat, muscles, cartilage, bones, and capillary and venous blood (constant absorbers), thus rendering a highly processed and filtered final signal, which is displayed electronically as a plethysmographic wave form. Of the 2 wavelengths measured by the pulse oximeter, traditionally only the infrared signal is displayed because it is more stable over time, especially compared with the red signal, which is more susceptible to changes in the oxygen saturation. In addition, only the pulsatile component or AC portion of the infrared signal is displayed. The static or DC component (created mostly by the absorption of light by surrounding tissue) is eliminated by an autocentering routine used to ensure that the waveform remains on the display screen.

Wavelengths for Pulse Oximetry

The estimation of SpO_2 by pulse oximetry is based on the specific characteristics of oxygenated and deoxygenated hemoglobin (oxyhemoglobin and deoxyhemoglobin, respectively) with regard to light absorption in the red and infrared spectra. Deoxyhemoglobin is characterized by greater red-light absorption (wavelength range 600–750 nm), whereas oxyhemoglobin exhibits higher absorption in the infrared spectrum (850–1000 nm) **(Fig. 2)**.[9,13] Furthermore, the light absorption in vivo depends on the characteristics of the tissues across the site of measurement.[14,15] During short time periods, the absorption by the constant absorbers remains constant. Therefore, any change in light absorption should be attributed to the variations of the arterial blood volume related to the cardiac cycle.[15–18] By obtaining the ratio of light absorption in the red and infrared spectra and then calculating the ratio of these 2 ratios (ratio of absorption ratios), the SpO_2 can be calculated as follows[9,16]:

$$SpO_2 = \frac{f(AC_{red}/DC_{red})}{(AC_{infrared}/DC_{infrared})}$$

where, f is the calibration constant, which is manufacturer specific.

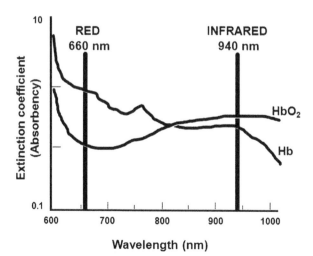

Fig. 2. Reference spectra exhibiting extinction coefficients (absorbency) of oxygenated hemoglobin (HbO_2) and deoxygenated hemoglobin (Hb) as a function of wavelength. The vertical lines indicate the wavelengths (red and infrared) commonly used in pulse oximetry.

Calibration of Pulse Oximeters

The Spo$_2$ is calculated using the ratio of absorption ratios by dedicated calibration algorithms stored in the microprocessor of the device. These algorithms are derived through arterial oxygen saturation measurements in healthy volunteers breathing mixtures of decreased oxygen concentrations and are usually unique for each manufacturer.[9,11,12,15,17,18] The displayed Spo$_2$ represents the mean of the measurements obtained during the previous 3 to 6 seconds, whereas the data are updated every 0.5 to 1.0 second.[9,11,17,18] The performance of each device is related to the reliability and complexity of the algorithms used in signal processing and to the speed and quality of the microprocessor. However, these results have been reported in patients with Spo$_2$ levels that exceed 80%[9,11,17-19]; the performance of pulse oximeters deteriorates when arterial oxygen saturation decreases to less than 80%.[15,20,21]

MORPHOLOGIC ANALYSIS OF PHOTOPLETHYSMOGRAPHIC WAVEFORM
Photoplethysmogram

Despite its simple appearance, the PPG waveform measured by pulse oximetry is a highly complex signal that contains an abundance of information in its shape, height, and timing. The time period between each of the successive intervals of the PPG waveform represents the repetition of the cardiac cycle, and is used to calculate the pulse rate. The intact and raw PPG waveforms are a projection of the hemodynamic output of the entire cardiovascular system.[22,23] As such, it contains more hemodynamic information than simply the Spo2 and heart rate. For instance, PPG is characterized by a second peak in each of its periods, which is referred to as the dicrotic notch and represents the closure of the aortic valve at the end of systole, thus causing a backlash and a momentary increase in blood volume of the arteries.[24] Also, as shown in the PPG morphology (**Fig. 3**), the amplitude of the PPG varies with the power of the left ventricular stroke and vasomotor tone. The changes in these and other morphologic details can be used to determine the hemodynamic status of the patient at any time point.

PPG measures changes in blood volume at the measured site. The larger the blood volume at the site (vasodilation), the more light gets absorbed, the less light passes through the site, and the resultant current generated by the photodetector is smaller. So, during systole, the amount of light transmitted through the site is less than during diastole, and the original PPG signal resembles a mirror image of an arterial blood pressure waveform. To make it easier for clinicians to interpret the PPG waveform, most devices invert the image on the display. In addition, the PPG waveform is frequently autoscaled to fit the display area. As a result, potential important

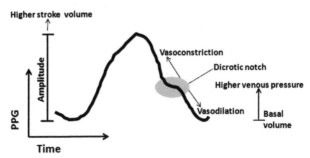

Fig. 3. Morphologic details of the PPG waveform with potential hemodynamic information that can be derived.

physiologic information that is contained in the AC and DC components of the signal is not used. Changes in the AC and DC components of the plethysmograph waveform have been related to vasomotor tone.[25–29] The DC component is also influenced by respiration and may contain information relating to the patients' fluid status.[30–33] Recent advances in pulse oximetry focusing on the morphologic analysis of the PPG waveform have defined new indices such as perfusion index (PI) and pleth variability index (PVI) that are capable of assessing hemodynamic status.

PI

PI is an assessment of the pulsatile strength at a specific monitoring site (eg, the hand, finger, or foot), and as such is an indirect and noninvasive measure of peripheral perfusion. It is calculated by expressing the pulsatile or AC component of the PPG signal (during arterial inflow) as a percentage of the nonpulsatile or DC component of PPG signal, both of which are derived from the amount of infrared (940 nm) light absorbed (**Fig. 4**):

$$PI = \frac{AC}{DC} \times 100\%$$

The PI value is relative to a particular monitoring site of each patient because physiologic conditions vary between monitoring sites and individual patients. The PI display ranges from 0.02% (very weak pulse strength) to 20% (very strong pulse strength). The Masimo signal extraction technology (Masimo Corporation, Irvine, CA) uses 5 signal processing algorithms to deliver high-precision sensitivity and specificity in the continuous measurement of the PI parameter, which can yield clinically useful information regarding the peripheral perfusion status of the patient.[34] The ability to trend PI is critical because only trends reveal the often subtle changes in perfusion that are otherwise missed by static displays. These subtle changes captured by the real-time trends provide immediate feedback on the perfusion status and/or efficacy of therapeutic interventions, thus guiding clinical management. Changes in PI can also occur as a result of local vasoconstriction (decrease in PI) or vasodilatation (increase in PI) in the skin at the monitoring site.[35] The measurement of PI is independent of other physiologic variables such as heart rate variability, arterial oxygen saturation, or oxygen consumption. However, PI is sensitive to several things such as

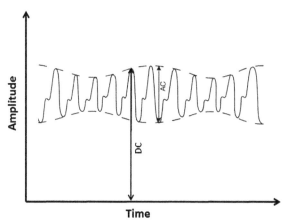

Fig. 4. Computation of PI from the pulsatile AC and nonpulsatile DC components of the infrared photoplethysmographic waveform.

temperature of the measurement site, exogenous vasoactive drugs, sympathetic nervous system tone (pain, anxiety), and stroke volume.[36]

PVI

Another variable that is derived from the PPG waveform is PVI. PVI is a new parameter that is currently provided by only 1 pulse oximeter manufacturer. PVI is a measure of the dynamic changes in the PPG waveform (ie, PI) that occur during the respiratory cycle and is thought to be a surrogate measure of intravascular volume. It is theorized that, with each inspiration, venous return to the heart is impeded, resulting in a temporary reduction in cardiac output. As a patient becomes volume depleted, with a resulting decrease in venous pressure, positive pressure ventilation has an exaggerated impact on the arterial blood pressure and the plethysmograph.[33,37,38] Monitoring the respiratory variability in the PPG waveform may be a useful method of evaluating fluid status.[39,40] The PVI reflects measurements of ventilation-induced respiratory changes in PI over a constant period of time and is calculated as follows[41,42]:

$$PVI = \left[\frac{(PI_{max} - PI_{min})}{PI_{max}}\right] \times 100\%$$

where PI_{max} and PI_{min} are the maximum and minimum values of PI (**Fig. 5**).

PVI therefore is displayed continuously as a percentage. The lower the number, the less variability there is in the PI over a respiratory cycle. Several similar parameters (pulse pressure variation, δ up/δ down, systolic blood pressure variability) have previously been derived from the invasive arterial blood pressure waveform. It is speculated that PVI has the potential to provide useful information concerning changes in the balance between intravascular fluid volume and intrathoracic airway pressure. For example, PVI may help clinicians noninvasively and continuously assess the fluid status of patients. An increasing PVI may indicate developing hypovolemia. In addition, the greater the PVI, the more likely the patient will respond to fluid administration. Trending of PVI may also be useful in monitoring patients with respiratory or cardiac failure, helping to evaluate the interrelationship between intrathoracic pressures and cardiac function.

Novel Applications

Photoplethysmographic waveform to assess microcirculation

The PI obtained from the PPG signal has been suggested to reflect changes in peripheral perfusion.[35,37] This ratio has recently been used as a noninvasive index of peripheral perfusion in critically ill patients.[43] Lima and colleagues[43] showed that PI with

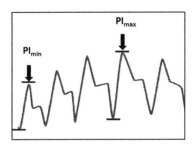

Fig. 5. PVI calculation from the PI_{max} and PI_{min} values of PI derived from the infrared plethysmographic waveform.

a threshold value of 1.4 can be used to detect abnormal peripheral perfusion in patients receiving intensive care. In particular, a PI value of less than or equal to 1.24 has been shown to be an accurate predictor of high illness severity in newborns.[44] PI monitoring has been shown to be helpful in identifying preterm and term neonates born to mothers with chorioamnionitis, a major predictor of morbidity and mortality in very low birth weight infants.[45–47] Moreover, PI values might be useful for early detection of ductus arteriosus–dependent systemic circulation (left heart obstructive disease).[48] Furthermore, PI is a useful index for detecting low superior vena cava flow, which is a risk factor for intraventricular hemorrhage in preterm infants.[49] In contrast, a decreased PI value in the preanesthesia phase of the elective cesarean section is a maternal predictor of increased neonatal morbidity, in particular early respiratory complications.[50] Higher values of PI are associated with prone sleeping position in low birth weight infants, presumably reflecting thermoregulatory adjustments in peripheral perfusion, and PI correlates significantly with other indirect measures of tissue perfusion such as heart rate and central-to-peripheral thermal gradients.[51]

Photoplethysmographic waveform to assess intravascular fluid volume

Estimation of intravascular volume is still a challenge in both adults and infants, in whom hypovolemia is a common cause of perioperative circulatory failure. In conjunction with clinical assessment, heart rate, mean arterial pressure, and central venous pressure are frequently used to guide fluid therapy in infants and neonates.[52] However, numerous studies have shown that values of preload, or change in preload to a fluid load, are poor indicators of whether a patient will benefit from additional fluid.[53–55] Investigations have progressed beyond static measurement of cardiac filling pressures to a more dynamic approach using invasive variables such as pulse pressure variation, stroke volume variation, and noninvasive measurements of PVI, which are based on heart-lung interaction induced by mechanical ventilation. These dynamic variables have been shown to predict reliably the response to a fluid load in adults in different clinical scenarios.[56–58] Cannesson and colleagues[41] showed that a PVI greater than or equal to 14% before volume expansion discriminates between responders and nonresponders with a sensitivity of 81% and specificity of 100% in adult patients under general anesthesia. Renner and colleagues[59] recently showed that PVI can predict fluid responsiveness in infants undergoing congenital heart surgery, with a threshold value of greater than or equal to 13% helping to discriminate between responders and nonresponders with an acceptable sensitivity but low specificity. We recently showed that PVI can predict ventricular preload and fluid responsiveness in mechanically ventilated infants with congenital heart disease; infants with transposition of great arteries showed superior postoperative fluid responsiveness compared with those with hypoplastic left heart syndrome, suggesting greater preload dependence.[60] These data suggest that PVI may have clinical applications for the noninvasive detection of hypovolemia and for monitoring the response to a fluid challenge.

LIMITATIONS OF THE METHODOLOGY

The quality of the PPG waveform can be affected by various factors inducing vasomotor tone, low cardiac output, and increased cutaneous vascular resistance.[61] Because the main purpose of pulse oximetry devices is to determine blood oxygen saturation, most oximeters have an autocentering algorithm and a high-pass filter that excludes frequencies below those of cardiac pulsations[62]; the goal is to optimize waveform resolution of the pulsatile signal rather than to facilitate assessment of respiration-induced changes. Valuable clinical information on fluid responsiveness may still be obtained from the plethysmographic signal even when other filters, such fixed bandpass filtering (for rejecting frequencies from confounding motion artifact, low peripheral perfusion, and most low signal-to-noise situations) and autogain filtering (for changing band noise in the physiologic window of interest) are used.[38] Pulse oximeters with autogain features remain valid in representing short cyclic variations in pulse volume, because percentage changes in PPG are displayed rather than absolute changes, and so the results are independent of scale. It is hoped that equipment manufacturers will consider adding features that will allow their devices to make accurate PPG waveforms analyses. These desirable characteristics should include the ability to turn off the autogain function, turn off the autocenter function, set the amplitude gain, and capture unprocessed signals by data collection equipment.

FUTURE DIRECTIONS

The availability of increasingly powerful methods of digital signal processing are allowing a renaissance in PPG research. Calculations that once required mainframe computers are now performed almost instantaneously with digital signal processing chips. This ability has allowed the detailed reexamination of the photoplethysmograph. Combined with improved understanding of the underlying physiology of the waveform, it is easy to predict the emergence of multifunction pulse oximeters. To uncover the true potential of this waveform, standardization and quantification of the photoplethysmograph as it is presented to the clinician are needed. What is viewed as an artifact from one perspective (ie, respiratory variation of the PPG while determining heart rate) becomes signal in another (ie, using the same respiratory variation of the PPG to predict fluid responsiveness). In addition, clinicians have a vital role to play in the discovery and verification of new uses of the waveform.

SUMMARY

Recent evidence suggests that photoplethysmography offers a productive avenue for technological developments in noninvasive circulatory monitoring. There is a need for better equipment generating waveforms that can be quantified in a standardized manner, well-designed prospective studies showing that clinically relevant information is being measured, and outcome studies showing that this information will help clinicians provide better care for their patients.

REFERENCES

1. Roberts VC. Photoplethysmography-fundamental aspects of the optical properties of blood in motion. Trans Inst Meas Control 1982;4:101–6.
2. Dorlas JC, Nijboer JA. Photo-electric plethysmography as a monitoring device in anaesthesia: application and interpretation. Br J Anaesth 1985;57:524–30.
3. Higgins JL, Fronek A. Photoplethysmographic evaluation of the relationship between skin reflectance and blood volume. J Biomed Eng 1986;8:130–6.
4. Lindberg LG, Oberg PA. Photoplethysmography: part 2. Influence of light source wavelength. Med Biol Eng Comput 1991;29:48–54.
5. Nijboer JA, Dorlas JC, Mahieu HF. Photoelectric plethysmography-some fundamental aspects of the reflection and transmission method. Clin Phys Physiol Meas 1981;2:205–15.
6. Webster JG. Design of pulse oximeters. New York: Taylor & Francis; 1997. p. 40–55.
7. Trafford J, Lafferty K. What does photoplethysmography measure? Med Biol Eng Comput 1984;22:479–80.

8. Spigulis J. Optical noninvasive monitoring of skin blood pulsations. Appl Opt 2005;44:1850–7.

9. Sinex JE. Pulse oximetry: principles and limitations. Am J Emerg Med 1999;17(1): 59–67.

10. Marr J, Abramo TJ. Monitoring in critically ill children. In: Baren JM, Rothrock SG, Brennan JA, et al, editors. Pediatric emergency medicine. Philadelphia: Saunders Elsevier; 2008. p. 50–2.

11. Jubran A. Pulse oximetry. Intensive Care Med 2004;30(11):2017–20.

12. Callahan JM. Pulse oximetry in emergency medicine. Emerg Med Clin North Am 2008;26(4):869–79.

13. Zijlstra WG, Buursma A, Meeuwsen-van der Roest WP. Absorption spectra of human fetal and adult oxyhemoglobin, de-oxyhemoglobin, carboxyhemoglobin and methemoglobin. Clin Chem 1991;37(9):1633–8.

14. Mannheimer PD. The light-tissue interaction of pulse oximetry. Anesth Analg 2007;105(Suppl 6):S10–7.

15. Zonios G, Shankar U, Iyer VK. Pulse oximetry theory and calibration for low saturations. IEEE Trans Biomed Eng 2004;51(5):818–22.

16. Aoyagi T. Pulse oximetry: its invention, theory, and future. J Anesth 2003;17(4): 259–66.

17. Hanning CD, Alexander-Williams JM. Pulse oximetry: a practical review. BMJ 1995;311(7001):367–70.

18. Hess DR, Branson RD. Noninvasive respiratory monitoring equipment. In: Branson RD, Hess DR, Chatburn RL, editors. Respiratory care equipment. Philadelphia: JP Lippincott; 1995. p. 193.

19. Salyer JW. Neonatal and pediatric pulse oximetry. Respir Care 2003;48(4): 386–96.

20. Nickerson BG, Sarkisian C, Tremper KK. Bias and precision of pulse oximeters and arterial oximeters. Chest 1988;93(3):515–7.

21. Severinghaus JW, Kelleher JF. Recent developments in pulse oximetry. Anesthesiology 1992;76(6):1018–38.

22. Murray WB, Foster PA. The peripheral pulse wave: information overlooked. J Clin Monit 1996;12:365–77.

23. Shelley K, Shelley S. Pulse oximeter waveform: photoelectric plethysmography (chapter 23). In: Lake C, Hines R, Blitt C, editors. Clinical monitoring: practical applications for anesthesia and critical care. Marrickville (Australia): Harcourt Brace; 2001. p. 420–8.

24. Hoeksel SA, Jansen JR, Blom A, et al. Detection of dicrotic notch in arterial pressure signals. J Clin Monit Comput 1997;13:309–16.

25. Shelley KH, Murray WB, Chang D. Arterial-pulse oximetry loops: a new method of monitoring vascular tone. J Clin Monit 1997;13:223–8.

26. Landsverk SA, Hoiseth LO, Kvandal P, et al. Poor agreement between respiratory variations in pulse oximetry photoplethysmographic waveform amplitude and pulse pressure in intensive care unit patients. Anesthesiology 2008;109: 849–55.

27. Hummler HD, Engelmann A, Pohlandt F, et al. Decreased accuracy of pulse oximetry measurements during low perfusion caused by sepsis: is the perfusion index of any value? Intensive Care Med 2006;32:1428–31.

28. Mowafi HA, Arab SA, Ismail SA, et al. Plethysmographic pulse wave amplitude is an effective indicator for intravascular injection of epinephrine-containing epidural test in sevoflurane-anesthetized pediatric patients. Anesth Analg 2008; 107:1536–41.

29. Mowafi HA, Ismail SA, Shafi MA, et al. The efficacy of perfusion index as an indicator for intravascular injection of epinephrine-containing epidural test dose in propofol-anesthetized adults. Anesth Analg 2009;108:549–53.

30. Cannesson M, Attof Y, Rosamel P, et al. Respiratory variations in pulse oximetry plethysmographic waveform amplitude to predict fluid responsiveness in the operating room. Anesthesiology 2007;106:1105–11.

31. Feissel M, Teboul JL, Merlani P, et al. Plethysmographic dynamic indices predict fluid responsiveness in septic ventilated patients. Intensive Care Med 2007;33: 993–9.

32. Shelley KH, Jablonka DH, Awad AA, et al. What is the best site for measuring the effect of ventilation on the pulse oximeter waveform? Anesth Analg 2006;103: 372–7.

33. Shelley KH. Photoplethysmography: beyond the calculation of arterial oxygen saturation and heart rate. Anesth Analg 2007;105:S31–6.

34. Goldman JM, Petterson MT, Kopotic RJ, et al. Masimo signal extraction pulse oximetry. J Clin Monit Comput 2000;16:475–83.

35. Hales JR, Stephens FR, Fawcett AA, et al. Observations on a new noninvasive monitor of skin blood flow. Clin Exp Pharmacol Physiol 1989;16:403–15.

36. Cannesson M, Talke P. Recent advances in pulse oximetry. F1000 Med Rep 2009; 1:66.

37. Partridge BL. Use of pulse oximetry as a noninvasive indicator of intravascular volume status. J Clin Monit 1987;3:263–8.

38. Natalini G, Rosano A, Franceschetti ME, et al. Variations in arterial blood pressure and photoplethysmography during mechanical ventilation. Anesth Analg 2006; 103:1182–8.

39. Monnet X, Lamia B, Teboul J. Pulse oximeter as a sensor of fluid responsiveness: do we have our finger on the best solution? Crit Care 2005;9:429–30.

40. Cannesson M, Besnard C, Durand PG, et al. Relation between respiratory variations in pulse oximetry plethysmographic waveform amplitude and arterial pulse pressure in ventilated patients. Crit Care 2005;9:562–8.

41. Cannesson M, Desebbe O, Rosamel P, et al. Pleth variability index to monitor the respiratory variations in the pulse oximeter plethysmographic waveform amplitude and predict fluid responsiveness in the operating theatre. Br J Anaesth 2008;101:200–6.

42. Zimmermann M, Feibicke T, Keyl C, et al. Accuracy of stroke volume variation compared with pleth variability index to predict fluid responsiveness in mechanically ventilated patients undergoing major surgery. Eur J Anaesthesiol 2010;27: 555–61.

43. Lima AP, Beelen P, Bakker J. Use of a peripheral perfusion index derived from the pulse oximetry signal as a noninvasive indicator of perfusion. Crit Care Med 2002; 30:1210–3.

44. De Felice C, Latini G, Vacca P, et al. The pulse oximeter perfusion index as a predictor for high illness severity in neonates. Eur J Pediatr 2002;161:561–2.

45. De Felice C, Del Vecchio A, Criscuolo M, et al. Early postnatal changes in the perfusion index in term newborns with subclinical chorioamnionitis. Arch Dis Child Fetal Neonatal Ed 2005;90:F411–4.

46. De Felice C, Toti P, Parrini S, et al. Histologic chorioamnionitis and severity of illness in very low birth weight newborns. Pediatr Crit Care Med 2005;5:298–302.

47. De Felice C, Goldstein MR, Parrini S, et al. Early dynamic changes in pulse oximetry signals in preterm newborns with histologic chorioamnionitis. Pediatr Crit Care Med 2006;7:138–42.

48. Granelli AW, Ostman-Smith I. Non-invasive peripheral perfusion index as a possible tool for screening for critical left heart obstruction. Acta Paediatr 2007;96:1455–9.
49. Takahashi S, Kakiuchi S, Nanba Y, et al. The perfusion index derived from a pulse oximeter for predicting low superior vena cava flow in very low birth weight infants. J Perinatol 2010;30:265–9.
50. De Felice C, Leoni L, Tommasini E, et al. Maternal pulse oximetry perfusion index as a predictor of early adverse respiratory neonatal outcome after elective caesarean delivery. Pediatr Crit Care Med 2008;9:203–8.
51. Sahni R, Schulze KF, Ohira-Kist K, et al. Interactions among peripheral perfusion, cardiac activity, oxygen saturation, thermal profile and body position in growing low birth weight infants. Acta Paediatr 2010;99(1):135–9.
52. Tibby SM, Hatherill M, Murdoch IA. Use of transesophageal Doppler ultrasonography in ventilated pediatric patients: derivation of cardiac output. Crit Care Med 2000;28:2045–50.
53. Kumar A, Anel R, Bunnell E, et al. Pulmonary artery occlusion pressure and central venous pressure fail to predict ventricular filling volume, cardiac performance, or the response to volume infusion in normal subjects. Crit Care Med 2004;32:691–9.
54. Michard F, Teboul JL. Predicting fluid responsiveness in ICU patients: a critical analysis of the evidence. Chest 2002;121:2000–8.
55. Renner J, Cavus E, Meybohm P, et al. Pulse pressure variation and stroke volume variation during different loading conditions in a paediatric animal model. Acta Anaesthesiol Scand 2008;52:374–80.
56. Cannesson M, Desebbe O, Lehot JJ. Fluid responsiveness using non-invasive predictors during major hepatic surgery. Br J Anaesth 2007;98:272–3.
57. Hofer CK, Muller SM, Furrer L, et al. Stroke volume and pulse pressure variation for prediction of fluid responsiveness in patients undergoing off-pump coronary artery bypass grafting. Chest 2005;128:848–54.
58. Michard F. Changes in arterial pressure during mechanical ventilation. Anesthesiology 2005;103:419–28.
59. Renner J, Broch O, Grueneald M, et al. Non-invasive prediction of fluid responsiveness in infants using pleth variability index. Anaesthesia 2011;66:582–9.
60. Sahni R, Harijith A, Bacha E, et al. Pleth variability index to monitor trends in postoperative ventricular preload and fluid responsiveness in infants with congenital heart disease. E-PAS2011 2927:322.
61. Awad AA, Haddadin AS, Tantawy H, et al. The relationship between the photoplethysmographic waveform and systemic vascular resistance. J Clin Monit Comput 2007;21:365–72.
62. Gesquiere MJ, Awad AA, Silverman DG, et al. Impact of withdrawal of 450 ml of blood on respiration-induced oscillations of the ear plethysmographic waveform. J Clin Monit Comput 2007;21:277–82.

Predictors of Bronchopulmonary Dysplasia

Andrea Trembath, MD, MPH[a],*, Matthew M. Laughon, MD, MPH[b]

KEYWORDS

- Bronchopulmonary dysplasia • Predictors/risk factors • Chronic lung disease
- Mechanical ventilation

KEY POINTS

- Bronchopulmonary dysplasia (BPD), also called chronic lung disease, is the most common serious pulmonary morbidity in premature infants.
- Premature infants with BPD have lifelong morbidities, including an increased risk of cerebral palsy and mental retardation.
- The incidence of BPD is inversely related to gestational age and birth weight.
- Prediction of BPD using parsimonious models by postnatal day is now possible.

INTRODUCTION

Although significant advances in respiratory care have been made in neonatal medicine, bronchopulmonary dysplasia (BPD) remains the most common serious pulmonary morbidity in premature infants. Premature infants with BPD have a longer initial hospitalization than their peers without BPD.[1] BPD remains a substantial lifelong burden. The costs of the disorder are both social and economic, and are measured in impaired childhood health and quality of life, family stress, economic hardship, and increased health care costs.[2–4]

Over the past 40 years, the definition, disease, and risk factors for BPD have changed.[5,6] BPD, as it was initially described by Northway and colleagues[7] in the 1960s, was based on clinical and radiographic evidence of pulmonary disease in moderately to late premature infants with a history of respiratory distress syndrome. The respiratory management of

Dr Laughon receives support from the U.S. government for his work in pediatric and neonatal clinical pharmacology (government contract HHSN267200700051C, PI: Benjamin under the Best Pharmaceuticals for Children's Act), and from the National Institute of Child Health & Human Development (1K23HL092225-01).

[a] Rainbow Babies & Children's Hospital, 11000 Euclid Avenue, RBC Suite 3100, Cleveland, OH 44106, USA; [b] Division of Neonatal-Perinatal Medicine, The University of North Carolina at Chapel Hill, 101 Manning Drive, CB 7596, Chapel Hill, NC 27599-7596, USA
* Corresponding author.
E-mail address: Andrea.Trembath@UHhospitals.org

these infants included exposure to prolonged mechanical ventilation and oxygen exposure. On histologic samples, the characteristic areas of hyperinflation alternating with areas of focal collapse were often noted, and hyperplasia of the bronchial epithelium.[8] Radiography of these infants showed areas of heterogeneity throughout the lung fields and coarse scattered opacities in the most severely affected of infants.[9]

The classical BPD described by Northway and colleagues has been replaced by a milder form of the disease. There is reason to believe that risk factors associated with the "new" BPD, compared with historical risk factors, may be distinct. This new BPD occurs in less mature infants exposed to antenatal steroids, who are often treated with exogenous surfactant therapy. They spend fewer days on positive pressure ventilation and have less exposure to supplemental oxygen. Animal studies suggest that the histology of new BPD shows more diffuse disease, fewer areas of hyperinflation, and a reduction in alveoli and capillaries, but little fibrosis.[10,11]

The incidence of BPD varies widely between centers, even after adjusting for potential risk factors. Data from 2010 from the Vermont Oxford Network show that the rates of BPD vary from 12% to 32% among infants born at less than 32 weeks' gestation. Although multiple trials have been aimed at reducing the incidence of BPD, the incidence seems to be stagnant, or even increasing. The rising absolute number of infants with BPD might be caused by the improvement in the survival of extremely low gestational age infants, the population most likely to have this diagnosis.[5,12,13] Compared with the pathology described by Northway and colleagues, the most common type of BPD today may be a less severe form of the disease.

This article reviews the definitions of BPD and the predictors of BPD by time period (before, at, and after birth). Several of the estimators that are available to quantify the risk of BPD, and to explain how this might affect clinicians, families, and researchers, are also reviewed.

DEFINING BPD

The definition of BPD most often uses receipt of oxygen therapy or positive pressure for a duration of time (usually in days) or on a specific day (eg, postnatal day 28 or at postmenstrual age [PMA] 36 weeks). The original definition was based on receipt of oxygen at 28 days of age. However, this definition does not take into account the various developmental considerations of infants born across the spectrum of susceptible gestational ages. Thus, attempts have been made to improve the definition through a corrected age "cut point," most commonly the need for supplemental oxygen therapy at 36 weeks' PMA. The National Institute of Child Health & Human Development (NICHD) divided the definition further using a severity scale. Because oxygen saturation targets vary among centers, a "physiologic definition" also has been proposed. These definitions are reviewed in more detail later.

A workshop to clarify the definition of BPD was held by the NICHD in June 2000 with the goal of distinguishing BPD from chronic lung disease (CLD), a condition that was believed to represent a group of heterogeneous diseases occurring later in life.[14] This workshop proposed a severity-based definition that classified BPD as mild, moderate, or severe based on either postnatal age or PMA (**Table 1**). Mild BPD was defined as a need for supplemental oxygen throughout the first 28 days but not at 36 weeks' PMA or at discharge; moderate BPD as a requirement for oxygen throughout the first 28 days plus treatment with less than 30% oxygen at 36 weeks' PMA; severe BPD as a requirement for oxygen throughout the first 28 days plus 30% oxygen or greater and/ or positive pressure at 36 weeks' PMA. Ehrenkranz and colleagues[15] validated the NICHD severity-based definition of BPD through comparing it with the more traditional

Table 1
NICHD severity-based definition of BPD

Gestational Age at Birth	Mild BPD	Moderate BPD	Severe BPD
<32 wk	Room air at 36 weeks' PMA or discharge[a]	<30% oxygen at 36 weeks' PMA or discharge[a]	≥30% oxygen and/or positive pressure at 36 weeks' PMA[a]
≥32 wk	Room air by 56 days' postnatal age or discharge[a]	<30% oxygen at 56 days' postnatal age or discharge[a]	≥30% oxygen and/or positive pressure at 56 days' postnatal age or discharge[a]

[a] All categories require treatment with >21% for at least 28 days, then assessment at PMA/postnatal day or discharge whichever comes first.

Adapted from Jobe AH, Bancalari E. Bronchopulmonary dysplasia. Am J Respir Crit Care Med 2001;163:1723–9; with permission.

definitions of BPD, such as supplemental oxygen at 28 days and at 36 weeks' PMA. The consensus NICHD severity-based scale better identified infants who are at most risk for poor pulmonary outcomes and neurodevelopment impairment than the traditional definitions.[15]

The physiologic definition of BPD was developed by Walsh and colleagues,[16] and defines BPD as a failure to maintain a saturation value greater than 90% when challenged with 21% oxygen at 36 weeks' PMA. Unit-specific rates of BPD using the physiologic-definition were compared with rates of BPD using the traditional definition of BPD (oxygen need at 36 weeks' PMA) for premature infants weighing 501 to 1249 g. The physiologic definition reduced the between-center variability in the diagnosis of BPD and reduced the diagnosis as much as 10% at individual centers. The physiologic definition has also been validated and shown to be independently predictive of cognitive impairment in infants with BPD.[17] The physiologic definition is used by the NICHD Neonatal Research Network centers throughout the United States.

Regardless of which definition of BPD is used, a period of time is required before the diagnosis is made. This delay makes identifying therapies for premature infants at risk of BPD challenging. An infant born at 23 weeks' gestation who needs mechanical ventilation at 34 weeks' PMA is likely to develop BPD, as defined as oxygen therapy at 36 weeks. That infant may benefit from strategies that improve short-term outcomes but that do not reduce the incidence of BPD. For example, in a Cochrane Systematic Review, Stewart and colleagues[18] found that the use of diuretics may transiently improve oxygenation and pulmonary function but did not reduce the development of BPD (relative risk [RR], 0.80; 95% CI, 0.18, 3.54). Recently, a prototype Proxy Reported Pulmonary Outcome Score (PRPOS) was developed to define nuances in pulmonary function as reported by caregivers. The PRPOS consists of 26 observations that can be made by a nurse before, during, and after providing routine care and feeding.[19] The goal is to make assessments about functional domains of infants that will help discriminate among infants with none, mild, moderate, and severe pulmonary dysfunction. This novel approach might allow testing of therapies (eg, diuretics) aimed at improving pulmonary outcomes that do not require waiting for the development of an outcome several days or weeks later.

UNDERSTANDING AND INTERPRETING THE PREDICTORS OF BPD

Predictors of disease are more commonly known as risk factors. In epidemiologic studies, risk is most often used synonymously with probability of disease occurrence; however, it may represent a wide variety of statistical measures that include incidence, prevalence, rate, or odds. A risk factor often implies an increase in the outcome of interest with exposure, although risk measures may also represent protective effects.[20]

In many studies, risks are often compared through relative measures, as in risk ratio, odds ratio, or rate ratio.[21] Relative measures are helpful for identifying risk factors but can be misleading when not accompanied by absolute measures such as the risk difference. For example, a relative risk of 2.0 indicates that the exposed group is twice as likely to develop the disease as the unexposed group. However, twice as likely may represent an absolute change in risk from 0.2 (20%) to 0.1 (10%; risk difference of 0.1 or 10%) or may represent an absolute change in risk from 0.002 (0.2%) to 0.001 (0.1%; risk difference of 0.001 or 0.1%). This is important because small changes in absolute risk differences might not be as amenable to change as a large risk difference.

Attributable risk proportion (ARP), also known as the etiologic fraction, represents the proportion of the incidence of disease among exposed persons that is caused by the exposure. The ARP is often useful when identifying risk factors in diseases that are multifactorial, such as BPD. As with all risk measures, however, caution should be used when inferring causality.[22] Most diseases such as BPD have many component causes, some of which remain either unknown or immeasurable. These component causes can occur at different times, and the sequence of their occurrence may be important in the development of the disease. In addition, risk measures cannot distinguish a necessary cause from a component cause. Removal of a single component cause can reduce disease burden, but removal of a necessary cause may prevent the disease entirely.[23] Several studies have shown that the retrospective examination of risk factors for BPD alone is difficult given the interrelation of true risk factors, the difficulty in distinguishing temporal relationships, and confounding factors.[24–26]

Traditionally, researchers identified risk factors for BPD through categorizing premature infants as having or not having BPD based on one of the definitions noted earlier, and then retrospectively examining all factors that influenced risk up to the time of diagnosis. As a result, each study has reached different conclusions regarding the risk factors for the development of BPD. In addition, most used some type of multivariate modeling to adjust for potential confounders and effect modifiers (eg, adjusting for gestational age).

For examples, in a study by Rojas and colleagues,[27] risk factors for BPD in ventilator-supported preterm infants weighing between 500 and 1000 g included low birth weight and the presence of a patent ductus arteriosus (PDA) and sepsis. Of these infants, 37% were diagnosed with BPD as defined as oxygen therapy at 28 days. In contrast, Marshall and colleagues[24] defined risk factors for BPD as nosocomial infection, magnitude of fluid intake on day 2, present of PDA, and need for ventilation at 48 hours of life. Of the 1244 infants between 500 and 1500 g included in the study, 26% developed CLD, defined as dependency on supplemental oxygen at 36 weeks' postmenstrual age. In a secondary analysis of the Neonatal Research Network Glutamine trial, the risk factors for infants who died or developed BPD (defined as oxygen therapy at 36 weeks' PMA) were lower birth weight and gestational age, male sex, lower 1- and 5-minute Apgar scores, higher oxygen requirement at 24 hours of age, longer duration of assisted ventilation, use of postnatal steroids, and the presence of severe intraventricular hemorrhage, necrotizing enterocolitis, PDA, and late-onset sepsis.[25] In preterm infants with respiratory failure enrolled in the Neonatal Research Network inhaled nitric oxide trial, the investigators found that the risk of death or BPD was associated with lower birth weight, higher oxygen requirement, male gender, additional surfactant doses, higher oxygenation index, and outborn status.[26] These examples show that in multifactorial diseases such as BPD, multiple definitions and confounding in retrospective studies can distort the exposure-outcome relationship.

RISK FACTORS BEFORE BIRTH
Antenatal Steroids

Antenatal steroids are associated with a decrease in both severity of respiratory distress syndrome and neonatal mortality.[28,29] Therefore, antenatal steroids were initially believed to decrease the risk of BPD.[30] In a multivariate analysis, Van Marter and colleagues[31] examined the independent effect of antenatal steroids on the risk of BPD. They found that treatment with either a partial or full course of antenatal steroids did not convey any additional benefit in reducing the likelihood of BPD after adjustment for other important confounders, such as gestational age, infection, and respiratory management strategies (odds ratio [OR], 0.98; 95% CI, 0.66, 1.5). In a Cochrane analysis[32] that included 818 infants from six studies, the risk of BPD (defined as oxygen at 36 weeks' PMA) was not significantly different in infants who were exposed to antenatal steroids and controls (RR, 0.86; 95% CI, 0.61, 1.22). Overall, these studies suggest that antenatal steroid exposure does not modify the risk of BPD; however, this may be because of an increase in survival of the most immature antenatal steroid-exposed infants.

Chorioamnionitis

Chorioamnionitis is one of the leading causes of very preterm delivery. The association between chorioamnionitis and BPD is difficult to assess because the diagnosis has several definitions. A clinical diagnosis of chorioamnionitis is commonly made based on maternal symptoms and is subject to significant variability among providers. Furthermore, clinical chorioamnionitis may only reflect acute inflammatory changes. Histologic evidence of chorioamnionitis is the gold standard and may reflect chronic infection, but placental pathology is not always available. Antenatal inflammation, such as chorioamnionitis, has been associated with an increased rate of lung maturation.[33] In a retrospective study by Dempsey[34] of 392 infants born at less than 30 weeks' PMA, histologic chorioamnionitis was associated with a higher incidence of premature deliveries and an increased risk of sepsis. However, chorioamnionitis was also associated with a significant decrease in the incidence of respiratory distress syndrome (OR, 0.43; P value = .001), a finding that has been repeatedly shown in multiple other studies.

The presence of chorioamnionitis is also associated with a disturbance in the normal lung maturation and growth that may affect the development of BPD.[35–37] A recent meta-analysis suggested that even when adjusted for other confounding factors, an association remains between chorioamnionitis and an increased risk for BPD.[38] However, other studies aimed at identifying predictive factors for the development of BPD using a histologic diagnosis suggest that a true association with chorioamnionitis may not exist.[39,40]

Fetal Growth Restriction

Fetal growth restriction, defined as a birth weight less than 1 SD below the median, is associated with an increased risk of BPD among premature infants. In a study by Bose and colleagues,[39] characteristics and potential risk factors for BPD were evaluated among 1241 infants enrolled in the Extremely Low Gestational Age Newborn (ELGAN) study. The authors examined the role of prenatal factors, such as preeclampsia and fetal indications for delivery, the microbiology and histology of the placenta, and neonatal characteristics, including fetal growth restriction (FGR). Among these infants, FGR was highly predictive of the development of BPD in all gestational ages except the lowest (23–24 weeks), after adjustment. The investigators speculated that the biologic mechanisms leading to FGR also lead to vulnerability of the developing lung, rendering infants with FGR at higher risk for the development of BPD.

RISK FACTORS AT BIRTH
Infant Demographics: Gestational Age, Birth Weight, and Sex

Extreme prematurity and extremely-low-birth-weight have been well established as risk factors for BPD. Gestational age and birth weight are inversely proportional to the incidence of BPD and the severity of the disease. Among infants meeting the physiologic definition of BPD at 36 weeks', 95% are very-low-birth-weight (VLBW).[16] In the NICHD network, the incidence of BPD at 23 weeks' PMA (as defined as oxygen at 36 weeks' PMA) was 73%, with 56% of infants having severe BPD. In comparison, at 28 weeks' PMA, the incidence of BPD was 23%, with only 8% of infants having severe BPD.[41] Male infants have a higher risk of developing BPD compared with females.[27,39,42]

RISK FACTORS AFTER BIRTH
Respiratory Patterns

Describing the early respiratory patterns of extremely low gestational age newborns may provide insight into early risk factors for BPD. Among these infants, three distinct patterns of lung disease typically emerge in the first 2 weeks of life.[43–47] The first pattern includes infants with little lung disease, who progressively recover. The second group of infants experiences early persistent pulmonary dysfunction and requires significant and prolonged respiratory support from birth. The third group experiences an initial improvement in lung disease in the first week of life, followed by a respiratory decompensation that often requires mechanical ventilation and increased supplemental oxygen. This group is described as having pulmonary deterioration.

Almost half of infants who have pulmonary deterioration develop BPD, which makes pulmonary deterioration an important early marker.[48] The characteristics and exposure history of infants from the ELGAN study were evaluated for associations with pulmonary deterioration.[49] Of the 1340 infants who were enrolled, approximately 40% developed pulmonary deterioration. Risk factors that may contribute to pulmonary deterioration include late surfactant deficiency,[50] sepsis, and PDA. The authors found that the most important markers of pulmonary deterioration were lower gestational age, lower birth weight, increased severity of illness (as defined as neonatal acute physiology II score), and need for higher levels of respiratory support. Other factors previously associated with pulmonary deterioration, including male sex, multiple pregnancy, cesarean section, antenatal steroids, and infection, were not statistically significant in multivariate regression models.[43,46] Among infants who had rapid resolution of their respiratory disease, 17% (n = 249) developed BPD (defined as supplemental oxygen at 36 weeks) compared with 51% (n = 484) in infants with pulmonary deterioration and 67% (n = 576) among infants with early persistent pulmonary dysfunction (**Fig. 1**).

Mechanical Ventilation

Mechanical ventilation is life-saving for premature infants with respiratory failure. However, mechanical ventilation uses positive pressure that produces ventilator-initiated lung injury.[51,52] The development of surfactant therapy led to many extremely premature infants receiving obligatory mechanical ventilation after surfactant

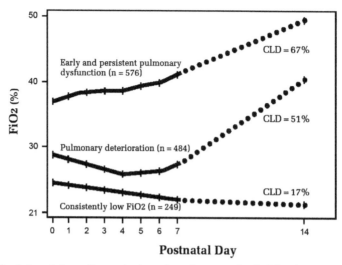

Fig. 1. Risk of chronic lung disease (or bronchopulmonary dysplasia) among 1340 extremely low gestational age newborns with three patterns of respiratory disease. (*Reprinted from* Laughon M, Allred EN, Bose C, et al. Patterns of respiratory disease during the first 2 postnatal weeks in extremely premature infants. Pediatrics 2009;123:1124–31; with permission from the American Academy of Pediatrics.)

replacement therapy. However, reports emerged about substantial differences in BPD rates; infants born in centers that used mechanical ventilation more frequently had a higher risk of BPD.[53,54] For example, the risk of BPD ranges from less than 10% to greater than 40% among the Neonatal Research Network centers in infants with birth weights of less than 1250 g.[55] This variation is not explained by differences in birth weight, gestational age, race, frequency of prenatal steroid use, or incidence of respiratory distress syndrome.

Avoidance of mechanical ventilation might decrease the risk of lung injury and BPD, and might explain some of the between-center differences in BPD rates.[54] Mechanical ventilation often begins shortly after birth; therefore, delivery room management strategies might influence the risk of BPD.[56,57] A full review of the association between delivery room management and BPD is presented in another article elsewhere in this issue. The use of nasal continuous positive airway pressure seems to be a successful strategy for avoiding the need for mechanical ventilation in some infants, with the presumptive benefit of decreasing the risk of BPD.[58]

Postnatal Steroids

The use of corticosteroids for the prevention or treatment of BPD has been examined in numerous clinical trials. Two Cochrane reviews provide information about the effect of treatment with systemic steroids on the incidence of CLD.[59,60] Early treatment was defined as beginning before postnatal day eight[59]; late treatment was defined as beginning after 7 days of postnatal age.[60] Twelve trials examined the neurodevelopmental impact of early corticosteroids and showed an increased risk of cerebral palsy (RR, 1.45; 95% CI, 1.06, 1.98), with impairment of motor function a risk associated with early treatment. Benefits of late treatment included decreased risks of BPD at 28 days and at 36 weeks' PMA (RR, 0.72; 95% CI, 0.61, 0.85) and death or CLD at 28 days and at 36 weeks' PMA (RR, 0.72; 95% CI, 0.63, 0.82). An increased risk of abnormal neurologic examination was seen, but not an increase in neurosensory impairment or cerebral palsy.

The Dexamethasone: A Randomized Trial (DART) study identified patients at high risk for BPD based on gestational age or birth weight (<28 weeks' PMA or <1000 g) and the need for mechanical ventilation after postnatal day 7.[61] Study infants were randomized to dexamethasone or placebo; 60% of those who received dexamethasone (21 of 35) were extubated by the 10th day of treatment compared with 12% (4 of 34) in the placebo group. Rates of mortality before follow-up, major disability, cerebral palsy, or the combined outcomes of death or cerebral palsy were not substantially different between groups. Furthermore, the incidence of BPD was 85% in the dexamethasone group and 91% in the placebo group.[62]

For infants at high risk of developing BPD, corticosteroids might reduce the risk of BPD and cerebral palsy. In a meta-regression analysis, Doyle and colleagues[63] reviewed the results of available randomized controlled trials of postnatal corticosteroids and determined the risk of BPD and cerebral palsy in the control groups. They found that the risk of cerebral palsy increased with the use of corticosteroids; however, a significant effect measure modification was seen among the groups with BPD. As the risk of BPD increased (>65%), postnatal steroids reduced the risk of death or cerebral palsy.

Given the potential for risks and benefits to the neurodevelopment of premature infants, the American Academy of Pediatrics Committee[64] on Fetus and Newborn recently recommended in a revised policy statement:

"High-dose dexamethasone (0.5 mg/kg per day) does not seem to confer additional therapeutic benefit over lower doses and is not recommended. Evidence is insufficient to make a recommendation regarding other glucocorticoid doses and preparations. The clinician must use clinical judgment when attempting to balance the potential adverse effects of glucocorticoid treatment with those of bronchopulmonary dysplasia."

PDA

The role of the PDA in the development of BPD in preterm infants remains controversial. The presence of a PDA has been associated with the need for prolonged mechanical ventilation, increased mortality, and a higher risk of BPD.[65,66] However, the relationship between PDA and BPD is often distorted by confounding factors, such as gestational age and illness severity, and might not be causal.[67]

In a randomized clinical trial by Schmidt and colleagues[65] (Trial of Indomethacin Prophylaxis in Preterms [TIPP]), infants who received indomethacin prophylaxis had a decreased incidence of PDA (21% vs 49%; P value <.05); however, the incidence of BPD was similar between groups (45% vs 43%; P = .41). Indomethacin prophylaxis in this cohort increased the supplemental oxygen use from day 3 to day 7, decreased urine output during the first 4 days of life, and reduced weight loss by the end of the first week of life. Among infants who did not develop a PDA following prophylactic indomethacin, treatment was associated with a higher incidence of BPD (43% vs 30%; P = .015). These finding suggest that the early side effects of indomethacin may contribute to the increased risk of BPD in the treatment group.

Even when nonpharmacologic therapies are used to close the PDA, the risk for BPD is increased among treated infants. In a randomized trial of prophylactic PDA ligation among infants weighing less than 1000 g, Clyman and colleagues[68] found an increased incidence of BPD (defined as supplemental oxygen at 36 weeks) and need for mechanical ventilation at 36 weeks among infants who underwent surgical ligation within 24 hours of birth. In addition, the development of BPD in the control group was confined to infants who ultimately needed surgical ligation (after 24 hours). They concluded that closure of the PDA via surgical ligation increases the risk of BPD.

Previous studies to assess the role of ductal closure in the prevention of morbidities such as BPD have had small sample sizes. Meta-analysis has consistently shown no decrease in the risk of BPD with closure of the PDA.[69–71] In a recent systematic review, Benitz[67] reviewed all available randomized controlled trials to create a pooled point estimate for the associations between PDA closure and multiple morbidities. The pooled estimate showed a strong effect of ductal closure with pharmacologic therapies (OR, 0.23; 95% CI, 0.20, 0.26), but a nonsignificant effect on the incidence of BPD and BPD or death.[72] It is likely that the presence of a PDA is a marker for an increased risk of BPD. However, the large rate of crossover and the design of these studies makes the risks and benefits of strategies designed to close the PDA challenging to assess.

Supplemental Oxygen

For most infants, exposure to supplemental oxygen often begins in the delivery room. In a Cochrane meta-analysis of studies comparing resuscitation with 100% oxygen to resuscitation with room air in term and near-term infants, resuscitation performed with room air resulted in lower mortality than in those resuscitated with 100% oxygen (RR, 0.71).[73] However, among preterm infants the role of supplemental oxygen therapy in the delivery room is less clear. In a study of 78 infants born at 24–28 weeks gestation randomized to receive initial resuscitation with either 30% or 90% oxygen, Vento et al[74] found a lower incidence of BPD in infants randomized to receive initial resuscitation with 30% as compared to 90% oxygen (15.4% vs 31.7%, P<0.05). In a randomized controlled trials of room air versus oxygen administration for the delivery room resuscitation of preterm infants less than 32 weeks' gestation (Room Air vs Oxygen Administration During Resuscitation of Preterm Infants [ROAR] study), no difference was seen in the outcomes of BPD or death among infants treated with either room air, titrated oxygen therapy, or static 100% oxygen.[75] Although the use of oxygen for preterm infants in the delivery room does not seem to influence the development of BPD, limiting the use of supplemental oxygen when possible would seem prudent.

Supplemental oxygen has been implicated as a potential toxin for the developing lung and brain.[76] Infants who require high amounts of oxygen may represent a more ill group of infants for whom gas exchange is already impaired at the alveolar level. However, oxygen can also produce oxidative injury to capillary, endothelial, and alveolar membranes. Prior studies have indicated that high levels of oxygen exposure result in increased polymorphonuclear cell migration, increased proteolysis, and elevated levels of inflammatory cytokines.[77,78] Yet, oxygen therapy is often necessary in premature infants to prevent hypoxemia, and oxygen may be important for cell growth and development. In the Benefits Of Oxygen Saturation Targeting trial (BOOST-I), infants born at less than 30 weeks' gestation who were randomized to higher oxygen saturations (95%–98%) compared with standard oxygen saturations (92%–94%) at 32 weeks' corrected gestation remained on oxygen therapy at 36 weeks' corrected gestation more often (OR, 1.40; 95% CI, 1.15, 1.70). However, no difference was seen in the growth or development at 12 months between the groups.[79]

The need for supplemental oxygen therapy can be a marker of severe illness and is therefore associated with an increased risk of BPD. In the Surfactant, Positive Pressure, and Pulse Oximetry Randomized Trial (SUPPORT), one arm examined the effect of target ranges of oxygen saturations in extremely preterm infants. Infants who were randomized to lower oxygen saturations (85%–89%) and those who were randomized to higher oxygen saturations (91%–95%) had similar rates of BPD among survivors

(48.5% vs 54.2%; RR, 0.91; 95% CI, 0.83–1.01).[80] Furthermore, the SUPPORT trial reported increased mortality in the lower oxygen saturation group. These findings suggest that the role of oxygen in the development of BPD for preterm infants may be linked to the severity of illness rather than direct oxygen toxicity.

Vitamin A

Vitamin A is involved in multiple activities at the cellular level, including regulating gene transcription, signaling in embryonic development, and as a potent antioxidant. These functions are likely impaired in premature infants who exhibit vitamin A deficiency. Treatment with vitamin A replacement therapy decreases the risk of BPD or death by 36 weeks' PMA in infants weighing less than 1000 g who remain on respiratory support at 24 hours of life (RR, 0.89; 95% CI, 0.80–0.99).[81] The supplementation was noted to increase serum vitamin A levels without increasing the risk of toxicity. The use of vitamin A in VLBW infants has been hampered recently because of national shortages and lack of availability at many centers.[82]

Caffeine

The use of caffeine for the treatment of apnea of prematurity has been shown to decrease the risk of BPD, although the mechanisms of action are not clear. Caffeine has been shown to increase carbon dioxide chemoreceptor responsiveness, increase respiratory muscle performance, and generally increase central nervous system excitability.[83–85] In the Caffeine for Apnea of Prematurity (CAP) trial, the infants randomized to caffeine therapy had a lower incidence of BPD (36% vs 47%; adjusted OR, 0.64; 95% CI, 0.52–0.78), as defined by oxygen need at 36 weeks' PMA.[86]

Sepsis and the Systemic Inflammatory Response

Sepsis and the systemic inflammatory response increase the likelihood of BPD in premature infants. Several pathogens have been associated with the development of BPD, including *Ureaplasma urealyticum*, cytomegalovirus, and adenovirus.[87–89] The direct role that these pathogens play in the development of BPD is unclear, but is thought to be related to the systemic inflammatory response. The inflammatory response in the lung results in production of proinflammatory cytokines, migration of polymorphonuclear leukocytes, and changes in vascular permeability.[90,91] The presence of these factors likely causes immediate damage to alveoli and capillaries, but also may be related to the long-term arrest of alveolarization seen in infants with BPD.

PREDICTIVE MODELS OF BPD

In the past decade, researchers have developed predictive models for long-term morbidities, such as neurodevelopmental impairment. Schmidt and colleagues[92] examined the impact of BPD, brain injury, and severe retinopathy on 18-month outcomes and determined that the incidence of poor long-term outcomes increased with the presence of one, two, or all three neonatal morbidities. Tyson and colleagues[93] examined infants in the Neonatal Research Network and determined that exposure to antenatal corticosteroids, female sex, singleton birth, and higher birth weight (per 100-g increment) were each associated with reductions in the risk of death and the risk of death or neurodevelopmental impairment. The authors developed a simple Web-based predictive tool (www.nichd.nih.gov/neonatalestimates) that helps clinicians estimate the likelihood that intensive care will benefit individual infants.

Clinicians, parents, and researchers would benefit from an accurate predictive model of BPD risk based on readily available clinical information. Prediction scoring systems have been described for BPD and have included birthweight, gestational age, sex, PDA, sepsis, and exposure to mechanical ventilation, but until recently have not been readily available or adopted. In many of these scoring systems, death was not included as a competing outcome for BPD.[94–96] Some included radiographs as part of the scoring system, which introduces subjectivity and reduces generalizability.[97–100] Several used respiratory parameters that are not readily available to clinicians.[101,102] Despite generally good negative predictive values, the positive predictive values of these predictive models are low (range, 65%–75%).[97–104] Other significant problems were the absence of a contemporary cohort that included a high proportion of infants receiving antenatal corticosteroids and surfactant therapy.[98] None examined the risk of BPD based on the NICHD severity-based system.

An additional problem with previously reported analyses is a lack of detail regarding the change in BPD risk with advancing postnatal age.[94–96,98] Prior multivariable models included risk factors identifiable at birth, and exposures up to the time of diagnosis of BPD, but do not include postnatal age. The inclusion of postnatal age allows for the variable contribution of risk factors over time as potential preventative or therapeutic strategies that may be used to decrease the risk of BPD.

Laughon and colleagues[40] recently developed a predictive model using data from the NICHD Neonatal Research Network Benchmarking Trial, which is available online at https://neonatal.rti.org. This model incorporates gestational age, birthweight, race and ethnicity, sex, respiratory support, and fractional of inspired oxygen in a parsimonious model, providing estimates of severity of BPD or death by postnatal day. Several previously described risk factors—PDA, necrotizing enterocolitis, sepsis, and postnatal corticosteroids—did not significantly improve the prediction of BPD after adjustment for the other six factors. For example, a white male infant born at 26 weeks (birthweight, 750 g) who at day seven of life is on continuous positive airway pressure with an oxygen requirement of 35% has a 19.9% probability of having severe BPD, 34.2% probability for moderate BPD, 28.6% probability for mild BPD, and 10.2% probability for no BPD. An important feature of this model is that the relative contribution of each predicting factor changes with increasing postnatal age. In the postnatal day one and three models, gestational age provides the most information, whereas at later time points, mechanical ventilation conveys the most predictive information.

SUMMARY

The development of bronchopulmonary dysplasia is the result of the complex interactions between multiple perinatal and postnatal factors. Although predictive factors for BPD are easy to identify, they are often difficult to modify. Early identification of infants at the greatest risk of developing BPD through the use of estimators and models may allow a targeted approach for reducing BPD in the future.

REFERENCES

1. Cotten CM, Oh W, McDonald S, et al. Prolonged hospital stay for extremely premature infants: risk factors, center differences, and the impact of mortality on selecting a best-performing center. J Perinatol 2005;25:650–5.
2. Katz-Salamon M, Gerner EM, Jonsson B, et al. Early motor and mental development in very preterm infants with chronic lung disease. Arch Dis Child Fetal Neonatal Ed 2000;83:F1–6.
3. McAleese KA, Knapp MA, Rhodes TT. Financial and emotional cost of bronchopulmonary dysplasia. Clin Pediatr 1993;32:393–400.

4. Gough A, Spence D, Linden M, et al. General and respiratory health outcomes in adult survivors of bronchopulmonary dysplasia: a systematic review. Chest 2012;141(6):1554–67.

5. Hintz SR, Poole WK, Wright LL, et al. Changes in mortality and morbidities among infants born at less than 25 weeks during the post-surfactant era. Arch Dis Child Fetal Neonatal Ed 2005;90:F128–33.

6. Berger TM, Bachmann II, Adams M, et al. Impact of improved survival of very low-birth-weight infants on incidence and severity of bronchopulmonary dysplasia. Biol Neonate 2004;86:124–30.

7. Northway WH, Rosan RC, Porter DY. Pulmonary disease following respirator therapy of hyaline-membrane disease. N Engl J Med 1967;276:357–68.

8. Bancalari E. Barotrauma to the lung. In: Milunsky A, editor. Advances in perinatal medicine. New York: Plenum; 1982. p. 165.

9. Bancalari E, Gerhardt T. Bronchopulmonary dysplasia. Pediatr Clin North Am 1986;33:1–23.

10. Coalson JJ, Winter V, deLemos RA. Decreased alveolarization in baboon survivors with bronchopulmonary dysplasia. Am J Respir Crit Care Med 1995;152:640–6.

11. Jobe AJ. The new BPD: an arrest of lung development. Pediatr Res 1999;46: 641–3.

12. Stoelhorst GM, Rijken M, Martens SE, et al. Changes in neonatology: comparison of two cohorts of very preterm infants (gestational age <32 weeks): the Project On Preterm and Small for Gestational Age Infants 1983 and the Leiden Follow-Up Project on Prematurity 1996-1997. Pediatrics 2005;115:396–405.

13. Wadhawan R, Vohr BR, Fanaroff AA, et al. Does labor influence neonatal and neurodevelopmental outcomes of extremely-low-birth-weight infants who are born by cesarean delivery? Am J Obstet Gynecol 2003;189:501–6.

14. Jobe AH, Bancalari E. Bronchopulmonary dysplasia. Am J Respir Crit Care Med 2001;163:1723–9.

15. Ehrenkranz RA, Walsh MC, Vohr BR, et al. Validation of the National Institutes of Health consensus definition of bronchopulmonary dysplasia. Pediatrics 2005; 116:1353–60.

16. Walsh MC, Yao Q, Gettner P, et al. Impact of a physiologic definition on bronchopulmonary dysplasia rates. Pediatrics 2004;114:1305–11.

17. Natarajan G, Pappas A, Shankaran S, et al. Outcomes of extremely low birth weight infants with bronchopulmonary dysplasia: impact of the physiologic definition. Early Hum Dev 2012;88(7):509–15.

18. Stewart A, Brion LP, Soll R. Diuretics for respiratory distress syndrome in preterm infants. Cochrane Database Syst Rev 2011;(12):CD001454.

19. Massie SE, Tolleson-Rinehart S, DeWalt DA, et al. Development of a proxy-reported pulmonary outcome scale for preterm infants with bronchopulmonary dysplasia. Health Qual Life Outcomes 2011;9:55.

20. Fletcher R, Fletcher S. Clinical epidemiology. 4th edition. Philadelphia: Lippincott Williams & Wilkins; 2005.

21. Rothman K, Greenland S, Lash T. Modern epidemiology. 3rd edition. Philadelphia: Lippincott Williams & Wilkins; 2008. p. 51–70.

22. Greenland S, Robins JM. Identifiability, exchangeability, and epidemiological confounding. Int J Epidemiol 1986;15:413–9.

23. Bradford-Hill A. The environment and disease: association or causation? Proc R Soc Med 1965;58:295–300.

24. Marshall DD, Kotelchuck M, Young TE, et al. Risk factors for chronic lung disease in the surfactant era: a North Carolina population-based study of very

low birth weight infants. North Carolina Neonatologists Association. Pediatrics 1999;104:1345–50.

25. Oh W, Poindexter BB, Perritt R, et al. Association between fluid intake and weight loss during the first ten days of life and risk of bronchopulmonary dysplasia in extremely low birth weight infants. J Pediatr 2005;147:786–90.

26. Ambalavanan N, Van Meurs KP, Perritt R, et al. Predictors of death or bronchopulmonary dysplasia in preterm infants with respiratory failure. J Perinatol 2008; 28:420–6.

27. Rojas MA, Gonzalez A, Bancalari E, et al. Changing trends in the epidemiology and pathogenesis of neonatal chronic lung disease. J Pediatr 1995;126:605–10.

28. Crowley P. The effects of corticosteroid administration before preterm delivery: an overview of the evidence from controlled trials. Br J Obstet Gynaecol 1990;97:11–25.

29. Gilstrap LC, Christensen R, Clewell WH, et al. Effect of corticosteroids for fetal maturation on perinatal outcomes. JAMA 1995;273:413–8.

30. Van Marter LJ. Maternal glucocorticoid therapy and reduced risk of bronchopulmonary dysplasia. Pediatrics (Evanston) 1990;86:331–6.

31. Van Marter LJ, Allred EN, Leviton A, et al. Antenatal glucocorticoid treatment does not reduce chronic lung disease among surviving preterm infants. J Pediatrics 2001;138:198–204.

32. Roberts D, Dalziel S. Antenatal corticosteroids for accelerating fetal lung maturation for women at risk of preterm birth. Cochrane Database Syst Rev 2006;Jul 19(3):CD004454.

33. Been JV, Zimmermann LJ. Histological chorioamnionitis and respiratory outcome in preterm infants. Arch Dis Child Fetal Neonatal Ed 2009;94:F218–25.

34. Dempsey E. Outcome of neonates less than 30 weeks gestation with histologic chorioamnionitis. Am J Perinatol 2005;22:155–9.

35. Richardson BS. Preterm histologic chorioamnionitis: impact on cord gas and pH values and neonatal outcome. Am J Obstet Gynecol 2006;195:1357–65.

36. Mu SC. Impact on neonatal outcome and anthropometric growth in very low birth weight infants with histological chorioamnionitis. J Formos Med Assoc 2008;107:304–10.

37. De Felice C. Histologic chorioamnionitis and severity of illness in very low birth weight newborns. Pediatr Crit Care Med 2005;6:298–302.

38. Hartling L, Liang Y, Lacaze-Masmonteil T. Chorioamnionitis as a risk factor for bronchopulmonary dysplasia: a systematic review and meta-analysis. Arch Dis Child Fetal Neonatal Ed 2012;97:F8–17.

39. Bose C, Van Marter LJ, Laughon M, et al. Fetal growth restriction and chronic lung disease among infants born before the 28th week of gestation. Pediatrics 2009;124:e450–8.

40. Laughon MM, Langer JC, Bose CL, et al. Prediction of bronchopulmonary dysplasia by postnatal age in extremely premature infants. Am J Respir Crit Care Med 2011;183:1715–22.

41. Stoll BJ, Hansen NI, Bell EF, et al. Neonatal outcomes of extremely preterm infants from the NICHD Neonatal Research Network. Pediatrics 2010;126: 443–56.

42. Lemons JA, Bauer CR, Oh W, et al. Very low birth weight outcomes of the National Institute of Child health and human development neonatal research network, January 1995 through December 1996. Pediatrics 2001;107:e1.

43. Charafeddine L, D'Angio CT, Phelps DL. Atypical chronic lung disease patterns in neonates. Pediatrics 1999;103:759–65.

44. Panickar J, Scholefield H, Kumar Y, et al. Atypical chronic lung disease in preterm infants. J Perinat Med 2004;32:162–7.

45. Choi CW, Kim BI, Koh YY, et al. Clinical characteristics of chronic lung disease without preceding respiratory distress syndrome in preterm infants. Pediatr Int 2005;47:72–9.

46. Choi CW, Kim BI, Park JD, et al. Risk factors for the different types of chronic lung diseases of prematurity according to the preceding respiratory distress syndrome. Pediatr Int 2005;47:417–23.

47. Streubel AH, Donohue PK, Aucott SW. The epidemiology of atypical chronic lung disease in extremely low birth weight infants. J Perinatol 2008;28:141–8.

48. Kobaly K, Schluchter M, Minich N, et al. Outcomes of extremely low birth weight (<1 kg) and extremely low gestational age (<28 weeks) infants with bronchopulmonary dysplasia: effects of practice changes in 2000 to 2003. Pediatrics 2008;121:73–81.

49. Laughon M, Allred EN, Bose C, et al. Patterns of respiratory disease during the first 2 postnatal weeks in extremely premature infants. Pediatrics 2009;123:1124–31.

50. Merrill JD, Ballard RA, Cnaan A, et al. Dysfunction of pulmonary surfactant in chronically ventilated premature infants. Pediatr Res 2004;56:918–26.

51. Muscedere JG, Mullen JB, Gan K, et al. Tidal ventilation at low airway pressures can augment lung injury. Am J Respir Crit Care Med 1994;149:1327–34.

52. Meredith KS, deLemos RA, Coalson JJ, et al. Role of lung injury in the pathogenesis of hyaline membrane disease in premature baboons. J Appl Phys 1989;66:2150–8.

53. Avery ME, Tooley WH, Keller JB, et al. Is chronic lung disease in low birth weight infants preventable? A survey of eight centers. Pediatrics 1987;79:26–30.

54. Van Marter LJ, Allred EN, Pagano M, et al. Do clinical markers of barotrauma and oxygen toxicity explain interhospital variation in rates of chronic lung disease? The Neonatology Committee for the Developmental Network. Pediatrics 2000;105:1194–201.

55. Walsh M, Laptook A, Kazzi SN, et al. A cluster-randomized trial of benchmarking and multimodal quality improvement to improve rates of survival free of bronchopulmonary dysplasia for infants with birth weights of less than 1250 grams. Pediatrics 2007;119:876–90.

56. Leone TA, Rich W, Finer NN. A survey of delivery room resuscitation practices in the United States. Pediatrics 2006;117:e164–75.

57. Morley CJ, Davis PG, Doyle LW, et al. Nasal CPAP or intubation at birth for very preterm infants. N Engl J Med 2008;358:700–8.

58. Finer NN, Carlo WA, Duara S, et al. Delivery room continuous positive airway pressure/positive end-expiratory pressure in extremely low birth weight infants: a feasibility trial. Pediatrics 2004;114:651–7.

59. Halliday HL, Ehrenkranz RA, Doyle LW. Early (< 8 days) postnatal corticosteroids for preventing chronic lung disease in preterm infants. Cochrane Database Syst Rev 2009;(1):CD001146.

60. Halliday HL, Ehrenkranz RA, Doyle LW. Late (>7 days) postnatal corticosteroids for chronic lung disease in preterm infants. Cochrane Database Syst Rev 2009;(1):CD001145.

61. Doyle LW, Davis PG, Morley CJ, et al. Low-dose dexamethasone facilitates extubation among chronically ventilator-dependent infants: a multicenter, international, randomized, controlled trial. Pediatrics 2006;117:75–83.

62. Doyle LW, Davis PG, Morley CJ, et al. Outcome at 2 years of age of infants from the DART study: a multicenter, international, randomized, controlled trial of low-dose dexamethasone. Pediatrics 2007;119:716–21.

63. Doyle LW, Halliday HL, Ehrenkranz RA, et al. Impact of postnatal systemic corti-costeroids on mortality and cerebral palsy in preterm infants: effect modification by risk for chronic lung disease. Pediatrics 2005;115:655–61.

64. American Academy of Pediatrics. Policy Statement: Postnatal steroids to Prevent or Treat Bronchopulmonary Dysplasia. Committee on Fetus and Newborn. Pediatrics 2010;126:800–8.

65. Schmidt B, Davis P, Moddemann D, et al. Long-term effects of indomethacin prophylaxis in extremely-low-birth-weight infants. N Engl J Med 2001;344: 1966–72.

66. Brown ER. Increased risk of bronchopulmonary dysplasia in infants with patent ductus arteriosus. J Pediatr 1979;95:865–6.

67. Benitz WE. Patent ductus arteriosus: to treat or not to treat? Arch Dis Child Fetal Neonatal Ed 2012;97:F80–2.

68. Clyman R, Cassady G, Kirklin JK, et al. The role of patent ductus arteriosus liga-tion in bronchopulmonary dysplasia: reexamining a randomized controlled trial. J Pediatr 2009;154:873–6.

69. Fowlie PW, Davis PG. Prophylactic intravenous indomethacin for preventing mortality and morbidity in preterm infants. Cochrane Database Syst Rev 2002;(3):CD000174.

70. Cooke L, Steer P, Woodgate P. Indomethacin for asymptomatic patent ductus arteriosus in preterm infants. Cochrane Database Syst Rev 2003;(2):CD003745.

71. Shah SS, Ohlsson A. Ibuprofen for the prevention of patent ductus arteriosus in preterm and/or low birth weight infants. Cochrane Database Syst Rev 2006;(1):CD004213.

72. Benitz WE. Treatment of persistent patent ductus arteriosus in preterm infants: time to accept the null hypothesis? J Perinatol 2010;30:241–52.

73. Tan A, Schulze A, O'Donnell CP, et al. Air versus oxygen for resuscitation of infants at birth. Cochrane Database Syst Rev 2005;(2):CD002273.

74. Vento M, Moro M, Escrig R, et al. Preterm resuscitation with low oxygen causes less oxidative stress, inflammation, and chronic lung disease. Pediatrics 2009; 124:e439–49.

75. Rabi Y, Singhal N, Nettel-Aguirre A. Room-air versus oxygen administration for resuscitation of preterm infants: the ROAR study. Pediatrics 2011;128:e374–81.

76. Saugstad OD. Chronic lung disease: the role of oxidative stress. Biol Neonate 1998;74(Suppl 1):21–8.

77. Ogihara T, Hirano K, Morinobu T, et al. Raised concentrations of aldehyde lipid peroxidation products in premature infants with chronic lung disease. Arch Dis Child Fetal Neonatal Ed 1999;80:F21–5.

78. Delacourt C, d'Ortho MP, Macquin-Mavier I, et al. Oxidant-antioxidant balance in alveolar macrophages from newborn rats. Eur Respir J 1996;9:2517–24.

79. Askie LM, Henderson-Smart DJ, Irwig L, et al. Oxygen-saturation targets and outcomes in extremely preterm infants. N Engl J Med 2003;349:959–67.

80. Carlo WA, Finer NN, Walsh MC, et al. Target ranges of oxygen saturation in extremely preterm infants. N Engl J Med 2010;362:1959–69.

81. Tyson JE, Wright LL, Oh W, et al. Vitamin A supplementation for extremely-low-birth-weight infants. N Engl J Med 1999;340:1962–8.

82. Kaplan HC. Understanding variation in vitamin A supplementation among NICUs. Pediatrics (Evanston) 2010;126:e367–73.

83. Bairam A. Interactive ventilatory effects of two respiratory stimulants, caffeine and doxapram, in newborn lambs. Biol Neonate 1992;61:201–8.

84. Kassim Z. Effect of caffeine on respiratory muscle strength and lung function in prematurely born, ventilated infants. Eur J Pediatr 2009;168:1491–5.

85. Henderson-Smart DJ. Prophylactic methylxanthines for endotracheal extubation in preterm infants. Cochrane Database Syst Rev 2010;(12):CD000139.

86. Schmidt B, Roberts RS, Davis P, et al. Caffeine therapy for apnea of prematurity. N Engl J Med 2006;354:2112–21.

87. Hannaford K, Todd DA, Jeffery H, et al. Role of ureaplasma urealyticum in lung disease of prematurity. Arch Dis Child Fetal Neonatal Ed 1999;81:F162–7.

88. Ollikainen J, Heiskanen-Kosma T, Korppi M, et al. Clinical relevance of urea-plasma urealyticum colonization in preterm infants. Acta Paediatr 1998;87:1075–8.

89. Sawyer MH, Edwards DK, Spector SA. Cytomegalovirus infection and broncho-pulmonary dysplasia in premature infants. Am J Dis Child 1987;141:303–5.

90. Wynn J, Cornell TT, Wong HR, et al. The host response to sepsis and develop-mental impact. Pediatrics 2010;125:1031–41.

91. Cornell TT, Wynn J, Shanley TP, et al. Mechanisms and regulation of the gene-expression response to sepsis. Pediatrics 2010;125:1248–58.

92. Schmidt B, Asztalos EV, Roberts RS, et al. Impact of bronchopulmonary dysplasia, brain injury, and severe retinopathy on the outcome of extremely low-birth-weight infants at 18 months: results from the trial of indomethacin prophylaxis in preterms. JAMA 2003;289:1124–9.

93. Tyson JE, Parikh NA, Langer J, et al. Intensive care for extreme prematurity—moving beyond gestational age. N Engl J Med 2008;358:1672–81.

94. Ryan SW, Nycyk J, Shaw BN. Prediction of chronic neonatal lung disease on day 4 of life. Eur J Pediatr 1996;155:668–71.

95. Subhedar NV, Hamdan AH, Ryan SW, et al. Pulmonary artery pressure: early predictor of chronic lung disease in preterm infants. Arch Dis Child 1998;78:F20–4.

96. Romagnoli C, Zecca E, Tortorolo L, et al. A scoring system to predict the evolu-tion of respiratory distress syndrome into chronic lung disease in preterm infants. Intensive Care Med 1998;24:476–80.

97. Toce SS, Farrell PM, Leavitt LA, et al. Clinical and roentgenographic scoring systems for assessing bronchopulmonary dysplasia. Am J Dis Child 1984;138:581–5.

98. Corcoran JD, Patterson CC, Thomas PS, et al. Reduction in the risk of broncho-pulmonary dysplasia from 1980-1990: results of a multivariate logistic regres-sion analysis. Eur J Pediatr 1993;152:677–81.

99. Noack G, Mortensson W, Robertson B, et al. Correlations between radiological and cytological findings in early development of bronchopulmonary dysplasia. Eur J Pediatr 1993;152:1024–9.

100. Yuksel B, Greenough A, Karani J. Prediction of chronic lung disease from the chest radiograph appearance at seven days of age. Acta Paediatr 1993;82:944–7.

101. Bhutani VK, Abbasi S. Relative likelihood of bronchopulmonary dysplasia based on pulmonary mechanics measured in preterm neonates during the first week of life. J Pediatr 1992;120:605–13.

102. Kim YD, Kim EA, Kim KS, et al. Scoring method for early prediction of neonatal chronic lung disease using modified respiratory parameters. J Korean Med Sci 2005;20:397–401.

103. Sinkin RA, Cox C, Phelps DL. Predicting risk for bronchopulmonary dysplasia: selection criteria for clinical trials. Pediatrics 1990;86:728–36.
104. Rozycki HJ, Narla L. Early versus late identification of infants at high risk of developing moderate to severe bronchopulmonary dysplasia. Pediatr Pulmonol 1996;21:345–52.

Clinical Effectiveness and Safety of Permissive Hypercapnia

Julie Ryu, MD[a], Gabriel Haddad, MD[b], Waldemar A. Carlo, MD[c],*

KEYWORDS

- Hypercapnia/physiopathology • Infant, premature
- Positive-pressure respiration/methods • Respiration, artificial
- Respiratory distress syndrome, newborn/therapy • Respiratory mechanics/physiology • Ventilator-induced lung injury/physiopathology
- Ventilator-induced lung injury/prevention & control

KEY POINTS

- Ventilator–induced lung injury remains an important cause of neonatal morbidity.
- Permissive hypercapnia is a ventilatory strategy that may reduce injury to the developing lung through a variety of mechanisms. Literature on physiology rationale, experimental research, and clinical trials suggest that permissive hypercapnia may be beneficial in preterm neonates.
- Taken together, 7 trials suggest that a strategy of permissive hypercapnia started early, before the initiation of mechanical ventilation, combined with prolonged permissive hypercapnia during mechanical ventilation optimizes pulmonary/survival benefits and seems to be safe in neonates.
- Data from clinical trials support the use of permissive hypercapnia as an alternative to traditional ventilator support strategies that aim to maintain normocapnia.
- Further research is necessary to elucidate better strategies of permissive hypercapnia such as target carbon dioxide levels, duration of the intervention, and minimal tidal volume ventilation.

INTRODUCTION

Advances in perinatal care, such as antenatal steroids, surfactant replacement, and improvement in ventilatory support, have reduced mortality of preterm infants.[1] However, improved survival has also resulted in an increase in bronchopulmonary

The authors have nothing to disclose and no potential conflicts of interest.
[a] Department of Pediatrics, Rady Children's Hospital, University of California San Diego, 9500 Gilman Drive, MC 0735, La Jolla, CA 92093, USA; [b] Department of Pediatrics, Rady Children's Hospital, University of California San Diego, 9500 Gilman Drive, La Jolla, CA 92093-0735, USA; [c] Division of Neonatology, Department of Pediatrics, Women and Infants Center, University of Alabama at Birmingham, 1700 6th Avenue South, 176F Suite 9380, Birmingham, AL 35249-7335, USA
* Corresponding author.
E-mail address: wcarlo@peds.uab.edu

dysplasia (BPD).[1] Lung injury, including ventilator-induced lung injury, remains an important cause of neonatal morbidity and may lead to the development of BPD.[2] Ventilator strategies that minimize lung injury may improve respiratory outcomes in preterm infants and increase survival. One such strategy to reduce lung injury, called *permissive hypercapnia*, depends on the use of higher carbon dioxide tension (Pco$_2$) targets while using lower tidal volumes.[3] Permissive hypercapnia may reduce the risk of lung injury by multiple mechanisms as discussed later.

PHYSIOLOGIC ADVANTAGES OF HYPERCAPNIC ACIDOSIS

A ventilator management strategy that permits hypercapnia has several physiologic effects on gas exchange, cardiac output, and respiratory drive that together may be beneficial. The increase in alveolar CO_2 that occurs during permissive hypercapnia increases CO_2 elimination for the same minute ventilation based on the equation $K \cdot VCO_2 = PaCO_2 \cdot Va$.

In this equation, K is a constant, VCO_2 is CO_2 elimination, Pa_{CO_2} is alveolar CO_2, and Va is alveolar ventilation. If the Pa_{CO_2} is allowed to increase and alveolar ventilation is kept constant, CO_2 elimination will increase. Therefore, a clinician can use lower tidal volumes and peak inspiratory pressures (decreasing alveolar ventilation) and allow the Pa_{CO_2} to increase, yet maintain effective CO_2 removal. The hyperbolic relationship between Pa_{CO_2} and minute ventilation permits effective CO_2 removal at a lower-than-expected amount of alveolar ventilation.[4] Aside from increasing the efficiency of CO_2 removal, therapeutic hypercapnia can improve ventilation-perfusion matching in the lung.[5,6] In addition, hypercapnic acidosis permits more unloading of oxygen to the tissues because of the rightward shift of the oxygen dissociation curve (Bohr effect). Another physiologic advantage is stabilization or increase in respiratory drive, resulting in less apnea[7] that can facilitate weaning an infant off the ventilator.[8,9] In animals and humans, both therapeutic hypercapnia and permissive hypercapnia have been shown to increase overall cardiac output[10,11] probably because of an increase in peripheral vascular resistance.[12] Furthermore, as tidal volume and peak inspiratory pressure are lowered, mean airway pressure decreases, which may also improve preload and cardiac output.[13–15]

EXPERIMENTAL STUDIES IN SUPPORT OF HYPERCAPNIA

Experimental studies demonstrate that mechanical ventilation can cause lung injury both in adult and infant lungs. Regardless of the pressures used, markers of lung injury (pulmonary edema, epithelial injury, hyaline membranes, filtration coefficient, and lymphatic flow) are increased with the use of high tidal volumes but not with the use of low tidal volumes (**Table 1**).[16–19] Ventilation of immature animals with large tidal volumes immediately after birth decreases lung compliance.[20,21] Inflation of the lung to volumes higher than total lung capacity can lead to lung injury.[22] Repeated collapse and reopening of the alveoli during the breath cycle can also result in lung injury.[23] Ventilatory strategies that focus on avoiding large tidal volumes as well as repeated collapse and reopening of alveoli may minimize lung injury (**Fig. 1**). However, decreasing tidal volume decreases minute ventilation for a given ventilatory rate and leads to an increase in Pco$_2$. Experimental and clinical research is being conducted to determine if permissive hypercapnia is a safe and effective strategy in preterm infants.

Several experimental studies support the evaluation of hypercapnia in the clinical setting, not only as a consequence of volutrauma minimizing strategies but also as a therapeutic tool to reduce lung injury. Thus, it is important to distinguish between permissive hypercapnia (the presence of hypercapnia in the setting of ventilated patients being managed with low minute ventilation) and therapeutic hypercapnia

Table 1
Tidal volume as a cause of lung injury

	Ventilation Mode		Symptoms of Lung Injury		
	Tidal Volume	Peak Pressure	Pulmonary Edema	Epithelial Injury	Hyaline Membrane
Control	High	High	Yes	Yes	Yes
Iron lung	High	Low	Yes	Yes	Yes
Chest Strapping	Low	High	No	No	No

(deliberate induction of hypercapnia by adding CO_2 to inspired gases).[24] Each intervention produces hypercapnic acidosis, but therapeutic hypercapnia allows researchers to experimentally test the independent effects of hypercapnic acidosis. For example, in an in vivo rabbit model of high tidal volume, ventilator-induced lung injury (25 mL/kg tidal volume in both experimental groups), therapeutic hypercapnia ($Paco_2$ 80–100 mm Hg vs 40 mm Hg) attenuated various measures of lung injury.[25] Similarly, in a rat model of endotoxin-induced lung injury in which lower volumes were used (4.5 mL/kg), therapeutic hypercapnia either before or after instillation of intratracheal endotoxin also reduced lung injury indices.[26] It is interesting to note that buffering hypercapnic acidosis to maintain normal pH may abrogate the protective effects of hypercapnic acidosis.[27] These studies demonstrate some of the potential benefits of hypercapnic acidosis per se in adult animal models in vivo. This finding is important because permissive hypercapnia, although decreasing the risk of lung injury caused by mechanical reasons (lung stretch), may also be beneficial because of the additive effects of hypercapnia independent of acidosis. Li and associates[28] investigated the effect of hypercapnia on overall growth characteristics, lung structure, and global gene expression in lungs of newborn mice exposed to 8% or 12% CO_2 for 2 weeks. Their research demonstrated a substantial number of genes with altered expression in mice exposed to 8% CO_2 but not in those exposed to 12% CO_2. Of particular interest was an increase in transcription of the genes encoding surfactant-associated protein A and B. These proteins, expressed in bronchial epithelial and type II alveolar cells, may contribute to host defense mechanisms in the lung. Overall growth (body weight), hemoglobin concentration, and lung alveolar development were normal in both the hypercapnia and control

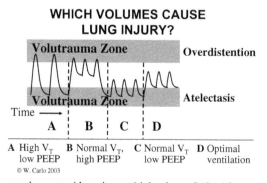

Fig. 1. Volutrauma may be caused by a large tidal volume (V_T) with or without low positive end expiratory pressure (PEEP) (A). A normal tidal volume with high PEEP (B) may also cause lung overdistention and volutrauma. A low PEEP (A, C) may cause repeated collapse and reopening of the alveoli, which also causes lung injury.

groups. Ryu and colleagues[29–31] have also demonstrated that exposure to hypercapnia alters lung structure and lung matrix composition independent of hypoxia or stretch exposure, a finding that has not been previously reported in adults, thus demonstrating that studies performed on the mature animal may not translate identically to the immature animal. Indeed, studies have also demonstrated that hypercapnia may attenuate hyperoxia-induced fibrosis in neonatal mice.

Studies that have investigated the effect of hypercapnia on the immune system have been mainly performed in animals or in vitro experiments using human cell lines. In vitro studies using exposure to high levels of CO_2 have been shown to suppress immune function through various mechanisms, including suppressing macrophage and neutrophil phagocytic function and cytokine signaling.[32,33] In vitro studies using human bronchial epithelial cells and alveolar type II cells also demonstrated poor wound healing when exposed to hypercapnia alone in a neutral pH environment.[34]

Innate immune signaling can inhibit structural lung development in experimental animal models.[35,36] Hypercapnic acidosis may enhance host defense mechanisms through altered gene expression and promote alveolar development in the developing lung. One of the benefits of hypercapnic acidosis demonstrated by in vivo animal studies is reduced neutrophil influx into the lung and reduced inflammatory cytokine production.[25,26,37] Such antiinflammatory effects of hypercapnic acidosis have also been studied in vitro using neutrophils and endothelial cells. Hypercapnia can affect various neutrophil functions, such as chemotaxis, by altering the ability of neutrophils to regulate intracellular pH.[38] Hypercapnic acidosis can also alter neutrophil adherence to pulmonary endothelial cells by decreasing the endothelial expression of the adhesion molecule intercellular adhesion molecule 1 (ICAM-1) and of the chemoattractant interleukin 8.[39] Furthermore, hypercapnic acidosis can decrease lipopolysaccharide (LPS)-stimulated secretion of the acute proinflammatory cytokine tumor necrosis factor alpha in isolated rat macrophages.[40] The proposed mechanism of decreased expression of ICAM-1 and inflammatory cytokines seems to be related to decreased activation of nuclear factor kappa beta, a key early regulator of gene expression in the innate immune response.[41] The ability of hypercapnic acidosis to modulate the innate immune response has important implications for lung development. Thus, hypercapnic acidosis also may be beneficial to the developing lung via its antiinflammatory and immune-modulating capabilities. However, more experimental research is needed to determine how hypercapnic acidosis can be optimized to protect the preterm lung.

Despite data that support hypercapnic acidosis as beneficial, some studies have reported neutral or negative results. Possible negative effects of hypercapnia on gas exchange include a small reduction in Pao$_2$ concentration caused by the increased Paco$_2$. This negative effect can be overcome with slight increases in the fraction of inspired oxygen to increase the alveolar oxygen concentration. Lang and associates[42] used intravenous LPS injection to mimic sepsis-related lung injury in adult rabbits and demonstrated that permissive hypercapnia contributed to lung injury via amplified oxidative injury. Hypercapnia may impair cell repair mechanisms after injury[43] and induce injury to alveolar epithelial cells by potentiating tissue nitration.[40] In an adult rabbit lung-injury model using saline lavage to cause surfactant deficiency, therapeutic hypercapnia did not improve oxygenation or attenuate lung injury (edema, compliance, airway pressure, or cytokine production) after high-volume ventilation (12 mL/kg vs 5 mL/kg of tidal volume).[28] Although a recent preliminary report suggested that therapeutic hypercapnia (5.5% inspired CO_2) could protect the neonatal rat lung from hyperoxic injury,[44] other investigators who used higher CO_2 concentrations (8% CO_2) did not report this benefit.[30]

Because of the beneficial results in adult randomized trials[45] and the association between hypocapnia and poor pulmonary and neurodevelopmental outcomes, permissive hypercapnia has emerged as a potential strategy to improve morbidity in neonates. Two retrospective studies in preterm neonates reported that higher $Paco_2$ values were associated with lower bronchopulmonary dysplasia rates.[46,47] Peak levels of $Paco_2$ greater than 50 mm Hg in the first 4 postnatal days and greater than 40 mm Hg before the administration of surfactant were associated with a lower incidence of BPD in these two studies. A population-based study of 407 infants younger than 28 weeks or less than 1000 g using historic controls also suggested that permissive hypercapnia resulted in a decreased rate of BPD.[48] Low $Paco_2$ values may reflect ventilator management strategies that result in overventilation in infants who have favorable lung compliance. This mechanism could be an important cause of lung injury, particularly in neonates who have less-severe lung disease. Thus, it is possible that ventilatory strategies that target mild hypercapnia or prevent hypocapnia result in reduced incidence or severity of lung injury.[49] Retrospective studies in neonates who have congenital diaphragmatic hernia, including the data on 1210 neonates from 53 centers of the Congenital Diaphragmatic Study Group, reported that permissive hypercapnia was associated with an increase in survival[50] and a decreased need for extracorporeal membrane oxygenation.[51]

Hypercapnia has been associated with an increased risk of impaired cerebral blood flow autoregulation and intracranial hemorrhage in neonates.[52] However, hypercapnic acidosis increases cerebral oxygen delivery,[53] and the CO_2-induced alterations in cerebral blood flow seem to be reversible.[54] A recent retrospective study of 849 infants weighing 1250 g or less revealed that severe hypocapnia, severe hypercapnia, and wide fluctuations in $Paco_2$ were associated with an increased risk of hemorrhage.[55] However, the randomized controlled trials of permissive hypercapnia in neonates have not reported an increase in intracranial hemorrhage.

ADULT CLINICAL STUDIES

The literature on the effect of permissive hypercapnia in adult humans is not uniform. There are many reasons why this is so. First, it is not evident what constitutes hypercapnia. Normal CO_2 levels range from 35 to 45 mm Hg, whereas CO_2 levels as extreme as 375 mm Hg for brief intervals (minutes)[56] have been reported without long-term consequences. The range from 45 to 375 mm Hg is vast, and the consequences are not equal and may not be linearly related. Furthermore, the timing and duration of hypercapnia varies. Thus, studies that use various strategies of hypercapnia may present different clinical findings depending on the level of hypercapnia used.

Treatment with low-tidal-volume (producing CO_2 levels of ~50 mm Hg) versus conventional ventilation (resulting CO_2 levels ranged from 35–38 mm Hg) had variable effects on survival rates in adults with acute respiratory distress syndrome (ARDS).[7,57,58] However, in a much larger randomized controlled trial, mortality was reduced by 22% in patients with ARDS who were ventilated with 6 mL/kg instead of 12 mL/kg, allowing the Pco_2 to increase to 45 ± 10 mm Hg.[59] In a Cochrane meta-analysis, outcomes from using tidal volumes of 7 versus 10 to 15 mL/kg in patients were inconclusive, but there was a trend toward decreased mortality at 28 days in the low-tidal-volume group.[45] In nature, hypercapnia is always associated with hypoxia and acidosis. However, with supplemental oxygen and medications, hypercapnia can exist independently or in conjunction with hypoxia and/or acidosis. When patients with ARDS were treated with low-tidal-volume ventilation but acidosis was corrected, the protective effects of stretch-limiting ventilation on mortality were lost.[60] In fact, it was suggested that hypercapnic acidosis may help attenuate stretch injury associated with the higher-tidal-volume group, as shown in experimental models.

NEONATAL CLINICAL STUDIES

Following controlled nonrandomized studies in neonates that suggested benefits of hypercapnia, 7 randomized controlled trials of permissive hypercapnia have been performed in preterm neonates. Permissive hypercapnia has been tested before initiation of mechanical ventilation, during ventilation, or both before and during ventilation. Various levels of permissive hypercapnia have been used, usually limited by a pH of at least 7.20.

The 3 trials (total of 1514 neonates) in which permissive hypercapnia was used before the initiation of mechanical ventilation reported trends for a reduction of BPD/death in the range of 5% to 7%.[61–63] In contrast, the 3 small trials (total of 334 neonates) in which permissive hypercapnia was used for a limited time period (4–10 days) during mechanical ventilation had heterogeneous results,[8,64,65] with only the longer intervention (10 days) showing a trend for a reduction in BPD/death.[65]

The largest trial of permissive hypercapnia (1316 neonates) used a strategy of continuous positive airway pressure started within 1 hour after birth and permissive hypercapnia before intubation and for 14 days while on mechanical ventilation.[66] The target $Paco_2$ was higher than 65 mm Hg with a pH higher than 7.20 compared with $Paco_2$ targets less than 50 mm Hg and a pH higher than 7.30 in the control group. The incidence of BPD/death tended to be lower in the permissive hypercapnia group (47.8% vs 51.0%) but this difference did not reach statistical significance. In the most immature infants (24–25 weeks), death occurred significantly less often in the permissive hypercapnia group (23.9% vs 32.1%, $P = .03$). In addition, for the whole cohort, infants randomized to permissive hypercapnia received mechanical ventilation and surfactant supplementation less often, had less days of mechanical ventilation, and were less often treated with postnatal corticosteroids for BPD (all $P<.05$). There was no harm or adverse effects of permissive hypercapnia reported.

SUMMARY

Permissive hypercapnia is a ventilatory strategy that may reduce injury to the developing lung through a variety of mechanisms. Data based on the current literature, pertinent physiologic rationale, and experimental research suggest that permissive hypercapnia may be beneficial. Taken together, 7 trials suggest that a strategy of permissive hypercapnia started early, before initiation of mechanical ventilation, combined with prolonged permissive hypercapnia during mechanical ventilation optimizes pulmonary/survival benefits and seems to be safe in neonates. These data support the use of permissive hypercapnia as an alternative to traditional ventilator support strategies that aim to maintain normocapnia. Further research is necessary to elucidate better strategies of permissive hypercapnia, such as target CO_2 levels, duration of the intervention, and minimal tidal volume ventilation.

REFERENCES

1. Fanaroff A, Stoll J, Wright L, et al. Trends in neonatal morbidity and mortality for very low birth weight infants. Am J Obstet Gynecol 2007;196:147.e1–8.
2. Attar M, Donn S. Mechanisms of ventilator-induced lung injury in premature infants. Semin Neonatol 2002;7:353–60.

3. Miller J, Carlo W. Safety and effectiveness of permissive hypercapnia in the preterm infant. Curr Opin Pediatr 2007;191:142–4.
4. Boynton B, Hammond M. Pulmonary gas exchange: basic principles and the effects of mechanical ventilation. In: Boynton B, Carlo WA, Jobe A, editors. New therapies for neonatal respiratory failure: a physiologic approach. Cambridge (England): Cambridge University Press; 1994. p. 115–29.
5. Brogan T, Robertson H, Lamm W, et al. Carbon dioxide added late in inspiration reduces ventilation perfusion heterogeneity without causing respiratory acidosis. J Appl Physiol 2004;96:1894–8.
6. Sinclair S, Kregenow D, Star I, et al. Therapeutic hypercapnia and ventilation-perfusion matching in acute lung injury. Chest 2006;130:85–92.
7. Alvaro R, Khalil M, Qurashi, et al. CO_2 inhalation as a treatment for apnea of prematurity: a randomized double-blind controlled trial. J Pediatr 2012;160: 252–7.
8. Mariani G, Cifuentes J, Carlo W. Randomized trial of permissive hypercapnia in preterm infants. Pediatrics 1999;104:1082–8.
9. Sovik S, Lossius K. Development of ventilatory response to transient hypercapnia and hypercapnic hypoxia in term neonates. Pediatr Res 2004;55:302–9.
10. Walley R, Lewis T, Wood L. Acute respiratory acidosis decreases left ventricular contractility but increases cardiac output in dogs. Circ Res 1990;67:628–35.
11. Weber T, Tschernich H, Sitzwohl C, et al. Tromethamine buffer modifies the depressant effect of permissive hypercapnia on myocardial contractility in patients with acute respiratory distress syndrome. Am J Respir Crit Care Med 2000;162:1361–5.
12. Cardenas V Jr, Zwischenberger J, Tao W, et al. Correction of blood pH attenuates changes in hemodynamics and oxygen blood flow during permissive hypercapnia. Crit Care Med 1996;5:827–34.
13. Weiner J, Chatburn R, Carlo W. Ventilation and hemodynamic effects of high-frequency jet ventilation following cardiac surgery. Respir Care 1987;32:332–8.
14. Gullberg N, Winberg P, Sellden H. Changes in stroke volume cause changes in cardiac output in neonates and infants when mean airway pressure is altered. Acta Anaesthesiol Scand 1999;43:999–1004.
15. Gullberg N, Winberg P, Sellden H. Changes in mean airway pressure during HFOV influences cardiac output in neonates and infants. Acta Anaesthesiol Scand 2004;48:218–23.
16. Peevy K, Hernandez L, Moise A, et al. Barotrauma and microvascular injury in lungs of nonadult rabbits: effect of ventilation pattern. Crit Care Med 1990;18: 634–7.
17. Carlton D, Cummings J, Scheerer R, et al. Lung overexpansion increases pulmonary microvascular protein permeability in young lambs. J Appl Physiol 1990;9: 577–83.
18. Hernandez L, Peevy K, Moise A, et al. Chest wall restriction limits high airway pressure-induced lung injury in young rabbits. J Appl Physiol 1999;66:2364–8.
19. Parker J, Hernandez L, Peevy K. Mechanisms of ventilator-induced lung injury. Crit Care Med 1993;21:131–43.
20. Bjorklund L, Ingimarsson J, Curstedt T, et al. Manual ventilation with a few large breaths at birth compromises the therapeutic effect of subsequent surfactant replacement in immature lambs. Pediatr Res 1997;42:348–55.
21. Ingimarsson J, Bjorklund L, Curstedt T, et al. Incomplete protection by prophylactic surfactant against the adverse effects of large lung inflations at birth in immature lambs. Intensive Care Med 2004;30:1446–53.

22. Jobe A. Antenatal factors and development of bronchopulmonary dysplasia. Semin Neonatol 2003;8:9–17.
23. Muscedere J, Mullen J, Gan K, et al. Tidal ventilation at low airway pressures can augment lung injury. Am J Respir Crit Care Med 1994;149:1327–34.
24. Rotta A, Steinhorn D. Is permissive hypercapnia a beneficial strategy for pediatric acute lung injury? Respir Care Clin 2006;12:371–87.
25. Sinclair S, Dregenow D, Lamm W, et al. Hypercapnic acidosis is protective in an in vivo model of ventilator-induced lung injury. Am J Respir Crit Care Med 2002; 166:403–8.
26. Laffey J, Honan D, Hopkins N, et al. Hypercapnic acidosis attenuates endotoxin induced acute lung injury. Am J Respir Crit Care Med 2004;169:46–56.
27. Nichol A, Naughton F, O'Cronin D, et al. Buffered hypercapnia worsens lung injury in endotoxin-induced pneumonia. In: Abstracts of the American Thoracic Society (ATS). San Francisco, 2007. p. A784.
28. Rai S, Engelberts D, Laffey J, et al. Therapeutic hypercapnia is not protective in the in vivo surfactant-depleted rabbit lung. Pediatr Res 2004;55:42–9.
29. Ryu J, Sukkarieh M, Heldt G, et al. Effect of chronic hypercapnia on lung development. In: Abstracts of the American Thoracic Society (ATS). San Francisco, 2007. p. A87.
30. Vicencio A, Du Z, Haddad G. Chronic hypercapnia attenuates hyperoxia-induced fibrosis in neonatal mice. In: Abstracts of the American Thoracic Society (ATS). San Francisco, 2007. p. A92.
31. Vicencio A, Du Z, Morrow B. Chronic hypercapnia accelerates alveolar formation and maturation in the neonatal mouse. Pediatric Academic Societies' 2007 Annual Meeting. 2007. EPAS61: 8035.3. Available at: www.aps_spr.org. Accessed July 12, 2012.
32. Wang N, Gates K, Trejo H, et al. Elevated CO2 selectively inhibits interleukin-6 and tumor necrosis factor expression and decreases phagocytosis in the macrophage. FASEB J 2010;24:2178–90.
33. Coakley R, Taggart C, Greene C, et al. Ambient pCO2 modulates intracellular pH, intracellular oxidant generation, and interleukin-8 secretion in human neutrophils. J Leukoc Biol 2002;714:603–10.
34. O'Toole D, Hassett P, Contreras M, et al. Hypercapnic acidosis attenuates pulmonary epithelial wound repair by an NF-kappaB dependent mechanism. Thorax 2009;64:976–82.
35. Prince L, Dieperink H, Okoh V, et al. Toll-like receptor signaling inhibits structural development of the distal fetal mouse lung. Dev Dynam 2005;233:553–61.
36. Benjamin J, Smith R, Halloran B, et al. FGF-10 is decreased in bronchopulmonary dysplasia and suppressed by toll-like receptor activation. Am J Physiol Lung Cell Mol Physiol 2007;292:550–8.
37. Laffey J, Tanaka M, Engelberts D, et al. Therapeutic hypercapnia reduces pulmonary and systemic injury follow in vivo lung reperfusion. Am J Respir Crit Care Med 2000;162:2287–94.
38. O'Croinin D, Chonghaile M, Higgins B, et al. Bench-to bedside review: permissive hypercapnia. Crit Care 2005;9:51–9.
39. Takeshita K, Suzuki Y, Nishio K, et al. Hypercapnic acidosis attenuates endotoxin-induced nuclear factor-kappa-beta activation. Am J Respir Cell Mol Biol 2003;29: 124–32.
40. Lang J, Chumley P, Eiserich J, et al. Hypercapnia induces injury to alveolar epithelial cells via a nitric oxide-dependent pathway. Am J Physiol Lung Cell Mol Physiol 2000;279:994–1002.

41. Watterberg K, Demers L, Scott S, et al. Chorioamnionitis and early lung inflammation in infants in whom bronchopulmonary dysplasia develops. Pediatrics 1996; 97:210–5.
42. Lang J, Figueroa M, Sanders K, et al. Hypercapnia via reduced rate and tidal volume contributes to lipopolysaccharide-induced lung injury. Am J Respir Crit Care Med 2005;171:147–57.
43. Doerr C, Gajic O, Berrios J, et al. Hypercapnic acidosis impairs plasma membrane wound resealing in ventilator-injured lungs. Am J Respir Crit Care Med 2005;171:1371–7.
44. Masood A, Jankov R, Yi M, et al. Therapeutic hypercapnia protects against chronic neonatal lung injury and prevents vascular remodeling in the neonatal rat. In: Abstracts of the Pediatric Academic Societies' 2007 Annual Meeting. Toronto, May 5–8, 2007. Abstract 6291.7.
45. Petrucci N, Lacovelli W. Ventilation with lower tidal volumes versus traditional tidal volumes in adults for acute lung injury and acute respiratory distress syndrome. Cochrane Database Syst Rev 2004;(2):CD003844. Update in: Cochrane Database Syst Rev 2007. CD003844.
46. Kraybill E, Runyun D, Bose C, et al. Risk factors for chronic lung disease in infants with birth weights of 751 to 1000 grams. J Pediatr 1989;115:115–20.
47. Garland J, Buck R, Allred E, et al. Hypocarbia before surfactant therapy appears to increase bronchopulmonary dysplasia risk in infants with respiratory distress syndrome. Arch Pediatr Adolesc Med 1995;149:617–22.
48. Kamper J, Feilberg J, Jonsbo F, et al. The Danish national study in infants with extremely low gestational age and birth weight (the ETFOL study): respiratory morbidity and outcome. Acta Paediatr 2004;93:225–32.
49. Carlo W. Permissive hypercapnia and permissive hypoxemia in neonates. J Perinatol 2007;27(Suppl 1):S64–70.
50. Bagolan P, Casaccia G, Crescenzi F, et al. Impact of a current treatment protocol on outcome of high-risk congenital diaphragmatic hernia. J Pediatr Surg 2004;39: 313–8.
51. Dudell G, CDH Study Group. Are permissive strategies now standard of care for neonates with congenital diaphragmatic hernia (CDH) [abstract]? Pediatric Academic Societies 2006 Annual Meeting. 2006. E-PAS59:453. Available at: www.aps_spr.org. Accessed July 12, 2012.
52. Kaiser J, Gauss C, Williams D. The effects of hypercapnia on cerebral autoregulation in ventilated very low birth weight infants. Pediatr Res 2005;58:931–5.
53. Hare G, Kavanagh B, Mazer D, et al. Hypercapnia increases cerebral tissue oxygen tension in anesthetized rats. Can J Anesth 2003;50:1061–8.
54. Hino J, Short B, Rais-Bahrami K, et al. Cerebral blood flow and metabolism during and after prolonged hypercapnia in newborn lambs. Crit Care Med 2000;10:3505–10.
55. Fabres J, Carlo W, Phillips V, et al. Both extremes of $PaCO_2$ and the magnitude of fluctuations are associated with severe intraventricular hemorrhage in preterm infants. Pediatrics 2007;2:299–305.
56. Potkin R, Swenson E. Resuscitation from severe acute hypercapnia. Determinants of tolerance and survival. Chest 1992;102:1742–5.
57. Amato M, Barbas C, Medeiros D, et al. Effect of a protective-ventilation strategy on mortality in the acute respiratory distress syndrome. N Engl J Med 1998;338: 347–54.
58. Stewart T, Meade M, Cook D, et al. Evaluation of a ventilation strategy to prevent barotrauma in patients at high risk for acute respiratory distress syndrome.

Pressure- and Volume-Limited Ventilation Strategy Group. N Engl J Med 1998; 338:355–61.

59. The Acute Respiratory Distress Syndrome Network. Ventilation with lower tidal volumes as compared with traditional tidal volumes for acute lung injury and the acute respiratory distress syndrome. N Engl J Med 2000;342:1301–8.

60. Kregenow D, Rubenfeld G, Hudson L, et al. Hypercapnic acidosis and mortality in acute lung injury. Crit Care Med 2006;34:1–7.

61. Morley C, Davis P, Doyle L, et al. Nasal CPCP or intubation at birth for very preterm infants. N Engl J Med 2008;358:700–8.

62. Dunn M, Kaempf J, DeKlerk A, et al. Randomized trial comparing 3 approaches to the initial respiratory management of preterm neonates. Pediatrics 2011;128: e1069.

63. Tapia J, Urzua S, Bancalari A, et al. Randomized trial of early bubble continuous positive airway pressure for very low birth weight infants. J Pediatr 2012 July; 161(1):75–80.e1.

64. Thome U, Carroll W, Wu T, et al. Outcome of extremely preterm infants randomized at birth to different PaCO2 targets during the first seven days of life. Biol Neonate 2006;90:21–5.

65. Carlo W, Stark A, Wright L, et al. Minimal ventilation to prevent bronchopulmonary dysplasia in extremely-low-birthweight infants. J Pediatr 2002;141:370–4.

66. Finer N, Carlo W, Walsh M, et al. Early CPAP versus surfactant in extremely preterm infants. N Engl J Med 2010;362:1970–9.

Can Nitric Oxide–Based Therapy Prevent Bronchopulmonary Dysplasia?

Thomas M. Raffay, MD[a], Richard J. Martin, MD[a,*],
James D. Reynolds, PhD[b,c]

KEYWORDS

- Inhaled nitric oxide (iNO) • Bronchopulmonary dysplasia (BPD) • Neonate
- Prematurity • S-nitrosylation • S-nitrosothiol (SNO) • Ethyl nitrite (ENO)

KEY POINTS

- Nitric oxide (NO) plays a role in cellular signaling, inflammation, growth and differentiation, and metabolism and has specifically shown an ability to decrease pulmonary vascular resistance.
- Animal models of the major pulmonary morbidity of prematurity, bronchopulmonary dysplasia (BPD), have shown that inhaled NO (iNO) improved pulmonary function, promoted lung development, and prevented much of the disease associated with BPD.
- Multiple clinical trials have examined the use of iNO in preterm infants to prevent BPD; despite differing protocols, iNO has not proved to be of clear, unequivocal benefit in this at-risk population.
- In 2010, the National Institutes of Health Consensus Development Conference provided therapeutic guidelines for the use of iNO; their primary conclusion was that apart from occasional instances of pulmonary hypertension or hypoplasia, routine or rescue use of iNO cannot be recommended in preterm infants with respiratory failure.
- Much of the bioactivity of NO is mitigated through S-nitrosylation of proteins, and this may be a better therapeutic target.
- Inhaled ethyl nitrite could be a superior therapeutic agent to iNO because it more efficiently S-nitrosylates proteins, does not create potentially harmful by-products like peroxynitrite, and improves tissue blood flow and oxygen delivery.
- Future investigations of the role that NO plays in lung development and pulmonary function are needed.

Supported in part by: NIH Grants HL 56470, R01HL095463, R01HL091876, and UL1RR024989, and by DARPA Contract N66001-10-C-2015.
[a] Division of Neonatology, Department of Pediatrics, Rainbow Babies & Children's Hospital, Case Medical Center/University Hospitals, 11100 Euclid Avenue, Cleveland, OH 44106-6010, USA; [b] Institute for Transformative Molecular Medicine, Case Western Reserve University, 10900 Euclid Avenue, Cleveland, OH 44106-6010, USA; [c] Department of Anesthesia and Perioperative Medicine, Case Medical Center/University Hospitals, 11100 Euclid Avenue, Cleveland, OH 44106-6010, USA
* Corresponding author. Rainbow Babies and Children's Hospital, 11100 Euclid Avenue, RBC Suite 3100, Cleveland, OH 44106-6010.
E-mail address: rxm6@case.edu

OVERVIEW

In 1999, the initial approved clinical indication for inhaled nitric oxide (iNO) issued by the US Food and Drug Administration (FDA) was limited to: "...treatment of term and near-term (>34 weeks) neonates with hypoxic respiratory failure associated with clinical or echocardiographic evidence of pulmonary hypertension." At the time, anticipation was high that iNO would receive subsequent clearance as a therapeutic intervention for a variety of pediatric and adult respiratory conditions. Thirteen years, multiple clinical trials, and millions of dollars later the FDA-approved indication for iNO is the same as it was last century. This outcome has been particularly disappointing with respect to bronchopulmonary dysplasia (BPD). It was predicted that iNO-mediated improvements in neonatal oxygenation would hasten resolution of acute respiratory distress and thus lead to a significant decline in BPD incidence rates. Instead, a series of well-designed multicenter clinical trials have at best shown inconsistent equivocal benefits of iNO therapy to prevent or treat BPD.

Inhaled NO is not a panacea for pulmonary diseases. However, future respiratory therapies directed toward NO bioactivity may confer therapeutic benefit in the prevention or treatment of BPD, but the agents may be in a different form from a free radical gas. A growing understanding of endogenous NO biology is helping to explain how and when exogenous NO may confer benefit or harm; this knowledge is also helping to identify new better-targeted NO-based therapies. In this review, results of the BPD clinical trials that used iNO in the preterm population are placed in context, the biologic basis for novel NO therapeutics are considered, and possible future directions for NO-focused clinical and basic research in developmental lung disease are identified.

THE CLINICAL PROBLEM

Concomitant in the 1960s with the development of ventilatory strategies to oxygenate newborns in respiratory distress was the recognition that these interventions could produce lung disease.[1] The original characterization of BPD was based on chest radiographic findings (cysts and pulmonary fibrosis) and a need for prolonged oxygen support resulting from oxygen toxicity and mechanical trauma; it typically applied to neonates older than 30 weeks' postmenstrual age, the lower age threshold for survival at the time. In the ensuing decades, as additional interventions were developed to help distressed neonates survive (most notably surfactant and antenatal steroid therapy), the cause of BPD has evolved such that it is currently viewed as a disease of prematurity.

The concept of BPD resulting from lung injury (old definition) has been replaced with the view that it arises from aberrant development of immature lungs exposed to the ex uterine milieu (new definition). This concept is borne out by epidemiologic data. In the current neonatal intensive care environment, rarely would the average patient in Northway and colleagues' cohort (1900 g at 33 weeks' gestation) develop BPD. Instead, the disease is concentrated amongst what are now considered low-birth-weight and very-low-birth-weight but viable populations. From an overall incidence of 20% for infants weighing less than 1500 g, the BPD rate increases to 30% when the birth weight is between 750 and 1000 g and to 50% for infants born weighing less than 750 g.[2] The sickest infants are now surviving, but with lung dysfunction, keeping the overall incidence rate essentially constant.

BPD has a multifactorial cause through a combination of hyperoxia and barotrauma or volutrauma superimposed on a structurally and biochemically immature lung. The acute lung injury in the vulnerable infant results in airway remodeling, decreased alveolarization, alveolar simplification, and lung fibrosis.[3,4] Many other factors are contributory, notably antenatal and postnatal infection and inflammation, along with nutritional deficiencies. In addition, BPD may have a genetic component.[5] One of the major therapeutic challenges is to identify which specific pathophysiologic process or processes to target. An even greater challenge is to determine the appropriate timing of any therapy to optimize potential benefit and minimize both unnecessary treatment and untoward side effects (**Fig. 1**).

BPD continues to be the major pulmonary morbidity of prematurity,[6,7] with annual care costs in the United States estimated to be upwards of $26 billion.[8] Equally important is the emerging concept that BPD may be a chronic condition. After their initial care, 50% of patients with low-birth-weight and very-low-birth-weight are rehospitalized for respiratory distress during early childhood. Although some lung parameters can normalize in later childhood, exacerbated regression in function may occur as these individuals age. When Northway and colleagues[9] reassessed their original (pre-surfactant era) patients, most had some degree of airway obstruction, airway hyper-reactivity, or hyperinflation. This finding was replicated in a different cohort of BPD survivors who have undergone serial pulmonary testing into midadulthood[10]; at their most recent testing (mean age of 38 years), these individuals showed "increasing static pulmonary hyperinflation with age indicative of bronchiolar dysfunction or early emphysematous changes."

Longitudinal assessments of BPD survivors who received surfactant are scant, so the full scope of adult respiratory disease that can be traced to aberrant neonatal lung development or overly aggressive therapeutic intervention remains unclear. Nonetheless, the possibility of chronic pulmonary disease adds impetus to finding effective therapies to prevent and treat BPD.

PRECLINICAL SUPPORT FOR NO GAS IN NEONATAL LUNG DISEASE

The development of iNO for persistent pulmonary hypertension of the newborn followed a course of positive preclinical[11] and case series[12,13] results that led to multi-center clinical trials.[14–16] Preclinical results from animal models of BPD have also shown benefits with iNO therapy.

In a premature baboon preparation, inhalation of 5 ppm of NO during the first 14 days of life was compared with a standard ventilatory arm[17]; animals in both cohorts were administered surfactant. At the end of the study, animals in the iNO group had

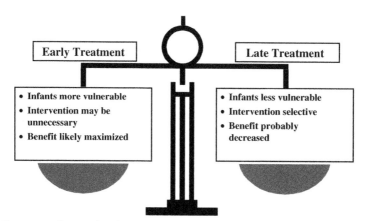

Fig. 1. The pros and cons of early versus late therapeutic intervention in the course of BPD.

improved pulmonary function (increased compliance and decreased expiratory resistance) compared with baboons in the control arm. Continuous iNO therapy was also associated with preservation of lung growth, normalization of elastin deposition, and stimulation of secondary crest development. The investigators proposed that iNO corrected dysfunctions in NO-mediated biosynthetic pathways and suggested that this dysfunction contributes to the pathogenesis of BPD. Dysregulation of NO activities in the lungs have also been observed in rodents[18] and were again found to be responsive to iNO.[19]

Positive results were also seen in sheep. Chronically ventilated preterm lambs received 5 to 15 ppm iNO for 21 days; comparisons were again made to animals that received standard ventilatory support.[20] Lung development was measured by radial alveolar counts and lung capillary surface density, parameters that were significantly better in the iNO treatment group. In addition, the treated lambs had markedly lower expiratory resistance, with a significant decrease in airway smooth muscle mass. Inhaled NO also produced decreases in pulmonary vascular resistance and pulmonary arterial smooth muscle, but these benefits were modest compared with the other end points.

The preclinical data point to an impairment of endogenous NO signaling in neonatal lung injury, an impairment that can be addressed with iNO (**Fig. 2**). As detailed in the next section, these positive animal findings have not translated into clear clinical benefits of iNO therapy for human preterm neonates.

CLINICAL TRIAL RESULTS FOR USE OF INHALED NO IN PRETERM INFANTS

Fourteen randomized, controlled clinical trials[21–34] have been conducted to test the ability of iNO to reduce mortality or the incidence of BPD in preterm infants (a total study population of 3430). The methodology, dosage, and duration of iNO treatment, as well as timing of the intervention, have varied amongst these trials (as shown in **Fig. 3**), leading to conflicting and equivocal results (**Table 1**; the reader is referred to the individual reports or the articles describing the group analyses for detailed descriptions of the methodologic differences). In addition to the conclusions reached by the individual clinical research teams, the current study population of more than 3400 has allowed for post hoc testing of pooled results.

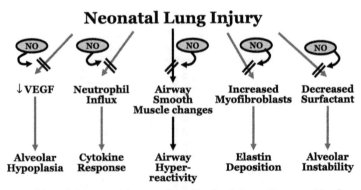

Fig. 2. Neonatal lung injury may trigger a diversity of cellular pathways with adverse effects on lung development. Based on available animal data, NO seemed to have the potential to block these pathways and downstream consequences.

Dose and Duration of Inhaled Nitric Oxide (iNO) Therapy

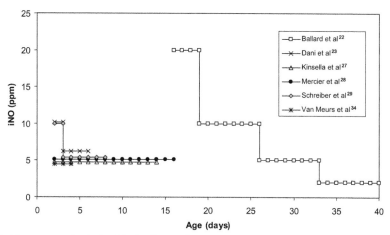

Fig. 3. The temporal relationship in the median initiation, dose, and duration of inhaled NO treatment among 6 major trials. (*Adapted from* Truog WE. Inhaled nitric oxide for the prevention of bronchopulmonary dysplasia. Expert Opin Pharmacother 2007;8:1505–13; with permission.)

In a 2010 Cochrane review,[35] Barrington and Finer determined that the wide variations in patient age, illness severity, and control group mortalities precluded pooling and analyzing the results as a single data set. Instead, these investigators organized the 14 clinical trials into cohorts based on the entry criteria and the timing of iNO administration. Three distinct groups were identified:

1. Nine of the trials[21,23–25,27,30,31,33,34] were defined as early-rescue treatment (<3 days of life) based on oxygenation criteria
2. Three of the trials[26,28,29] were given the designation of routine early use for intubated infants (<3 days of life)
3. Two of the trials[22,32] were defined as later use (>3 days of life) for infants at increased risk for BPD

There were trends toward improved outcomes with iNO treatment, most notably in group 2, in which the effect size (typical relative risk of 0.93 with 95% confidence interval of 0.86–1.01) approached significance, but they remained only trends. Analyses found no statistically significant effect of iNO on rates of BPD or mortality; however, 1 large multicenter trial using later use, longer duration, and higher initial dose did document benefit.[22] In addition, the investigators found no effect of iNO on the incidence of neurologic impairment and there were no clear effects on the frequency or severity of intraventricular hemorrhage. Barrington and Finer summarized their findings this way: "iNO as rescue therapy for the very ill preterm infant does not appear to be effective. Early routine use of iNO in preterm infants with respiratory disease does not affect serious brain injury or improve survival without BPD. Later use of iNO to prevent BPD might be effective, but requires further study."

Using different methodology, Askie and colleagues[36] performed a meta-analysis on 12[22–30,32–34] of the 14 trials for which individual patient data (IPD) were available. The investigators tested multiple subgroups, which can be linked under 3 categories:

Therapeutic: starting dose and duration of iNO treatment, antenatal or postnatal steroid use, administration of surfactant, and ventilation mode at randomization.

Table 1
Study protocols of randomized, controlled trials using iNO in preterm infants

Author, Year	Number	Gestational Age (wk)	Age at Enrollment	Birth Weight (g)	Start→Titration (Maximum) iNO, ppm	Weaning Protocol	Planned Duration of iNO	Relative Risk of Death or BPD (95% Confidence Interval)[a]
Subhedar et al,[32] 1997	42	<32	>4 d	—	20→5 (20)[b]	Attempt at 72 h; iNO stopped with extubation	72 h	1.04 (0.92, 1.19)
Franco-Belgian Collaborative,[21] 1999	85	<33	<7 d	—	10→5 (20)[b]	Practitioner's discretion; 5 ppm and then off	—	0.84 (0.54, 1.31)
Kinsella et al,[27] 1999	80	≤34	≤7 d	—	5→0 (5)[b]	Attempt at 7 d; iNO stopped with extubation	7–14 d	0.85 (0.70, 1.03)
Srisuparp et al,[30] 2002	34	<32	<3 d	<2000	20→5 (20)[b]	Down to 5 ppm over 24–48 h, iNO stopped with extubation	Maximum: 7 d	BPD rates not reported
Schreiber et al,[29] 2003	207	<34	<3 d	<2000	10→5 (10)	10 ppm for 1 d, 5 ppm for 6 d, then off; iNO stopped 1 h before extubation	7 d	0.76 (0.60, 0.97)
Van Meurs et al,[34] 2005	420	<34	>4 h	401–1500	5→10 (10)	Attempt at 10–14 h; iNO stopped if no response at 10 ppm or with extubation	Maximum: 14 d	0.99 (0.90, 1.09)
Field et al,[24] 2005	108	<34	<28 d	—	5→40 (40)[b]	iNO doses doubled until response achieved to a maximum of 40 ppm; iNO stopped before extubation	48 h to 3 d	0.98 (0.87, 1.12)

Study	N	Gestational age	Age at entry	Birth weight (g)	iNO dose (ppm)	Weaning protocol	Duration	Risk ratio (95% CI)
Hascoet et al,[25] 2005	145	<32	6–48 h	—	5→10 (10)[b]	iNO stopped when the alveolar-arterial oxygen gradient (aAo₂) >0.22 or with extubation	Median: 28 h	1.04 (0.77, 1.41)
Dani et al,[23] 2006	40	<30	<7 d	—	10→6 (10)	10 ppm for 4 h, then 6 ppm. Attempt at 72 h; iNO stopped with extubation	Mean: 4.1 d	0.56 (0.35, 0.88)
Kinsella et al,[26] 2006	793	≤34	<48 h	500–1250	5 (5)	None; iNO stopped with extubation	Maximum: 21 d	0.95 (0.87, 1.03)
Ballard et al,[22] 2006	582	<32	7–21 d	500–1250	20→2 (20)	20 ppm for 48–96 h, then decreased to 10, 5, and 2 ppm at weekly intervals. Continued for duration of therapy regardless of respiratory support	Minimum: 24 d	0.89 (0.78, 1.02)
Van Meurs et al,[33] 2007	29	<34	>4 h	>1500	5→10 (10)[b]	Attempt at 10–14 h. iNO stopped if no response at 10 ppm or with extubation	Maximum: 14 d	0.83 (0.43, 1.62)
Su and Chen,[31] 2008	65	<32	Mean: 2.4–2.5 d	≤1500	5→20 (20)[b]	Attempt at 6 h	Mean: 4.9 d	0.79 (0.51, 1.21)
Mercier et al,[28] 2010	800	24–28 6/7	<24 h	>500	5 (5)	None; iNO continued for ≥7 d, then discontinued with extubation for maximum of 21 days	7–21 d	0.98 (0.81, 1.18)
Total (14 randomized controlled trials)	3430	≤34	Birth to 27 d	401–2000	Start 5–20 (Max 5–40)	—	<24 h to 24 d	—

a Risk ratio and 95% confidence intervals reported as calculated in Barrington and Finer's Cochrane review.[35]
b Changes to iNO dose made based on physiologic response in patient.

Demographic: gestational age at birth, postnatal age at time of randomization, birth weight, multiplicity, and ethnicity.

Pathology: severity of hypoxemia (in terms of oxygen index), presence of a patent ductus arteriosus, and pulmonary hypertension.

In patients of multiple births, the researchers also analyzed for correlations between siblings.

Of a study population of 3298 infants, the incidence of mortality or chronic lung disease was 59% in the iNO treatment group and 61% in the control cohort for a relative risk of 0.96 with a 95% confidence interval of 0.92 to 1.01 ($P = .11$). The incidence of neurologic injury was also similar at 25% and 23% for iNO-treated infants and controls, respectively (relative risk of 1.12 and 95% confidence interval of 0.98 to 1.28; $P = .09$). In addition, iNO was found to have no statistically significant benefit when tested with respect to the demographic variables.

In trials that started with an iNO dose greater than 5 ppm, there was a 9% absolute risk reduction in the composite outcome of death or BPD (relative risk of 0.83 and 95% confidence interval of 0.74–0.95). However, translating this positive finding into a therapeutic recommendation is not straightforward, for 2 reasons:

1. The relevant low-dose trials, although starting at less than 5 ppm, subsequently exceeded this concentration during the course of therapy because iNO dosing was based on (and titrated to) the patient's response
2. The relevant higher-dose trials used protocols that reduced the iNO dose over the course of therapy

The investigators' conclusions: "...[R]esults of this IPD meta-analysis of all available worldwide data indicate that routine use of iNO for treatment of respiratory failure in preterm infants cannot be recommended. The use of a higher starting dose might be associated with improved outcome, but because there were differences in the designs of the trials included in the analyses, it requires further examination."

A third group analysis of the available iNO data was conducted by Donohue and colleagues.[37] These investigators combined the results of the 14 randomized trials with those from 7 follow-up assessments[38–45] and 1 observational study.[46] Their meta-analyses were broken down into short-term and long-term outcomes:

Short-Term Outcomes
Survival/death in the neonatal intensive care unit (NICU)
BPD at 36 weeks' postmenstruation age
Death or BPD composite at 36 weeks' postmenstruation age
Brain injury
Patent ductus arteriosus
Sepsis
Necrotizing enterocolitis
Retinopathy of prematurity
Pulmonary hemorrhage
Air leak

Long-term outcomes
Survival/death after NICU discharge
Cerebral palsy
Mental development index
Neurodevelopmental impairment

The investigators reported 1 positive finding in that there was no evidence that treatment of preterm infants with iNO influences the incidence rates for other complications of prematurity. The same lack of influence was found to be true for the beneficial parameters. Inhaled NO therapy did not alter the incidence of:

NICU mortality (risk ratio of 0.97 with 95% confidence interval at 0.82–1.15);
BPD in survivors at 36 weeks (risk ratio of 0.93 with 95% confidence interval at 0.86–1.003);
Cerebral palsy (risk ratio of 1.36 with 95% confidence interval at 0.88–2.10)
Neurodevelopmental impairment (risk ratio of 0.91 with 95% confidence interval at 0.77–1.12); or
Cognitive impairment (risk ratio of 0.72 with 95% confidence interval at 0.35–1.45).

A small difference was identified in the composite outcome of death or BPD at 36 weeks' postmenstrual age, which favored iNO therapy over the control group (risk ratio of 0.93 with 95% confidence interval at 0.87–0.99). However, this 7% reduction in death or BPD was not enough for the investigators to accept iNO as a viable therapy for preterm infants: "There is currently no evidence to support the use of iNO in preterm infants with respiratory failure outside the context of rigorously conducted randomized clinical trials." Although some have criticized this conclusion,[47] Donohue and colleagues' findings[37] are consistent with the results of the other 2 analyses.

THE NATIONAL INSTITUTES OF HEALTH WEIGHS-IN

National Institutes of Health (NIH) Consensus and State-of-the-Science Statements are prepared by independent panels of health professionals and public representatives. The goal of such efforts is to provide health care workers, patients, and the general public with a responsible (presumably free of bias) assessment of currently available data regarding a particular medical condition, practice, or therapy. Such statements are an independent report of the panel; they are not considered policy statements of the NIH or the Federal Government.

To assess the risks and benefits of treating premature infants with iNO, the Eunice Kennedy Shriver National Institute of Child Health and Human Development, the National Heart, Lung, and Blood Institute, and the NIH Office of Medical Applications of Research convened a Consensus Development Panel that met between October 27 and 29, 2010.[8] The 16-member Consensus Development Panel comprised physicians and caregivers active in the areas of neonatology, pediatric pulmonology and neurology, and perinatal epidemiology. An additional 18 experts from relevant medical fields (many of whom had been involved in one or more of the iNO preterm infant clinical trials) participated by presenting data to the panel and the conference attendees.

To develop the consensus statement the panel was charged with answering 6 questions:

1. Does iNO therapy increase survival or reduce the occurrence or severity of BPD among premature infants who receive respiratory support?
2. Are there short-term risks of iNO therapy among premature infants who receive respiratory support?
3. Are there effects of iNO therapy on long-term pulmonary or neurodevelopmental outcomes among premature infants who receive respiratory support?
4. Does the effect of iNO therapy on BPD or death or neurodevelopmental impairment vary across subpopulations of premature infants?

5. Does the effect of iNO therapy on BPD or death or neurodevelopmental impairment vary by timing of initiation, mode of delivery, dose and duration, or concurrent therapies?
6. What are the future research directions needed to better understand the risks, benefits, and alternatives to iNO therapy for premature infants who receive respiratory support?

In attempting to answer these questions the panel generated a 5-part consensus statement:

1. The available evidence does not support use of iNO in early-routine, early-rescue, or later-rescue regimens in the care of premature infants of less than 34 weeks' gestation who require respiratory support.
2. There are rare clinical situations, including pulmonary hypertension or hypoplasia, that have been inadequately studied in which iNO may have benefit in infants of less than 34 weeks' gestation. In such situations, clinicians should communicate with families regarding the current evidence on its risks and benefits as well as remaining uncertainties.
3. Future research should seek to understand the gap between benefits on lung development and function in infants at high risk of BPD suggested by basic research and animal studies and the results of clinical trials to date.
4. Predefined subgroup and post hoc analyses of previous trials showing potential benefit of iNO have generated hypotheses for future research for clinical trials. Previous strategies shown to be ineffective are discouraged unless new evidence emerges. Future trials should attempt to quantify the individual effects of each of these treatment-related variables (timing, dose, and duration), ideally by randomly assigning them separately.
5. From assessment of currently available data, hospitals, clinicians, and the pharmaceutical industry should avoid marketing iNO for premature infants of less than 34 weeks' gestation.

Taken together, it is obvious iNO is not a panacea for preterm infants. However, given the vital roles NO plays in lung development and oxygen delivery, it is difficult to rationalize why it has been so difficult to show therapeutic benefit in these patients. In this regard, the answer may lie not so much in how or when to start iNO therapy as in how administration of NO as a nitrogen monoxide radical differs from how the body generates and deploys endogenous NO bioactivity.

BIOLOGY OF NO AND S-NITROSYLATION

Over the last 2 decades, there has been great interest in and delineation of the multiple roles NO has in cellular signaling, inflammation, growth and differentiation, and metabolism. NO-based signaling classically involves the binding of NO to hemes in soluble guanylate cyclase (sGC) to increase cyclic guanosine monophosphate (cGMP). This pathway explains how NO bioactivity derived from the endothelium produces vascular relaxation (and how iNO may chiefly act). However, it is now recognized that most of the effects of NO on cellular signaling are elicited by S-nitrosylation,[48] the ubiquitous modification of cysteine thiol side chains to produce S-nitrosothiols (SNOs) (Fig. 4). Rather than mediate cellular signaling that involves posttranslational modifications, protein hemes seem to promote the requisite redox chemistry of NO. Thousands of proteins have been identified as targets of S-nitrosylation, in which activity can increase or decrease in response to the addition (or removal) of the NO group.[49]

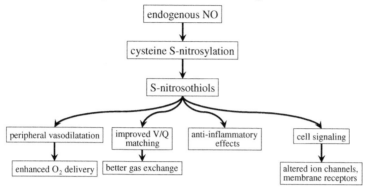

Fig. 4. The multiple roles of endogenous NO bioactivity in affecting respiratory and gas exchange via SNO-mediated signaling.

The breadth of cellular activities regulated by *S*-nitrosylation is reminiscent of phosphorylation. These activities include the developing lung and encompass maturational changes in lung parenchymal, vascular, and airway structures.[50] In vivo SNO homeostasis is a balance between *S*-nitrosylation and denitrosylation, and both the addition and removal of NO are key components in the transduction of SNO-based signaling. NO/SNO regulation is tied to oxygenation. Nitroso-redox balance refers to the interplay between reactive oxygen species (ROS) and NO at critical regulatory cysteine thiols. Irreversible thiol oxidation of cysteine residues by ROS can lead to losses in *S*-nitrosylation control of protein function. The balance between NO bioactivity and ROS production plays a pivotal role in cellular and organ function.[51–54]

By direct analogy to dysregulated phosphorylation, aberrant *S*-nitrosylation is increasingly acknowledged as a causal factor in disease.[55,56] Typically, these states are associated with hyponitrosylation or hypernitrosylation of key proteins that play essential roles in disease (patho)physiology. In several acute and chronic conditions in which SNO levels are altered, administration of an *S*-nitrosylating agent or an exogenous SNO was determined to be beneficial.[57–62] A few aspects of protein *S*-nitrosylation are highlighted in the following section. For more in-depth coverage, the reader is referred to several reviews that have been published in the last few years.[55,63–67]

SNOs IN THE PULMONARY SYSTEM

The major sources/producers of endogenous NO are the 3 NO synthases (NOSs): neuronal NOS (nNOS, NOS1), inducible NOS (iNOS, NOS2), and endothelial NOS (eNOS, NOS3). All 3 isoforms are expressed and active throughout the lungs. In many areas, NOS is colocalized with its target protein(s), providing for tight control of activity under normal physiologic conditions. SNOs have integral roles in respiratory biology from regulating pulmonary vascular tone to ventilation-perfusion matching to central control of breathing.[63] Dysregulation of SNO homeostasis is a common theme in several lung diseases, including cystic fibrosis,[68,69] asthma,[70,71] and pulmonary arterial hypertension (PAH).[72]

SNOs and Oxygenation

Hemoglobin (Hb) is the prototypical S-nitrosylated protein in that it can deploy NO bioactivity as the red blood cells (RBCs) transit the circulatory system.[73,74] In this setting, NO binds to heme iron of deoxy, T-state Hb mainly in the venous circulation to generate HbFeNO.[75,76] In response to oxygenation within the lungs and the transition of Hb from T-state to R-state, the NO group can transfer to the cysteine residue at position 93 on the Hb β chain to form SNO-Hb. The transition from high to low oxygen tension in the arterial periphery promotes the release of SNO-based vasodilatory activity from the RBCs.[77,78] Under normal physiologic conditions, tissue Po_2 (partial pressure of oxygen) is low and falls further with local increases in metabolism. Thus, the release of vasodilatory NO bioactivity by RBCs subserves the graded increases in blood flow that are coupled to progressive decreases in Hb oxygen saturation.[79]

The uptake of oxygen by RBCs within the lungs is similarly controlled to match flow to ventilation, with SNO-Hb entering the lung positioned to influence ventilation-perfusion matching.[79] Local hypoxic pulmonary vasoconstriction occurs to divert blood to better-oxygenated areas within the lungs; NO trapping by Hb is an important contributor to this vasoconstriction.[74,80] In essence, the binding and release of NO bioactivity in the form of SNOs is a central component of the physiologic response to local hypoxia.[74]

The reconceptualization of the respiratory cycle as a 3-gas system[74] (NO, oxygen, and carbon dioxide), provides the explanation for why increasing blood oxygen content can fail to improve tissue oxygenation.[81] Tissue blood flow not blood oxygenation is the primary determinant of oxygen delivery.[73,74]

Tissue perfusion is primarily regulated by hypoxic vasodilation, which couples metabolic demand to local blood flow.[82–84] Work by Guyton, Saltin, and Stamler[85–87] have identified the RBC as the principal transducer of hypoxic vasodilation. Both acute and chronic reductions in oxygenation produce profound declines in circulating NO bioactivity. In healthy human volunteers, a 60-minute exposure to hypobaric hypoxia (0.56 atm) reduced circulating RBC SNO-Hb levels by ~80%.[88] This response helps to rationalize the reductions in systemic vascular resistance that occur with acute hypoxia (ie, SNO unloading in the hypoxic periphery), as well as the exaggerated increases in pulmonary vascular resistance and pulmonary arterial pressure that are produced by SNO-depleted RBCs.

SNOs and Inflammation

SNOs have broad-based antiinflammatory actions, from inhibition of toll-like receptor (TLR) signaling, to regulating expression of various cytokines[89–91] and antiinflammatory mediators[92,93] to modulating a myriad of signal transduction pathways including the mitogen-activated protein kinases. Diverse mechanisms have been proposed to account for these actions,[55] including attenuation of nuclear factor κB (NF-κB) p50-p65 activity.[94,95] Under basal conditions, upstream S-nitrosylation acts to reduce the amount of inflammatory interleukins (ILs) (eg, IL-1β, IL-6) and chemokines and enhance the antiinflammatory ILs such as IL-10. Protein S-nitrosylation by NO generated from NOS2 (iNOS) can be proinflammatory but it occurs downstream of TLR activation (ie, it first requires a loss of SNO regulatory inhibition of TLR-mediated signaling or NOS2 expression).[55] In addition, S-nitrosylation has been found to regulate the activities of other mediators of lung inflammation, including surfactant protein D,[96] c-Jun NH2-terminal kinase 1,[97] and cyclooxygenase 2.[98]

SNOs and Cell Signaling

A broad range of membrane receptors and ion channels have their activity or expression regulated by S-nitrosylation. These membrane receptors and ion channels include but are not limited to G-protein–coupled receptors, voltage-gated potassium and sodium channels, L-type calcium channels, intracellular second messengers such as G-protein and tyrosine kinases, and intracellular regulators of receptor function such as β-arrestin and dynamin. Again, colocalization is important. For instance, NOS isoforms associate directly with the ion channels or with neighboring scaffolding proteins that place the NO source close to the channel. NOSs can thereby selectively S-nitrosylate critical thiols to influence channel activity. In addition to effecting post-translational protein modification within cells, S-nitrosylation also has major regulator roles and control over the other methods of posttranslational modification (eg, phosphorylation, acetylation, ubiquitylation, sumoylation).[66]

Endogenous NO production both acts on and is acted on by factors that regulate the growth and development of the lung, notably vascular endothelial growth factor (VEGF) and hypoxia-inducible factor 1 α (HIF-1α). Other factors regulated by S-nitrosylation (either directly or through upstream effectors) include angiopoietins, metalloproteinases, intracellular adhesion molecules, transforming growth factor (TGF) β1, tumor necrosis factor α, caspases, lactoferrin, and endothelin 1. Although S-nitrosylation control has not been shown to occur within the lungs for all of this disparate group, several of these factors (along with the inflammatory mediators identified earlier) have been proposed as potential biomarkers for diagnosing and assessing the severity of BPD.[99]

RELEVANCE FOR LUNG DEVELOPMENT

Human lung development can be viewed as progressing through 5 stages; each stage is identified by the appearance, growth, and differentiation of various structures in the airway and pulmonary vasculature.[100]

  Stage 1: embryonic (between weeks 3 and 7 of gestation): budding of the foregut endodermal epithelium into the adjacent primitive mesoderm.
  Stage 2: pseudoglandular (weeks 7–17 of gestation): repeated dichotomous branching of epithelial-lined airways.
  Stage 3: canalicular (weeks 17–27): differentiation of the alveolar cells in concert with proliferation of the vasculature and epithelial thinning to start forming functional gas exchange units.
  Stage 4: Saccular (weeks 28–36 of gestation): additional branching and lengthening of the acinar tubules and buds into thin-walled alveolar saccules and ducts.
  Stage 5: Alveolar (from week 36 into the postnatal period): extensive proliferation of the alveolar ducts and alveoli.

Preterm infants at high risk for BPD are bridging stages 3 and 4, with viability dictated by the presence of functional gas exchange units. Surfactant therapy (along with antenatal steroids) has increased survival by acting to accelerate mesenchyme thinning, thus improving gas diffusion and exchange as well as initiating endogenous surfactant production. However, although this intervention improves survival, it may not affect the development of BPD. Lungs obtained at autopsy from preterm infants with severe BPD showed the same pattern of alveolar simplification and interstitial fibrosis immaterial of whether or not the patients had received surfactant before death.[101]

Except for the latter parts of stage 5 (ie, postnatal), pulmonary development occurs under conditions of low oxygen tension[102] and high pulmonary vascular resistance with reduced blood flow (<20% of ventricular output).[103] It is under these conditions that the growth factors linked to low oxygen are optimized to direct lung development and vascularization, and from this perspective even room air (Fio_2 [fraction of inspired oxygen] of 21%) can be considered hyperoxic. As a result, when the immature lung is exposed to air after preterm delivery hypoxic growth factors (VEGF, HIF-1α, platelet-derived growth factor) decline and factors that limit cell growth and alveolarization (eg, TGF-α and TGF-β, connective tissue growth factor) are subsequently overexpressed and thus act to arrest pulmonary development early in stage 4.[104]

ABERRANT PROTEIN S-NITROSYLATION IN THE IMMATURE LUNG

The 3 NOS isoforms are present in fetal pulmonary tissues by the time of ex uterine viability (>24 weeks' gestation).[105,106] In the healthy developing lung, NOS1 (nNOS) is mostly associated with large blood vessels and with the lining of the airway. NOS1 can also be found in smaller blood vessels, but not generally in the lung parenchyma. NOS3 (eNOS) is mostly localized to the pulmonary epithelium. There is only a modest amount of inducible NOS2 (iNOS) found in healthy lung and it is mostly limited to the epithelium in large airways.

As noted earlier, dysregulation of NO bioactivity in the mature lung is a common theme for several pulmonary diseases.[68–72] There is also clear evidence that pulmonary SNO homeostasis and protein S-nitrosylation are disrupted in the immature lung with BPD. Within autopsied lungs of infants who died of severe BPD, there is a significant increase in protein nitrosylation[107] as well as significant increases in the levels of NOS2[106]; both consistent with a loss of upstream SNO control of inflammation. Others have reported significant amounts of nitrotyrosine (a stable marker of nitrosative stress) distributed throughout the lungs of infants with chronic lung disease of prematurity, with the amount directly correlating with disease severity[105] (however, these investigators did not identify differences in NOS levels).

Consistent with dysregulation of SNO homeostasis, levels of proangiogenic factors activated by S-nitrosylation (notably VEGF) are reduced[108–110] whereas levels of antiangiogenic agents repressed by S-nitrosylation (eg, TGF-β, endoglin) are increased[111,112] in lung tissues and tracheal aspirates of infants with BPD. A similar effect is seen with endothelial colony-forming cells (ECFC), in which hyperoxia significantly disrupts VEGF-NO signaling, leading to impaired growth, a disruption that can be corrected by addition of exogenous VEGF and NO.[113] ECFCs from the cord blood of premature infants are significantly more sensitive to hyperoxic disruption of VEGF-NO activity than cells from term infants.

Other medical manipulations conducted on preterm infants (independent of ventilator strategies) may also affect SNO homeostasis and contribute to BPD; chief among these is blood transfusion. Upwards of 80% of extremely preterm infants receive RBCs during their stay in the NICU,[114] typically to correct anemia resulting from multiple phlebotomies.[115] Administration of RBCs has been identified as a risk factor for developing BPD,[116,117] with relative risk coincident with the number of transfusions.[118] The processing and storage of blood leads to significant depletion of SNO-Hb, such that banked RBCs have reduced ability to effect hypoxic vasodilation[119]; this defect is directly linked to the impaired ability of banked blood to increase tissue oxygenation. As a result, infused SNO-Hb–depleted RBCs can act as overall sinks for NO bioactivity, leading to disruptions in oxygen uptake within the lungs and reduced oxygen delivery in the periphery.[120] In this setting, transfusion can be additive to (rather than corrective of) the other disrupters of pulmonary SNO homeostasis.

Based on the preceding information, resolution of aberrant S-nitrosylation provides an attractive therapeutic target for BPD prevention or amelioration. There is significant support for the postulate that S-nitrosylating therapy could ameliorate several of the inflammatory and other injurious cellular processes that adversely effect ex uterine development of the premature lung. What is not so clear is whether or not restoration/supplementation of S-nitrosylation is best accomplished with iNO.

WHY iNO SHOULD WORK FOR BPD (AND WHY IT MIGHT NOT)

NO dilates pulmonary resistance vessels by primarily acting on sGC to increase cGMP levels.[121] Inhaled NO was originally viewed as a selective pulmonary vasodilator because of its rapid metabolism by Hb as RBCs transit the lung. This view is now changing, because various studies indicate that iNO can exert peripheral effects on blood flow in addition to the oxygenation benefit gained by improved ventilation-perfusion matching.[122–128] This list includes a study involving 8 infants (0–38 months) in acute respiratory distress who showed increases in microcirculatory blood flow 60 minutes after starting iNO therapy at 20 ppm.[127] These blood flow effects of iNO seem to occur via SNO-based mechanisms, as reflected by increases in the concentrations of circulating SNO-Hb and other SNO moieties.[124,128,129]

This triple combination of reducing pulmonary resistance, increasing blood oxygenation, and peripheral improvements in end-organ blood flow should, on the surface, make iNO an ideal agent to improve the physiologic status of preterm infants. However, there are several factors that alone or in combination can reduce the therapeutic efficacy of NO gas:

- There are several pathways by which iNO can generate SNO-Hb (and other SNOs), but these reactions are not efficient. These pathways entail higher dosages or longer exposure periods to iNO (although this could account for the dose-related trend for improvement noted by Askie and colleagues[36]). In the pediatric study by Top and colleagues,[127] microcirculatory blood flow increased with an iNO dose of 20 ppm.
- NO gas has a predilection to react with oxygen to generate tissue damaging, higher-order nitrogen oxides (NOx), including peroxynitrite. The generation of NOx by iNO is enhanced in the presence of supplemental oxygen and at higher iNO doses.
- RBC Hb interacts with iNO to form met-Hb. Fetal Hb is more sensitive to oxidation than adult Hb and preterm infants have significantly less met-Hb reductase.[130]
- To effect relaxation in pulmonary vessels, iNO needs to interact with sGC. It is not clear how much functional sGC is present in the immature lung nor is it certain that there is sufficient reserve activity for iNO to increase formation of cGMP.
- Hyperoxia or inflammation can lead to increases in phosphodiesterase activity, which in turn results in faster breakdown of cGMP.[131] Hyperoxia has also been shown to increase arginase expression and activity, which diverts the substrate arginine from NO synthase (**Fig. 5**).[132]
- Discontinuation of iNO therapy can induce rebound pulmonary hypertension.

The impact of these limitations probably varies based on the patient's physiologic status and developmental state. However, collectively, they point to the need for alternatives to iNO. One obvious alternative is to identify S-nitrosylating agents that are more efficient than NO gas in correcting dysregulations in SNO homeostasis.

POTENTIAL SOURCES OF EXOGENOUS NO/SNO BIOACTIVITY

Organic nitrates and organic nitrites can S-nitrosylate proteins.[133] However, the intravenous use of such NO-donor compounds to treat preterm infants is limited by

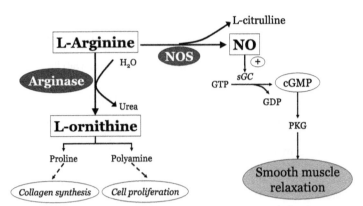

Fig. 5. Arginine serves as a common substrate for the enzymes NOS and arginase. Upregulation of arginase may divert arginine away from NOS, resulting in deficient NO/cGMP signaling and potential detrimental lung effects.

nonspecific vasodilation and significant systemic hypotension can impair oxygenation by reducing flow to the right heart. In addition, most of these agents also impair hypoxic vasoconstriction that can further disrupt ventilation-perfusion matching, resulting in enhanced blood flow to poorly ventilated lung areas. Drug efficacy is also limited by tolerance development and accumulation of toxic metabolites (eg, cyanogen/cyanide radical from sodium nitroprusside).

Inhalation of aerosolized formulations of various organic nitrates and nitrites can relax the pulmonary vasculature,[134] but they have seen little use in neonatology; this is despite some agents' long history in adult therapy (eg, inhaled amyl nitrite has been used to treat angina since the 1860s[135]). Administration of sodium nitroprusside through the ventilation circuit was reported to improve oxygenation status of 10 critically ill neonates (between 28 and 40 weeks' gestational age).[136] However, the report suggests the infants desaturated when drug administration ceased (the article does not provide outcome information). In addition, only 2 infants were less than 33 weeks, which makes predicting effects in a preterm cohort impracticable. In a study involving older children (9–53 months) with congenital heart disease and PAH, inhaled nitroglycerin acutely decreased pulmonary arterial pressure.[137] Extrapolating this finding to preterm care in the NICU is difficult. The exposure time was brief because the drug was administered during a diagnostic right heart catheterization, precluding the collection of data on effect duration or appearance of tachyphylaxis.

Outside potential financial savings, it is unclear if inhalation of an organic nitrate/nitrite currently in clinical use would offer appreciable benefit over iNO, especially because the aerosolized forms that have been tested (nitroglycerin and sodium nitroprusside) can still lower systemic blood pressure after inhalation.[138] The consummate nitrosylating agent would work via S-nitrosylation mechanisms to improve oxygenation, stimulate alveolar growth and differentiation, and reduce inflammation. It would preferentially react with thiols, be biocompatible (both drug and metabolites), resist decomposition in a gaseous medium, be unreactive with oxygen, and yet be highly volatile so that it can be inhaled to act in the lungs. One agent that meets these criteria is ethyl nitrite (ENO).

ENO AS AN EXOGENOUS S-NITROSYLATING AGENT

ENO is a low-molecular-weight (75.07), colorless organic nitrite with a density of 0.9. It can be stored as a liquid, but with a low boiling point (16.5–17°C) it is volatile at room temperature, which allows for inhalation or other gaseous routes of delivery. On exposure to biologic media (including blood), ENO preferentially reacts with thiols to form stable adducts with endocrine activity. Further, it does not form toxic NOx when mixed with oxygen.[139] ENO (like SNO-Hb itself[140]) has potent systemic (blood flow-increasing) as well as pulmonary vascular effects. A series of preclinical translational studies with this agent showed that ENO:

- Are highly selective for thiols
- Can rapidly restore RBC SNO-Hb levels[139]
- Decreases pulmonary pressures in animal models[72,139]
- Produces SNOs, which are known to increase circulating stem cells[141]
- Effectively attenuates pneumoperitoneum-induced reductions in splanchnic blood flow and insufflation-induced markers of tissue injury[142,143]
- Improves outcome in a mouse model of subarachnoid hemorrhage[144]
- Reduces both hyperoxic[59] and immunologic[60] pulmonary inflammatory responses and associated pulmonary cell damage in rodent models of lung injury

ENO has been tested clinically in 2 high-risk patient populations. In the first trial, ENO was administered by ventilator to infants with persistent pulmonary hypertension of the newborn (the 7 patients ranged between 38 and 40 weeks' gestational age).[145] The drug produced sustained dose-dependent improvements in postductal arterial oxygen saturation and in systemic hemodynamics. There was no evidence of rebound pulmonary hypertension when drug administration was abruptly terminated after 4 hours of exposure.

The second trial was conducted on adults with pulmonary hypertension.[72] These patients were found to have low amounts of circulating SNO-Hb, which negatively affected the ability of their RBCs to elicit hypoxic vasodilation. In addition, RBC SNO levels were inversely correlated with pulmonary artery pressure. Inhaled ENO

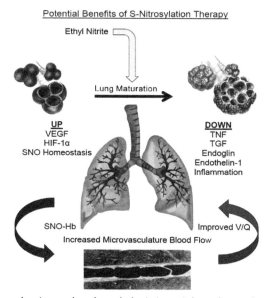

Potential Benefits of S-Nitrosylation Therapy

Ethyl Nitrite

Lung Maturation

UP
VEGF
HIF-1α
SNO Homeostasis

DOWN
TNF
TGF
Endoglin
Endothelin-1
Inflammation

SNO-Hb

Improved V/Q

Increased Microvasculature Blood Flow

Fig. 6. Potential mechanisms whereby ethyl nitrite might enhance lung maturation and improve ventilation/perfusion matching.

produced immediate salutary effects: pulmonary arterial pressure and pulmonary vascular resistance declined, and arterial Po_2 increased. These effects were accompanied by increases in SNO-Hb. Moreover, ENO corrected the impairments in RBC hypoxic vasodilatory activity. Studies in large animals have shown that effects of ENO are mediated primarily via RBCs (and not through direct effects of ENO in the lungs).

As of this writing, no preterm infant has been administered ENO, but the results compiled to date are supportive for conducting a clinical trial for preventing or ameliorating BPD in this patient population. In addition, it is reasonable to predict that ENO therapy could confer multiple benefits by addressing other organ injuries of prematurity that are believed to result from impaired blood flow and oxygen delivery (eg, acute kidney injury, necrotizing enterocolitis, periventricular leukomalacia; administration of ENO can correct flow deficiencies to multiple internal organs) (**Fig. 6**).[143] The mechanism of action of ENO differs fundamentally from the major action of iNO (or phosphodiesterase inhibitors). Phosphodiesterase inhibitors act mainly on the sGC pathway within the pulmonary vasculature and have limited ability to increase SNO-Hb (ie, improve peripheral oxygen delivery) or to correct other aspects of SNO-based signaling that are disrupted in the immature lung.

SUMMARY

Over the last decade there has been remarkable interest in the potential ability of inhaled NO to decrease the incidence or severity of BPD. As we have detailed, this interest has been driven by a solid body of experimental data primarily in animal models, documenting a diversity of biologically based beneficial effects on lung development. These encouraging experimental data were followed up by a considerable number of well-designed, randomized, clinical trials, blinded for experimental versus control groups. As a result of these clinical trials, initial enthusiasm has been greatly diminished by a series of negative results. Systematic meta-analysis of the available data are complicated by the variable study designs. Furthermore, there is no currently available biomarker to indicate potential for selective benefit.

Further studies addressing the combination of patient population, dose, duration, and timing of inhaled NO exposure are needed. These studies need to be appropriately powered to detect an effect on BPD or mortality as well as monitor for adverse outcomes of treatment. At the time of this writing, 4 active clinical trials[146–149] are under way that will add to the growing fund of knowledge and it is hoped will identify a dosing regimen most beneficial in this at-risk population of preterm infants. Nonetheless, based on available data, it was possible to convene a consensus conference in late 2010 to provide therapeutic guidelines from leading clinical and basic investigators in the field.[8] Their primary conclusion is that apart from occasional instances of pulmonary hypertension or hypoplasia, routine or rescue use of inhaled NO cannot be recommended in preterm infants with respiratory failure. As for preterm infants with BPD, although promising results derived from basic studies have not been realized, future investigation of the role of NO in lung development should proceed.

REFERENCES

1. Northway WH Jr, Rosan RC, Porter DY. Pulmonary disease following respirator therapy of hyaline-membrane disease. Bronchopulmonary dysplasia. N Engl J Med 1967;276:357–68.
2. Fanaroff AA, Stoll BJ, Wright LL, et al. Trends in neonatal morbidity and mortality for very low birthweight infants. Am J Obstet Gynecol 2007;196(147):e1–8.

3. D'Angio CT, Maniscalco WM. Bronchopulmonary dysplasia in preterm infants: pathophysiology and management strategies. Paediatr Drugs 2004;6:303–30.

4. Gien J, Kinsella JP. Pathogenesis and treatment of bronchopulmonary dysplasia. Curr Opin Pediatr 2011;23:305–13.

5. Bancalari E, Polin RA. The newborn lung. 1st edition. Philadelphia: Saunders/Elsevier; 2008.

6. Baraldi E, Filippone M. Chronic lung disease after premature birth. N Engl J Med 2007;357:1946–55.

7. Jobe AH, Bancalari E. Bronchopulmonary dysplasia. Am J Respir Crit Care Med 2001;163:1723–9.

8. Cole FS, Alleyne C, Barks JD, et al. NIH Consensus Development Conference statement: inhaled nitric-oxide therapy for premature infants. Pediatrics 2011; 127:363–9.

9. Northway WH Jr, Moss RB, Carlisle KB, et al. Late pulmonary sequelae of bronchopulmonary dysplasia. N Engl J Med 1990;323:1793–9.

10. Trachsel D, Brutsche MH, Hug-Batschelet H, et al. Progressive static pulmonary hyperinflation in survivors of severe bronchopulmonary dysplasia by mid-adulthood. Thorax 2011. [Epub ahead of print].

11. Frostell C, Fratacci MD, Wain JC, et al. Inhaled nitric oxide. A selective pulmonary vasodilator reversing hypoxic pulmonary vasoconstriction. Circulation 1991;83:2038–47.

12. Roberts JD, Polaner DM, Lang P, et al. Inhaled nitric oxide in persistent pulmonary hypertension of the newborn. Lancet 1992;340:818–9.

13. Kinsella JP, Neish SR, Shaffer E, et al. Low-dose inhalation nitric oxide in persistent pulmonary hypertension of the newborn. Lancet 1992;340:819–20.

14. Inhaled nitric oxide in full-term and nearly full-term infants with hypoxic respiratory failure. The Neonatal Inhaled Nitric Oxide Study Group. N Engl J Med 1997; 336:597–604.

15. Clark RH, Kueser TJ, Walker MW, et al. Low-dose nitric oxide therapy for persistent pulmonary hypertension of the newborn. Clinical Inhaled Nitric Oxide Research Group. N Engl J Med 2000;342:469–74.

16. Davidson D, Barefield ES, Kattwinkel J, et al. Inhaled nitric oxide for the early treatment of persistent pulmonary hypertension of the term newborn: a randomized, double-masked, placebo-controlled, dose-response, multicenter study. The I-NO/PPHN Study Group. Pediatrics 1998;101:325–34.

17. McCurnin DC, Pierce RA, Chang LY, et al. Inhaled NO improves early pulmonary function and modifies lung growth and elastin deposition in a baboon model of neonatal chronic lung disease. Am J Physiol Lung Cell Mol Physiol 2005;288: L450–9.

18. Iben SC, Dreshaj IA, Farver CF, et al. Role of endogenous nitric oxide in hyperoxia-induced airway hyperreactivity in maturing rats. J Applied Physiology 2000;89:1205–12.

19. Lin YJ, Markham NE, Balasubramaniam V, et al. Inhaled nitric oxide enhances distal lung growth after exposure to hyperoxia in neonatal rats. Pediatr Res 2005;58:22–9.

20. Bland RD, Albertine KH, Carlton DP, et al. Inhaled nitric oxide effects on lung structure and function in chronically ventilated preterm lambs. Am J Respir Crit Care Med 2005;172:899–906.

21. Early compared with delayed inhaled nitric oxide in moderately hypoxaemic neonates with respiratory failure: a randomised controlled trial. The Franco-Belgium Collaborative NO Trial Group. Lancet 1999;354:1066–71.

22. Ballard RA, Truog WE, Cnaan A, et al. Inhaled nitric oxide in preterm infants undergoing mechanical ventilation. N Engl J Med 2006;355:343–53.

23. Dani C, Bertini G, Pezzati M, et al. Inhaled nitric oxide in very preterm infants with severe respiratory distress syndrome. Acta Paediatr 2006;95:1116–23.

24. Field D, Elbourne D, Truesdale A, et al. Neonatal ventilation with inhaled nitric oxide versus ventilatory support without inhaled nitric oxide for preterm infants with severe respiratory failure: the INNOVO multicentre randomised controlled trial (ISRCTN 17821339). Pediatrics 2005;115:926–36.

25. Hascoet JM, Fresson J, Claris O, et al. The safety and efficacy of nitric oxide therapy in premature infants. J Pediatr 2005;146:318–23.

26. Kinsella JP, Cutter GR, Walsh WF, et al. Early inhaled nitric oxide therapy in premature newborns with respiratory failure. N Engl J Med 2006;355:354–64.

27. Kinsella JP, Walsh WF, Bose CL, et al. Inhaled nitric oxide in premature neonates with severe hypoxaemic respiratory failure: a randomised controlled trial. Lancet 1999;354:1061–5.

28. Mercier JC, Hummler H, Durrmeyer X, et al. Inhaled nitric oxide for prevention of bronchopulmonary dysplasia in premature babies (EUNO): a randomised controlled trial. Lancet 2010;376:346–54.

29. Schreiber MD, Gin-Mestan K, Marks JD, et al. Inhaled nitric oxide in premature infants with the respiratory distress syndrome. N Engl J Med 2003;349:2099–107.

30. Srisuparp P, Heitschmidt M, Schreiber MD. Inhaled nitric oxide therapy in premature infants with mild to moderate respiratory distress syndrome. J Med Assoc Thai 2002;85(Suppl 2):S469–78.

31. Su PH, Chen JY. Inhaled nitric oxide in the management of preterm infants with severe respiratory failure. J Perinatol 2008;28:112–6.

32. Subhedar NV, Ryan SW, Shaw NJ. Open randomised controlled trial of inhaled nitric oxide and early dexamethasone in high risk preterm infants. Arch Dis Child Fetal Neonatal Ed 1997;77:F185–90.

33. Van Meurs KP, Hintz SR, Ehrenkranz RA, et al. Inhaled nitric oxide in infants >1500 g and <34 weeks gestation with severe respiratory failure. J Perinatol 2007;27: 347–52.

34. Van Meurs KP, Wright LL, Ehrenkranz RA, et al. Inhaled nitric oxide for premature infants with severe respiratory failure. N Engl J Med 2005;353:13–22.

35. Barrington KJ, Finer N. Inhaled nitric oxide for respiratory failure in preterm infants. Cochrane Database Syst Rev 2010;12:CD000509.

36. Askie LM, Ballard RA, Cutter GR, et al. Inhaled nitric oxide in preterm infants: an individual-patient data meta-analysis of randomized trials. Pediatrics 2011;128: 729–39.

37. Donohue PK, Gilmore MM, Cristofalo E, et al. Inhaled nitric oxide in preterm infants: a systematic review. Pediatrics 2011;127:e414–22.

38. Hibbs AM, Walsh MC, Martin RJ, et al. One-year respiratory outcomes of preterm infants enrolled in the Nitric Oxide (to prevent) Chronic Lung Disease trial. J Pediatr 2008;153:525–9.

39. Walsh MC, Hibbs AM, Martin CR, et al. Two-year neurodevelopmental outcomes of ventilated preterm infants treated with inhaled nitric oxide. J Pediatr 2010;156: 556–561.e1.

40. Watson RS, Clermont G, Kinsella JP, et al. Clinical and economic effects of iNO in premature newborns with respiratory failure at 1 year. Pediatrics 2009;124: 1333–43.

41. Hamon I, Fresson J, Nicolas MB, et al. Early inhaled nitric oxide improves oxidative balance in very preterm infants. Pediatr Res 2005;57:637–43.

42. Huddy CL, Bennett CC, Hardy P, et al. The INNOVO multicentre randomised controlled trial: neonatal ventilation with inhaled nitric oxide versus ventilatory support without nitric oxide for severe respiratory failure in preterm infants: follow up at 4-5 years. Arch Dis Child Fetal Neonatal Ed 2008;93:F430–5.
43. Hintz SR, Van Meurs KP, Perritt R, et al. Neurodevelopmental outcomes of premature infants with severe respiratory failure enrolled in a randomized controlled trial of inhaled nitric oxide. J Pediatr 2007;151:16–22.e1–3.
44. Mestan KK, Marks JD, Hecox K, et al. Neurodevelopmental outcomes of premature infants treated with inhaled nitric oxide. N Engl J Med 2005;353:23–32.
45. Bennett AJ, Shaw NJ, Gregg JE, et al. Neurodevelopmental outcome in high-risk preterm infants treated with inhaled nitric oxide. Acta Paediatr 2001;90:573–6.
46. Tanaka Y, Hayashi T, Kitajima H, et al. Inhaled nitric oxide therapy decreases the risk of cerebral palsy in preterm infants with persistent pulmonary hypertension of the newborn. Pediatrics 2007;119:1159–64.
47. Steinhorn RH, Shaul PW, deRegnier RA, et al. Inhaled nitric oxide and bronchopulmonary dysplasia. Pediatrics 2011;128:e255–6 [author reply: e6–7].
48. Lima B, Forrester MT, Hess DT, et al. S-Nitrosylation in cardiovascular signaling. Circ Res 2010;106:633–46.
49. Hess DT, Foster MW, Stamler JS. Assays for S-nitrosothiols and S-nitrosylated proteins and mechanistic insights into cardioprotection. Circulation 2009;120:190–3.
50. Martin RJ, Walsh MC. Inhaled nitric oxide for preterm infants–who benefits? N Engl J Med 2005;353:82–4.
51. Khan SA, Lee K, Minhas KM, et al. Neuronal nitric oxide synthase negatively regulates xanthine oxidoreductase inhibition of cardiac excitation-contraction coupling. Proc Natl Acad Sci U S A 2004;101:15944–8.
52. Saavedra WF, Paolocci N, St John ME, et al. Imbalance between xanthine oxidase and nitric oxide synthase signaling pathways underlies mechanoenergetic uncoupling in the failing heart. Circ Res 2002;90:297–304.
53. Landmesser U, Spiekermann S, Dikalov S, et al. Vascular oxidative stress and endothelial dysfunction in patients with chronic heart failure: role of xanthine-oxidase and extracellular superoxide dismutase. Circulation 2002;106:3073–8.
54. Hilenski LL, Clempus RE, Quinn MT, et al. Distinct subcellular localizations of Nox1 and Nox4 in vascular smooth muscle cells. Arterioscler Thromb Vasc Biol 2004;24:677–83.
55. Foster MW, Hess DT, Stamler JS. Protein S-nitrosylation in health and disease: a current perspective. Trends Mol Med 2009;15:391–404.
56. Wei W, Li B, Hanes MA, et al. S-Nitrosylation from GSNOR deficiency impairs DNA repair and promotes hepatocarcinogenesis. Sci Transl Med 2010;2:19ra3.
57. Prasad R, Giri S, Nath N, et al. GSNO attenuates EAE disease by S-nitrosylation-mediated modulation of endothelial-monocyte interactions. Glia 2007;55:65–77.
58. Savidge TC, Newman P, Pothoulakis C, et al. Enteric glia regulate intestinal barrier function and inflammation via release of S-nitrosoglutathione. Gastroenterology 2007;132:1344–58.
59. Auten RL, Mason SN, Whorton MH, et al. Inhaled ethyl nitrite prevents hyperoxia-impaired postnatal alveolar development in newborn rats. Am J Respir Crit Care Med 2007;176:291–9.
60. Marshall HE, Potts EN, Kelleher ZT, et al. Protection from lipopolysaccharide-induced lung injury by augmentation of airway S-nitrosothiols. Am J Respir Crit Care Med 2009;180:11–8.
61. Que LG, Liu L, Yan Y, et al. Protection from experimental asthma by an endogenous bronchodilator. Science 2005;308:1618–21.

62. Snyder AH, McPherson ME, Hunt JF, et al. Acute effects of aerosolized S-nitrosoglutathione in cystic fibrosis. Am J Respir Crit Care Med 2002;165:922–6.

63. Gaston B, Singel D, Doctor A, et al. S-Nitrosothiol signaling in respiratory biology. Am J Respir Crit Care Med 2006;173:1186–93.

64. Daaka Y. S-Nitrosylation-regulated GPCR signaling. Biochim Biophys Acta 2012;1820(6):743–51.

65. Seth D, Stamler JS. The SNO-proteome: causation and classifications. Curr Opin Chem Biol 2011;15:129–36.

66. Hess DT, Stamler JS. Regulation by S-nitrosylation of protein post-translational modification. J Biol Chem 2012;287:4411–8.

67. Schulman IH, Hare JM. Regulation of cardiovascular cellular processes by S-nitrosylation. Biochim Biophys Acta 2012;1820(6):752–62.

68. Grasemann H, Gaston B, Fang K, et al. Decreased levels of nitrosothiols in the lower airways of patients with cystic fibrosis and normal pulmonary function. J Pediatr 1999;135:770–2.

69. Zaman K, Carraro S, Doherty J, et al. S-Nitrosylating agents: a novel class of compounds that increase cystic fibrosis transmembrane conductance regulator expression and maturation in epithelial cells. Mol Pharmacol 2006;70:1435–42.

70. Gaston B, Sears S, Woods J, et al. Bronchodilator S-nitrosothiol deficiency in asthmatic respiratory failure. Lancet 1998;351:1317–9.

71. Que LG, Yang Z, Stamler JS, et al. S-Nitrosoglutathione reductase: an important regulator in human asthma. Am J Respir Crit Care Med 2009;180:226–31.

72. McMahon TJ, Ahearn GS, Moya MP, et al. A nitric oxide processing defect of red blood cells created by hypoxia: deficiency of S-nitrosohemoglobin in pulmonary hypertension. Proc Natl Acad Sci U S A 2005;102:14801–6.

73. Singel DJ, Stamler JS. Chemical physiology of blood flow regulation by red blood cells: the role of nitric oxide and S-nitrosohemoglobin. Annu Rev Physiol 2005;67:99–145.

74. Doctor A, Stamler JS. Nitric oxide transport in blood: a third gas in the respiratory cycle. In: Comprehensive Physiology. John Wiley & Sons, Inc; 2011. p. 541–68.

75. Luchsinger BP, Rich EN, Gow AJ, et al. Routes to S-nitroso-hemoglobin formation with heme redox and preferential reactivity in the beta subunits. Proc Natl Acad Sci U S A 2003;100:461–6.

76. Angelo M, Singel DJ, Stamler JS. An S-nitrosothiol (SNO) synthase function of hemoglobin that utilizes nitrite as a substrate. Proc Natl Acad Sci U S A 2006; 103:8366–71.

77. Pezacki JP, Ship NJ, Kluger R. Release of nitric oxide from S-nitrosohemoglobin. Electron transfer as a response to deoxygenation. J Am Chem Soc 2001;123: 4615–6.

78. McMahon TJ, Stone AE, Bonaventura J, et al. Functional coupling of oxygen binding and vasoactivity in S-nitrosohemoglobin. J Biol Chem 2000;275:16738–45.

79. Doctor A, Platt R, Sheram ML, et al. Hemoglobin conformation couples erythrocyte S-nitrosothiol content to O2 gradients. Proc Natl Acad Sci U S A 2005;102: 5709–14.

80. Deem S, Min JH, Moulding JD, et al. Red blood cells prevent inhibition of hypoxic pulmonary vasoconstriction by nitrite in isolated, perfused rat lungs. Am J Physiol Heart Circ Physiol 2007;292:H963–70.

81. Hodges AN, Delaney S, Lecomte JM, et al. Effect of hyperbaric oxygen on oxygen uptake and measurements in the blood and tissues in a normobaric environment. Br J Sports Med 2003;37:516–20.

82. Duling BR, Berne RM. Longitudinal gradients in periarteriolar oxygen tension. A possible mechanism for the participation of oxygen in local regulation of blood flow. Circ Res 1970;27:669–78.

83. Allen BW, Stamler JS, Piantadosi CA. Hemoglobin, nitric oxide and molecular mechanisms of hypoxic vasodilation. Trends Mol Med 2009;15:452–60.

84. Intaglietta M, Johnson PC, Winslow RM. Microvascular and tissue oxygen distribution. Cardiovasc Res 1996;32:632–43.

85. Roach RC, Koskolou MD, Calbet JA, et al. Arterial O2 content and tension in regulation of cardiac output and leg blood flow during exercise in humans. Am J Physiol 1999;276:H438–45.

86. Gonzalez-Alonso J, Olsen DB, Saltin B. Erythrocyte and the regulation of human skeletal muscle blood flow and oxygen delivery: role of circulating ATP. Circ Res 2002;91:1046–55.

87. Gonzalez-Alonso J, Mortensen SP, Dawson EA, et al. Erythrocytes and the regulation of human skeletal muscle blood flow and oxygen delivery: role of erythrocyte count and oxygenation state of haemoglobin. J Physiol 2006;572: 295–305.

88. McMahon TJ, Moon RE, Luschinger BP, et al. Nitric oxide in the human respiratory cycle. Nat Med 2002;8:711–7.

89. Schroeder RA, Cai C, Kuo PC. Endotoxin-mediated nitric oxide synthesis inhibits IL-1beta gene transcription in ANA-1 murine macrophages. Am J Physiol 1999;277:C523–30.

90. Xiong H, Zhu C, Li F, et al. Inhibition of interleukin-12 p40 transcription and NF-kappaB activation by nitric oxide in murine macrophages and dendritic cells. J Biol Chem 2004;279:10776–83.

91. Into T, Inomata M, Nakashima M, et al. Regulation of MyD88-dependent signaling events by S nitrosylation retards toll-like receptor signal transduction and initiation of acute-phase immune responses. Mol Cell Biol 2008;28:1338–47.

92. del Fresno C, Gomez-Garcia L, Caveda L, et al. Nitric oxide activates the expression of IRAK-M via the release of TNF-alpha in human monocytes. Nitric Oxide 2004;10:213–20.

93. Gonzalez-Leon MC, Soares-Schanoski A, del Fresno C, et al. Nitric oxide induces SOCS-1 expression in human monocytes in a TNF-alpha-dependent manner. J Endotoxin Res 2006;12:296–306.

94. Marshall HE, Stamler JS. Inhibition of NF-kappa B by S-nitrosylation. Biochemistry 2001;40:1688–93.

95. Kelleher ZT, Matsumoto A, Stamler JS, et al. NOS2 regulation of NF-kappaB by S-nitrosylation of p65. J Biol Chem 2007;282:30667–72.

96. Guo CJ, Atochina-Vasserman EN, Abramova E, et al. S-Nitrosylation of surfactant protein-D controls inflammatory function. PLoS Biol 2008;6:e266.

97. Park HS, Huh SH, Kim MS, et al. Nitric oxide negatively regulates c-Jun N-terminal kinase/stress-activated protein kinase by means of S-nitrosylation. Proc Natl Acad Sci U S A 2000;97:14382–7.

98. Kim SF, Huri DA, Snyder SH. Inducible nitric oxide synthase binds, S-nitrosylates, and activates cyclooxygenase-2. Science 2005;310:1966–70.

99. Thompson A, Bhandari V. Pulmonary biomarkers of bronchopulmonary dysplasia. Biomark Insights 2008;3:361–73.

100. Schwarz MA, Cleaver OB. Development of the pulmonary endothelium in development of the pulmonary circulation: vasculogenesis and angiogenesis. In: Voelkel NF, Rounds S, editors. The pulmonary endothelium: function in health and disease. Hoboken (NJ): John Wiley; 2009. p. 24.

101. Husain AN, Siddiqui NH, Stocker JT. Pathology of arrested acinar development in postsurfactant bronchopulmonary dysplasia. Hum Pathol 1998;29: 710–7.

102. Pardi G, Cetin I, Marconi AM, et al. Diagnostic value of blood sampling in fetuses with growth retardation. N Engl J Med 1993;328:692–6.

103. Gao Y, Raj JU. Regulation of the pulmonary circulation in the fetus and newborn. Physiol Rev 2010;90:1291–335.

104. Ahlfeld SK, Conway SJ. Aberrant signaling pathways of the lung mesenchyme and their contributions to the pathogenesis of bronchopulmonary dysplasia. Birth Defects Res A Clin Mol Teratol 2012;94:3–15.

105. Sheffield M, Mabry S, Thibeault DW, et al. Pulmonary nitric oxide synthases and nitrotyrosine: findings during lung development and in chronic lung disease of prematurity. Pediatrics 2006;118:1056–64.

106. Davis CW, Gonzales LW, Ballard RA, et al. Expression of nitric oxide synthases and endogenous NO metabolism in bronchopulmonary dysplasia. Pediatr Pulmonol 2008;43:703–9.

107. Gow AJ, Chen Q, Hess DT, et al. Basal and stimulated protein S-nitrosylation in multiple cell types and tissues. J Biol Chem 2002;277:9637–40.

108. Abman SH. Impaired vascular endothelial growth factor signaling in the pathogenesis of neonatal pulmonary vascular disease. Adv Exp Med Biol 2010;661: 323–35.

109. Bhatt AJ, Pryhuber GS, Huyck H, et al. Disrupted pulmonary vasculature and decreased vascular endothelial growth factor, Flt-1, and TIE-2 in human infants dying with bronchopulmonary dysplasia. Am J Respir Crit Care Med 2001;164: 1971–80.

110. Hasan J, Beharry KD, Valencia AM, et al. Soluble vascular endothelial growth factor receptor 1 in tracheal aspirate fluid of preterm neonates at birth may be predictive of bronchopulmonary dysplasia/chronic lung disease. Pediatrics 2009;123:1541–7.

111. Popova AP, Bozyk PD, Bentley JK, et al. Isolation of tracheal aspirate mesenchymal stromal cells predicts bronchopulmonary dysplasia. Pediatrics 2010; 126:e1127–33.

112. De Paepe ME, Patel C, Tsai A, et al. Endoglin (CD105) up-regulation in pulmonary microvasculature of ventilated preterm infants. Am J Respir Crit Care Med 2008;178:180–7.

113. Fujinaga H, Baker CD, Ryan SL, et al. Hyperoxia disrupts vascular endothelial growth factor-nitric oxide signaling and decreases growth of endothelial colony-forming cells from preterm infants. Am J Physiol Lung Cell Mol Physiol 2009;297:L1160–9.

114. Ohls RK. Transfusions in the preterm infant. Neoreviews 2007;8:e377–86.

115. Nunes dos Santos AM, Trindade CE. Red blood cell transfusions in the neonate. Neoreviews 2011;12:e13–9.

116. Cooke RW, Drury JA, Yoxall CW, et al. Blood transfusion and chronic lung disease in preterm infants. Eur J Pediatr 1997;156:47–50.

117. Valieva OA, Strandjord TP, Mayock DE, et al. Effects of transfusions in extremely low birth weight infants: a retrospective study. J Pediatr 2009;155:331–337.e1.

118. Zhang H, Fang J, Su H, et al. Risk factors for bronchopulmonary dysplasia in neonates born at ≤1500 g (1999-2009). Pediatr Int 2011;53:915–20.

119. Reynolds JD, Ahearn GS, Angelo M, et al. S-Nitrosohemoglobin deficiency: a mechanism for loss of physiological activity in banked blood. Proc Natl Acad Sci U S A 2007;104:17058–62.

120. Reynolds JD, Hess DT, Stamler JS. The transfusion problem: role of aberrant S-nitrosylation. Transfusion 2011;51:852–8.
121. Murad F. Shattuck Lecture. Nitric oxide and cyclic GMP in cell signaling and drug development. N Engl J Med 2006;355:2003–11.
122. Elrod JW, Calvert JW, Gundewar S, et al. Nitric oxide promotes distant organ protection: evidence for an endocrine role of nitric oxide. Proc Natl Acad Sci U S A 2008;105:11430–5.
123. Fox-Robichaud A, Payne D, Hasan SU, et al. Inhaled NO as a viable antiadhesive therapy for ischemia/reperfusion injury of distal microvascular beds. J Clin Invest 1998;101:2497–505.
124. Ibrahim YI, Ninnis JR, Hopper AO, et al. Inhaled nitric oxide therapy increases blood nitrite, nitrate, and s-nitrosohemoglobin concentrations in infants with pulmonary hypertension. J Pediatr 2012;160:245–51.
125. Minamishima S, Kida K, Tokuda K, et al. Inhaled nitric oxide improves outcomes after successful cardiopulmonary resuscitation in mice. Circulation 2011;124:1645–53.
126. Ng ES, Jourd'heuil D, McCord JM, et al. Enhanced S-nitroso-albumin formation from inhaled NO during ischemia/reperfusion. Circ Res 2004;94:559–65.
127. Top AP, Ince C, Schouwenberg PH, et al. Inhaled nitric oxide improves systemic microcirculation in infants with hypoxemic respiratory failure. Pediatr Crit Care Med 2011;12:e271–4.
128. Terpolilli NA, Kim SW, Thal SC, et al. Inhalation of nitric oxide prevents ischemic brain damage in experimental stroke by selective dilatation of collateral arterioles. Circ Res 2012;110(5):727–38.
129. McMahon TJ, Doctor A. Extrapulmonary effects of inhaled nitric oxide: role of reversible S-nitrosylation of erythrocytic hemoglobin. Proc Am Thorac Soc 2006;3:153–60.
130. Wind M, Stern A. Comparison of human adult and fetal hemoglobin: aminophenol-induced methemoglobin formation. Experientia 1977;33:1500–1.
131. Farrow KN, Groh BS, Schumacker PT, et al. Hyperoia increases phosphodiesterase 5 expression and activity in ovine fetal pulmonary artery smooth muscle cells. Circ Res 2008;102:226–33.
132. Ali NK, Jafri A, Sopi RB, et al. Role of arginase in impairing relaxation of lung parenchyma of hyperoxia-exposed neonatal rats. Neonatology 2012;101:106–15.
133. Janero DR, Bryan NS, Saijo F, et al. Differential nitros(yl)ation of blood and tissue constituents during glyceryl trinitrate biotransformation in vivo. Proc Natl Acad Sci U S A 2004;101:16958–63.
134. Schutte H, Grimminger F, Otterbein J, et al. Efficiency of aerosolized nitric oxide donor drugs to achieve sustained pulmonary vasodilation. J Pharmacol Exp Ther 1997;282:985–94.
135. Brunton TL. On the employment of nitrite of amyl in the collapse of cholera. Br Med J 1872;1:42–5.
136. Palhares DB, Figueiredo CS, Moura AJ. Endotracheal inhalatory sodium nitroprusside in severely hypoxic newborns. J Perinat Med 1998;26:219–24.
137. Goyal P, Kiran U, Chauhan S, et al. Efficacy of nitroglycerin inhalation in reducing pulmonary arterial hypertension in children with congenital heart disease. Br J Anaesth 2006;97:208–14.
138. Bando M, Ishii Y, Kitamura S, et al. Effects of inhalation of nitroglycerin on hypoxic pulmonary vasoconstriction. Respiration 1998;65:63–70.
139. Moya MP, Gow AJ, McMahon TJ, et al. S-Nitrosothiol repletion by an inhaled gas regulates pulmonary function. Proc Natl Acad Sci U S A 2001;98:5792–7.

140. Jia L, Bonaventura C, Bonaventura J, et al. S-Nitrosohaemoglobin: a dynamic activity of blood involved in vascular control. Nature 1996;380:221–6.
141. Lima B, Lam GK, Xie L, et al. Endogenous S-nitrosothiols protect against myocardial injury. Proc Natl Acad Sci U S A 2009;106:6297–302.
142. Ali NA, Eubanks WS, Stamler JS, et al. A method to attenuate pneumoperitoneum-induced reductions in splanchnic blood flow. Ann Surg 2005;241:256–61.
143. Shimazutsu K, Uemura K, Auten KM, et al. Inclusion of a nitric oxide congener in the insufflation gas repletes S-nitrosohemoglobin and stabilizes physiologic status during prolonged carbon dioxide pneumoperitoneum. Clin Transl Sci 2009;2:405–12.
144. Sheng H, Reynolds JD, Auten RL, et al. Pharmacologically augmented S-nitrosylated hemoglobin improves recovery from murine subarachnoid hemorrhage. Stroke 2011;42:471–6.
145. Moya MP, Gow AJ, Califf RM, et al. Inhaled ethyl nitrite gas for persistent pulmonary hypertension of the newborn. Lancet 2002;360:141–3.
146. Inhaled nitric oxide and neuroprotection in premature infants (NOVA2). Available at: http://clinicaltrials.gov/ct2/show/NCT00515281. Accessed December 16, 2011.
147. Examining the use of non-invasive inhaled nitric oxide to reduce chronic lung disease in premature newborns. Available at: http://clinicaltrials.gov/ct2/show/NCT00955487. Accessed December 16, 2011.
148. Inhaled nitric oxide (INO) for the prevention of bronchopulmonary dysplasia (BPD) in preterm infants. Available at: http://clinicaltrials.gov/ct2/show/NCT00931632. Accessed December 16, 2011.
149. Trial of late surfactant to prevent BPD: a pilot study in ventilated preterm neonates receiving inhaled nitric oxide (TOLSURF Pilot). Available at: http://clinicaltrials.gov/ct2/show/NCT00569530. Accessed December 16, 2011.

Pathophysiology of Aerodigestive Pulmonary Disorders in the Neonate

Sudarshan R. Jadcherla, MD, FRCPI, DCH, AGAF[a,b,c,]*

KEYWORDS

- Esophagus • Aerodigestive reflexes • Infant • Swallowing • Gastroesophageal reflux
- Dysphagia • Aspiration

KEY POINTS

- Embryologic origins and development, innervation, and functions of airway and pharyng-oesophageal segment (which together constitute the aerodigestive tract) are closely inter-related, and have codependent functions.
- The most important functions of the upper airway are facilitating ventilation, phonation, and lower airway protection; these functions are enabled by brain stem-mediated vagal reflexes that participate at multi-tier levels.
- The significant functions of the pharyngoesophageal segment include facilitating safe deglutition and esophageal transport of nutrients, volume clearance as in swallowing or emesis, and esophageal and airway protection.
- Aerodigestive symptoms and signs are not specific and can coexist.
- Nonpharmacologic approaches to manage gastroesophageal reflux disease are based on the physiology of esophago-gastric functions.
- Investigative methods to assess the aerodigestive tract have test-specific strengths and limitations.

Grant support from National Institutes of Health (NDDK) grants R01 DK 068158 (Jadcherla) and P01 DK 068051 (Jadcherla/Shaker) is acknowledged.

Conflict of interest: None.

[a] The Neonatal and Infant Feeding Disorders Program, Center for Perinatal Research, The Research Institute at Nationwide Children's Hospital, The Ohio State University Wexner College of Medicine, 700 Children's Drive, Columbus, OH 43205, USA; [b] Division of Neonatology, Department of Pediatrics, Center for Perinatal Research, The Research Institute at Nationwide Children's Hospital, The Ohio State University Wexner College of Medicine, 700 Children's Drive, Columbus, OH 43205, USA; [c] Division of Pediatric Gastroenterology and Nutrition, Center for Perinatal Research, Department of Pediatrics, The Research Institute at Nationwide Children's Hospital, The Ohio State University Wexner College of Medicine, 700 Children's Drive, Columbus, OH 43205, USA

* Division of Neonatology, Department of Pediatrics, Center for Perinatal Research, The Research Institute at Nationwide Children's Hospital, The Ohio State University Wexner College of Medicine, 700 Children's Drive, Columbus, OH 43205.

E-mail address: sudarshan.jadcherla@nationwidechildrens.org

INTRODUCTION TO AERODIGESTIVE PULMONARY DISORDERS

Technological advances in perinatal and neonatal care, respiratory management, and nutritional support have contributed to the increasing survival of high-risk neonates. Concomitantly, the prevalence of aerodigestive pathologies in survivors is also increasing. The exact prevalence of aerodigestive pulmonary disorders in the neonate is unknown. This fact may be related to increased survival of premature infants, changing definitions, and the heterogeneous nature of aerodigestive symptoms impeding accurate diagnosis. An estimate can be gleaned from the observations that 30% of preterm infants with birth weights less than 1000 g develop bronchopulmonary dysplasia (BPD),[1,2] and the estimated prevalence of swallowing problems in infants with BPD is 26%.[3]

Chronic lung disease of infancy (CLDI), a heterogeneous group of disorders, is associated with positive pressure mechanical ventilation and prolonged respiratory support requiring supplemental oxygen. The pathophysiology and management of BPD and CLDI are discussed elsewhere in this issue. Chronic aspiration, gastroesophageal reflux disease (GERD), reactive airway disease, and dysphagia may complicate or contribute to CLDI. An important therapeutic target directed at minimizing neonatal lung disease is management of feeding problems and aerodigestive symptoms. This article highlights the complexity and causes of aerodigestive symptoms and feeding problems (**Table 1**). Management of feeding problems in persistent CLDI requires further understanding of aerodigestive pathologies, which may aggravate and complicate recovery. The specific purposes of this article are to discuss

- Anatomy and physiology of the aerodigestive tract
- Maturation of basal and adaptive aerodigestive reflex mechanisms
- Gastroesophageal reflux (GER) and its implications
- Approaches to the evaluation of aerodigestive pathologies

Over the last decade, major advances in this field have led to clarification of aerodigestive pathophysiology, improved understanding of the symptoms, and development of newer multimodal, multidisciplinary clinical and translational approaches in

Table 1
Aerodigestive symptoms and related clinical mechanisms in neonates

Aerodigestive Symptoms	Related Clinical Mechanisms
Irritability and arching	Oromotor inertia, delayed swallowing, Dystonic neck muscles
Throat clearing and grunting	Poor pharyngeal clearance, nasopharyngeal reflux
Cough, stridor and wheeze, CLDI	Laryngeal penetration and airway microaspiration, airway Inflammation, macroaspiration
Regurgitation, reflux, and emesis	Gastroesophageal reflux, gastroesophageal reflux disease, gastroparesis, intestinal dysmotility, esophageal inflammation
Tachypnea, apnea and hyperpnoea, increased work of breathing, bradycardia and desaturations, apparent life-threatening events	Exaggerated airway protective and compensatory mechanisms, failed airway protective mechanisms, endurance and fatigue problems, lack of electrocortical arousal response

the human neonate. It is anticipated that improved understanding of areodigestive pathophysiology will result in appropriate evaluation and clarification, timely testing, and improved management of infants with CLDI.

ANATOMY OF AERODIGESTIVE TRACT

The complexities of the aerodigestive apparatus and functions confirm that it is much more than a conduit between the proximal airway, lungs and foregut. This section discusses the definition, developmental anatomy, and neuromuscular components of the aerodigestive apparatus.

Definition of the Aerodigestive Apparatus

For simplicity and clarity, the aerodigestive apparatus can be defined as the common pathway that facilitates safe breathing and safe swallowing. Broadly, this common pathway includes: nasopharynx, oropharynx, hypopharynx, esophagus, and stomach, in addition to supraglottic, glottic, and subglottic tubular airways (**Fig. 1**).

Developmental Anatomy and Embryology of the Aerodigestive Tract

The intricate relationship between the airway and foregut begins in embryonic life, and excellent articles pertinent to this section are available.[4–9] The aerodigestive organs are developed from adjacent segments of the primitive foregut.[6–9] The airway and the lung buds, the pharynx, the esophagus, the stomach, and the diaphragm are all derived from the primitive foregut and/or its mesenchyme, and share similar control systems.[6–9] By 4 weeks of embryologic life, the tracheobronchial diverticulum appears at the ventral wall of the foregut, with left vagus being anterior and right vagus posterior in position. At this stage of development, the stomach is a fusiform tube with the dorsal side growth rate greater than the ventral side, creating greater and lesser curvatures. At 7 weeks of embryonic life, the stomach also rotates 90° clockwise, and the greater curvature is now displaced to the left. The left vagus innervates the stomach

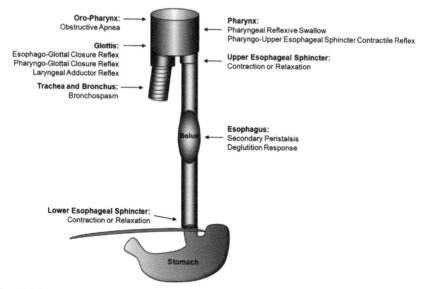

Fig. 1. Schematic representation of aerodigestive reflexes.

anteriorly, and the right vagus innervates the posterior aspect of the stomach. At 10 weeks, the esophagus and the stomach are in the proper position, with the circular and longitudinal muscle layers and the ganglion cells in place. The true vocal cords begin as glottal folds. By the 6th or 7th week of gestation, a structure superior to the true vocal cords evolves to protect the vocal cords and lower airway. This superior structure consists of epiglottis, aryepiglottic folds, false vocal cords, and the laryngeal ventricles. The epiglottis starts as a hypobranchial eminence behind the future tongue. By 7 weeks, the epiglottis is separated from the tongue. At the same time, 2 lateral folds connect to the base of the epiglottis, at the distal end of which develops the arytenoids cartilages. The larynx begins as a groove in the primitive foregut, which folds upon itself to become the laryngotracheal bud, the subsequent divisions of which form the bronchopulmonary segments. From this phase, 20 generations of conducting airways form. The first 8 generations constitute bronchi and acquire cartilaginous walls. The next 9 to 20 generations comprise the nonrespiratory bronchioles that are not cartilaginous, and contain smooth muscle; the subsequent divisions form the bronchopulmonary segments.[9]

Neuromuscular Components of the Aerodigestive Apparatus

Structurally, the pharynx is made of striated muscle, whereas the esophagus is a hollow tubular organ comprised of inner circular and outer longitudinal muscle layers with myenteric plexus in between. The proximal esophagus has striated muscle, whereas the distal esophagus has smooth muscle. The upper esophageal sphincter (UES), a constriction between the pharynx and the proximal esophagus, is characterized by a high-pressure zone generated by the cricopharyngeus (the principal muscle), proximal cervical esophagus, and inferior pharyngeal constrictor.[5] In contrast, the lower esophageal sphincter (LES) is an autonomous sphincter comprised chiefly of circular smooth muscle; the gastroesophageal junction integrity is further augmented by diaphragmatic crural fibers, intra-abdominal parts of the esophagus, and sling fibers of the stomach. The UES is innervated by: the vagus via the pharyngoesophageal, superior laryngeal, and recurrent laryngeal branches; the glossopharyngeal nerve; and the sympathetics via the cranial cervical ganglion. The distal end of the esophagus consists of the specialized smooth muscle, the LES, and an autonomous contractile apparatus that is tonically active and relaxes periodically to facilitate bolus transit. Although the LES is considered an important functional segment in preventing GER, other neighboring structures, including oblique sling fibers of stomach, musculofacial diaphragmatic sling, and the intra-abdominal esophagus, also contribute to this function.[4]

The musculature of the larynx is derived from the mesenchyme of the 4th and 6th pharyngeal arches. All laryngeal muscles are innervated by branches of the Xth cranial nerve. The superior laryngeal nerve innervates derivatives of the 4th pharyngeal arch (cricothyroid, levator palatini, and constrictors of pharynx), and the recurrent laryngeal nerve innervates derivatives of the 6th pharyngeal arch (intrinsic muscles of the larynx).

The airways and esophagus share common innervations.[4,5,10] Foregut afferents are derived from both vagal and dorsal root ganglions with cell bodies in the nodose ganglion. This afferent apparatus conveys signals to the neurons in the nucleus tractus solitarius, located in the dorsomedial medulla oblongata. These signals are integrated in a specific terminal site of the nucleus tractus solitarius, the subnucleus centralis, which is the sole point of termination of esophageal afferents. After sensory integration in the nucleus tractus solitarius, the signals in turn activate airway motor neurons in the nucleus ambiguous and the dorsal motor nucleus of the vagus, producing an efferent parasympathetic response and/or nonadrenergic noncholinergic response.

Thus, the sensory-motor components of aerodigestive tract innervations are as follows: (1) supraglottal mucosal areas from the 9th and 10th nerves, (2) supraglottal muscular areas from the 10th nerve, (3) infraglottal mucosal and muscular areas from the 10th nerve; and (4) pharynx and esophagus from the 9th and 10th nerves (**Tables 2** and **3**).

PHYSIOLOGY AND FUNCTIONS OF THE AERODIGESTIVE TRACT

The various organs within the aerodigestive tract have many functions; however, safe breathing and safe swallowing dominate regardless of age. The most important and highly relevant functions of the upper airway are

- Facilitating ventilation
- Phonation
- Lower airway protection

The significant functions of the pharyngoesophageal segment are

- Facilitating safe deglutition and esophageal transport of nutrients
- Volume clearance as in swallowing or emesis
- Airway protection

Glottal and esophageal functions vary depending on the stage of life.[1,5,11] For example, in fetal life, glottal and pharyngoesophageal transport functions in series, with lung fluid transported out of the primitive airway to the amniotic fluid pool, where it is swallowed by the fetal pharynx by 11 weeks of embryonic life. Primitive swallowing ability develops by 11 weeks; by 18 to 20 weeks, sucking movements appear, and by full-term gestation, the fetus can swallow and circulate nearly 500 mL of amniotic fluid in a day. Aspiration of amniotic fluid (comprised of fetal lung fluid, fetal urine, debris from skin cells, and particulate matter) can occur in utero, under conditions of fetal distress or asphyxia. Therefore, it is conceivable that the fetal larynx prevents aspiration under normal fetal conditions.

Table 2
Neuromuscular apparatus of the aerodigestive tract

Cranial Nerve (CN)	Location	Muscles Innervated
CN V (trigeminal)	Pons	Temporalis, masseter, medial pterygoid, lateral pterygoid, mylohyoid, digastric, tensor veli palatini
CN VII (facial)	Pons	Orbicularis oris, buccinators, stylohyoid, digastric
CN IX (glossopharyngeal)	Medulla	Stylopharyngeus, pharyngeal muscles
CN X (vagus)	Medulla	Thyroarytenoid, arytenoid, cricoarytenoid, aryepiglottic, thyroepiglottic, esophageal and stomach muscles
CN X and CN XI (accessory)	Medulla	Levator veli palatini, palatoglossus, uvular, palatopharyngeus, salpingopharyngeus, pharyngeal constrictors
CN XII (hypoglossal)	Medulla, C1	Intrinsic and extrinsic tongue muscles, geniohyoid
Ansa cervicallis/CN XII	C1, C2	Omohyoid, sternohyoid, thyrohyoid, sternothyroid

Table 3
Hierarchy of aerodigestive protection mechanisms in neonates

Organ	Reflexes	Physiologic Implications
Brain	• Arousals • Hypervigilant awake state	• Poor sleep patterns • Life-threatening events
Airway	• Glottal Closure • Bronchial muscle spasm • Reactive airway disease • Increase secretion in airway • Cough	• Obstructive apnea, desaturation, and bradycardia • Restrictive airway disease • Cough • Airway clearance
Pharynx	• Pharyngeal reflexive swallow • Phryngoglottal closure reflex • Deglutition apnea	• Pharyngeal clearance • Airway clearance and pharyngeal clearance • Airway protection
Esophageal	• Deglutition reflex • Secondary peristalsis • Upper esophageal sphincter contractile reflex • Lower esophageal sphincter relaxation reflex	• Swallowing esophageal clearance • Airway protection esophageal clearance

With the first breath at birth, the glottal airway and pharyngoesophageal segment functions in parallel and assume different roles. Immediately after birth, pharyngoesophageal functions continue as swallowing, whereas glottal opening and closure regulate the entry of air into and out of the lungs. Complete glottal adduction can occur as in the complex laryngeal chemoreflex, during which variable components of laryngeal adduction, apnea, repetitive swallowing, startle, hypertension and bradycardia, and hypoxia can be noted.[11] In fetal and neonatal life, laryngeal chemoreflex and glottal closure protect the airway from the potential hazard of aspiration, and repetitive swallowing clears the pharyngeal airway of any material. In premature and full term neonates, apnea contributes in part to the important airway protection mechanism. However, the consequences of exaggerated apnea and laryngospasm can be deleterious, during which there is an absence of airflow and lack of ventilation, thereby resulting in hypoxia. Subsequently, during infancy through adulthood, prolonged exhalations against partially closed glottis occur in the form of a cough reflex so as to steer irritants away from the airway.

Conditions that point toward malfunction or maladaptation of glottal reflexes across the age spectrum include: choking, anterograde and retrograde aspiration, life-threatening events or sudden deaths, dysphagia syndromes, GERD, intractable chronic lung disease, ventilator-associated pneumonias, and vocal cord paralysis. The underlying mechanisms of malfunction or maladaptation among these conditions are not well understood.

MATURATION OF BASAL AND ADAPTIVE AERODIGESTIVE REFLEX MECHANISMS

Pharyngeal swallowing and esophageal peristalsis constitute the principal methods used to drive the bolus away from the aerodigestive tract to the downstream digestive and absorptive organs of the gastrointestinal tract. This is called the peristaltic reflex, generated by coordination with the pharyngeal phase of swallowing, followed in sequence by relaxation of the UES, restoration of UES tone, ordered esophageal body peristalsis, coordinated relaxation of the LES, and restoration of LES tone.[12–15]

Peristaltic Reflexes

Pharyngeal swallowing is triggered by bolus movement from the oral cavity or by pharyngeal or esophageal stimulation. Esophageal peristalsis can be classified into primary and secondary peristalsis. Primary peristalsis or the deglutition response triggers the pharyngeal phase of swallowing followed by sequential reflexes that propagate distally into the stomach. This sequence is normally associated with a respiratory pause called deglutition apnea (**Fig. 2**). Secondary peristalsis is a swallow-independent sequence and is triggered by esophageal provocation. This reflex can occur due to esophageal distention, chemosensitive stimulation, or osmosensitive stimulation of the esophagus (**Fig. 3**).[16–18] Pharyngeal reflexive swallow is another important reflex evoked upon direct pharyngeal stimulation that facilitates pharyngeal clearance and bolus propagation distally (**Fig. 4**). Prolonged repetitive swallowing is associated with prolonged deglutition apnea and shallow breathing. Combined, these esophageal peristaltic functions participate in propulsion of a bolus presented during feeding and swallowing, and also during esophageal provocation caused by GER events.

Sphincteric Reflexes

Aerodigestive protection is also ensured by the UES and LES. UES and LES maintain a resting tone regardless of age or activity states, thus preventing any foregut luminal contents from reaching the airway. Furthermore, the UES contractile tone is triggered in response to esophageal provocation, the esophago-UES contractile reflex. During this occurrence, the proximal bolus movement of the bolus orad is halted by the vigilant esophago-UES contractile reflex (see **Fig. 3**). The UES contractile reflex is also triggered upon pharyngeal stimulation, pharyngo-UES contractile reflex. Often, the pharyngo-UES contractile reflex is accompanied by a pharyngeal reflexive swallow (see **Fig. 4**), thus the combination of these 2 reflexes results in robust swallowing, as is usually the case in adults.

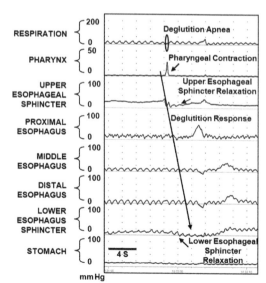

Fig. 2. An example of secondary peristaltic reflex along with esophago-UES contractile reflex, anterograde propagation (*long arrow*), and LES relaxation reflex (*arrow head*) evoked upon midesophageal stimulation (*shaded box*).

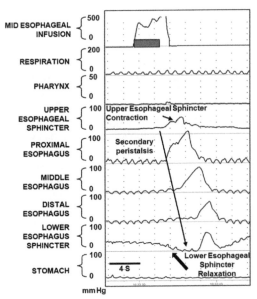

Fig. 3. An example of secondary peristaltic reflex along with esophago-UES contractile reflex, anterograde propagation (*long arrow*), and LES relaxation reflex (*arrow head*) evoked upon midesophageal stimulation (*shaded box*).

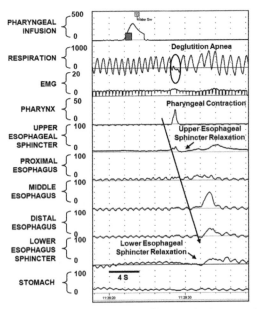

Fig. 4. An example of pharyngeal reflexive swallow evoked upon pharyngeal infusion (*shaded box*). Note the pharyngeal contraction (peak), UES relaxation, anterograde propagation (*long arrow*), LES relaxation, and deglutition apnea associated with this event.

Relaxation of the LES is equally important in facilitating bolus clearance distally. Esophageal provocation results in esophago-LES relaxation reflex (see **Fig. 3**), whereas pharyngeal provocation results in pharyngo-LES relaxation reflex (see **Fig. 4**).

Glottal Closure Reflexes

Adduction of the glottis via the laryngeal adductors shuts the glottis and protects any form of potential aspiration. Glottal adduction can occur upon pharyngeal stimulation, the pharyngoglottal closure reflex, or upon esophageal stimulation, the esophagoglottal closure reflex.[14,16–18] Prolonged glottal closure has physiologic consequences, however, and is associated with bradycardia and desaturation. Generally, either pharyngoglottal closure reflex or esophagoglottal closure reflex is associated with pharyngoesophageal peristalsis. Collectively, these reflexes prevent the ascending spread of the bolus, favor descending propulsion to ensure esophageal clearance, and enhance aerodigestive vigilance.

Laryngeal Chemo Reflex

A constellation of responses within the proximal aerodigestive tract is associated with laryngospasm, cessation of ventilation or airflow, repetitive pharyngeal contraction, and cardiorespiratory changes.[11] This reflex is also associated with stiffening of limbs and increased neuromuscular drive. This reflex is considered a brain stem arousal response.

Electrocortical Arousals

Electrocortical arousal, as an effect of visceral provocation or of its temporal relationships with aerodigestive reflexes in infants, is an important hypervigilant or protective state.[19,20] Sleep problems in aerodigestive pulmonary disorders alter the quality of life in infants. The author described the effects of esophageal provocation on esophageal reflex responses and electrocortical arousals during sleep, and found that electrocortical arousals are dependent on the frequency characteristics of esophageal neuromotor responses. Remarkably, swallow sequences were associated with arousals and sleep state changes, and arousals were associated with incomplete peristalsis, response delays to LES relaxation, and prolonged esophageal volume clearance. GER events (73.5%) provoked arousals. Arousals were associated with response delays to peristaltic reflexes or volume clearance, sleep state modification, and prolonged respiratory arousal. Midesophageal stimuli provoked arousals and were associated with increased frequency, prolonged latency, and prolonged response duration of peristaltic reflexes and UES contractile reflex, and increased frequency of sleep state changes and respiratory arousals. Electrocortical arousals add to the highest level of vigilance in response to an aerodigestive threat. Aerodigestive homeostasis is defended by multiple tiers of aerodigestive safety mechanisms, and when esophageal reflexes are delayed, cortical hypervigilance occurs.

Antireflux Mucosal Defenses

The refluxed material during GER events can be injurious to the esophagus and the aerodigestive tract. The properties of the refluxate or its presence in the esophagus contribute to the injury potential; this property can be related to acidity or alkalinity, enzymatic content, infective nature, or the physical composition of the refluxate. Often, the acidity is balanced by the esophageal mucosal protective mechanisms, also called the mucosal defenses. Mucosal HCO_3^- that neutralizes acidic reflux is a key element in preventing epithelial damage.[21] Additionally, GER events also increase the production of saliva. The increased secretion of saliva leads to peristalsis, which further aids in the clearance of the acidic gastric refluxate back into the stomach. The alkaline saliva also neutralizes the small amount of acidic refluxate that may still adhere to the esophageal mucosa after the bolus is cleared.

In summary (see **Fig. 1**), several tiers of aerodigestive protection exist in infants; there may be many other defensive reflexes that have not yet been discovered. Collectively, all these reflexes facilitate luminal clearance and maintain the respective functions of the airway and digestive tract.

GASTROESOPHAGEAL REFLEXES THAT CAUSE AND PROTECT AGAINST GER

Excellent recent articles are available pertinent to GERD and its management in neonates and infants, including a recent position statement from North American Society for Pediatric Gastroenterology, Hepatology, and Nutrition.[22–28] However, there is no focused guideline to help diagnose and manage GERD in the neonatal intensive care unit.

Symptomatology

Aerodigestive symptoms (see **Table 1**) provide clues to GER, and persistence of troublesome symptoms in the presence of chronic GER constitutes GERD. Dysphagia or abnormalities of swallowing in its various phases (oral, pharyngeal, esophageal, or gastric phase) can be related to esophageal pathology. GER or GERD are commonly suspected to be causes of swallowing problems. These entities range from simple regurgitation or physiologic reflux in asymptomatic thriving infants to troublesome symptoms seen in the pathologic form of GERD. GERD symptoms and its complications commonly include arching, irritability, throat clearing, autonomic signs such as facial flushing, tearing and cardiorespiratory changes, hoarse cry, choking, coughing and stridor, airway and respiratory compromise, retrograde aspiration, and bronchospasm. The symptoms in GERD syndrome can be due to abnormalities of refluxate clearance or abnormalities of aerodigestive protective functions.

Pathophysiological Basis for Symptoms in GERD

The pathophysiological basis for aerodigestive symptoms lie in sensory–motor modifications of the reflexes evoked in response to esophageal provocation from gastroesophageal refluxate. Owing to the variable composition of refluxed material, symptoms can vary and depend on the spatial and temporal characteristics of its spread and clearance.[23–25] For example, the refluxate may vary according to its:

- Physical characteristics: gas, liquid, mixed, or semisolid.
- Chemical characteristics: acid, weakly acid, nonacid or alkaline.
- Content: milk, partially digested milk, enzymes, bacteria, saliva, oral contents.
- Most proximal extent: distal esophagus, midesophagus, proximal esophagus, pharynx, nasopharynx, oropharynx.

Thus, the symptoms that occur from GER are the result of activation of afferent and efferent nerves subserving the route of spread of the refluxate. For example, when the most proximal extent is the pharynx, there is predominance of respiratory symptoms, in contrast to sensory symptoms when the most proximal extent is the distal esophagus.[24,25]

Furthermore, posture has an important bearing on GER and therefore with the symptoms associated with the events. This is because: (1) the angle at the gastroesophageal junction (angle of His) is obtuse (contrasting with an acute angle in adults), and is altered in different postures; (2) the relationship of the fundus to the esophageal body is modified; and (3) protective mechanisms can be recruited differently.[23,29–33] The effects of posture are summarized:

- Supine posture is recommended by the American Academy of Pediatrics to prevent sudden infant death syndrome (SIDS). However, GER is more frequent in this position, because the angle of His at the gastroesophageal junction becomes more obtuse. Importantly, airway protection mechanisms are also more favorable in supine position.[34–37]
- Prone posture is associated with more acute angulation at the gastroesophageal junction, thus preventing GER. However, aerodigestive clearance and protection mechanisms are impaired under these conditions. In extreme cases of GERD, this position is permissible under monitored, in-patient conditions.[29,38–40]
- Left lateral posture is associated with less GER.[27,29]
- Right lateral posture is associated with better gastric emptying, but more GER, implying that GER and gastric emptying may be unrelated.[31]

Causal Mechanisms of GER

GER is more frequent in neonates and young infants than at any other age owing to the following mechanisms

- Transient LES relaxation (TLESR): GER occurs most commonly due to transient LES relaxation in response to esophageal, gastric, or fundic distention.[41] This is a reflex mediated by the vagus nerve. The neurotransmitters implicated in increased TLESR include vasoactive intestinal peptide, nitric oxide, cholecystokinin, and acetylcholine. In contrast, gamma aminobutyric acid (GABA-B) receptors and opioids inhibit TLESR.[42–44] In addition, inflammation increases TLESR and decreases resting LES tone.
- Shorter esophageal length and intra-abdominal LES: LES length is shorter in premature infants. In addition, the intra-abdominal part of the LES develops in the postnatal period.[45]
- Smaller capacity of stomach: Premature infants have relatively small stomach capacity relative to the required volumes of feeding for optimal growth. This increases the predisposition to GER. Given the shorter esophageal length, the most proximal extent of GER also is higher.
- Role of diaphragm: The diaphragm and the phrenoesophageal ligaments or crural elements help to maintain the anatomic integrity of the gastroesophageal junction. With each inspiration there is an augmentation of LES resting tone. With TLESR, the crural diaphragm is inhibited concurrent with LES relaxation by the vagus nerve-mediated reflex, and thus the antireflux barrier is weakened.[13,46]

APPROACH TO EVALUATION OF AERODIGESTIVE PATHOLOGIES
Clinical Assessment

In a personalized program, detailed clinical assessment is a necessity before embarking on diagnostic testing.[47] Clinical aerodigestive assessment must include: predisposing risk factors, nutrition and growth details, review of anatomic defects, duration of illness, details of aerodigestive symptoms (see **Table 1**), feeding methods and symptom diary, as well as medication history. History of airway and digestive supportive therapies such as duration of respiratory support and feeding supportive methods can be helpful. Predisposing risk factors and alternate diagnoses must be excluded.[48]

Risk factors for aerodigestive problems, dysphagia, or GERD include: mechanical or functional obstruction; foregut dysmotility; anatomic malformations and congenital foregut anomalies, such as craniofacial birth defects, pharyngeal clefts, and webs; laryngeal clefts; postoperative esophageal strictures (following esophageal atresia or trachea–esophageal fistula repair), hiatus hernia, postoperative diaphragmatic hernia, intestinal malrotation, and hypertrophic pyloric stenosis. External compression of the esophagus due to pressure from trachea or left bronchus, left atrial enlargement, or postcardiothoracic surgery consequences should be considered on a case-by-case basis. Of importance, eosinophilic esophagitis is increasingly recognized in older infants and children.[49–52] In most of the previously mentioned circumstances, airway and digestive pathologies coexist.

Investigative Methods

Aerodigestive disorders require diverse approaches and strategies in diagnosing and correcting the problem. Esophageal pH-multichannel intraluminal impedance (pH-MII) monitoring, manometry, upper gastrointestinal fluoroscopy, and video–fluoroscopic swallow studies can be helpful in characterizing the esophageal structural and functional pathologies objectively. The advantages, limitations, and clinical relevance of these techniques are summarized in **Table 4**.

Table 4
Methods to investigate aerodigestive pathologies

Method	Advantages	Disadvantages
Upper gastrointestinal fluoroscopy[53,54]	Evaluates structural anatomy	Involves radiation exposure and transport
Video–fluoroscopic Swallow Study[55,56]	Clarifies oral bolus transit and anatomic abnormalities in the proximal aerodigestive tract	Involves radiation exposure, testing methods and conditions can contribute to variability in interpretation
Distal esophageal pH monitoring[57,58]	Smaller probe size, ambulatory, automated analysis available, user friendly	Feeds alter pH; nonacid GER and total GER are not measured; Cannot detect most proximal extent
pH-multichannel intraluminal impedance[23–25,59–64]	Ambulatory, detects liquid-, mixed-, gas- GER; detects acid and nonacid GER; reliable symptom documentation and analysis can increase objectivity; detects frequency, height, duration of reflux	Analysis cumbersome, semiautomated and labor-intensive, stiffer probes and malfunctions are frequent
Basal and adaptive esophageal manometry[12,16,17,45,65,66]	Provides mechanistic sensory–motor evaluation of esophageal peristaltic reflexes in response to provocation	Not commonly available; clinical correlation with direct observation is needed; analysis cumbersome and requires advanced training

SUMMARY

There is no single symptom or sign that is specific to aerodigestive pathologies, nor can a single test provide a definitive diagnosis for aerodigestive interactions. Therefore, clinicians need to cautiously weigh the benefits and weaknesses of different technologies and methods, scientific appropriateness of the testing conditions, clinico–pathologic correlation, and pharmacologic approaches. GERD symptoms and airway symptoms and disease can coexist, and cannot be distinguished without specific tests and direct observations. Important aerodigestive disorders include dysphagia, GERD, and aggravation of airway injury due to malfunctions of the swallowing or airway protection mechanisms. Application of consensus guidelines on GERD can be helpful in some circumstances.[28] In the evaluation of aerodigestive pathologies, assessment of structural, functional, and protective functions is important. Objective evaluation of aerodigestive reflexes and symptom correlation may provide support for evidence-based management of feeding and airway protection strategies.

ACKNOWLEDGMENTS

The author is grateful to Ms. Chin Yee Chan, MS, for the art and assistance with the manuscript.

REFERENCES

1. Allen J, Zwerdling R, Ehrenkranz R, et al. Statement on the care of the child with chronic lung disease of infancy and childhood. Am J Respir Crit Care Med 2003; 168:356–96.
2. Stevenson DK, Wright LL, Lemons JA, et al. Very low birth weight outcomes of the National Institute of Child Health and Human Development Neonatal Research Network, January 1993 through December 1994. Am J Obstet Gynecol 1998; 179:1632–9.
3. Mercado-Deane MG, Burton EM, Harlow SA, et al. Swallowing dysfunction in infants less than 1 year of age. Pediatr Radiol 2001;31:423–8.
4. Goyal R, Sivarao D. Functional anatomy and physiology of swallowing and esophageal motility. In: Castell DO, Ritcher JE, editors. The esophagus. 3rd edition. Philadelphia: Lippincott Williams & Wilkins; 1999. p. 1–31.
5. Lang IM, Shaker R. Anatomy and physiology of the upper esophageal sphincter. Am J Med 1997;103:50S–5S.
6. Mansfield LE. Embryonic origins of the relation of gastroesophageal reflux disease and airway disease. Am J Med 2001;111(Suppl 8A):3S–7S.
7. Miller JL, Sonies BC, Macedonia C. Emergence of oropharyngeal, laryngeal and swallowing activity in the developing fetal upper aerodigestive tract: an ultrasound evaluation. Early Hum Dev 2003;71:61–87.
8. Sadler TW. Special embryology, respiratory system. In: Sadler TW, editor. Langman's medical embryology. 7th edition. Baltimore (MD): Williams and Wilkins; 1995. p. 232–41.
9. Sadler TW. Special embryology, digestive system. In: Sadler TW, editor. Langman's medical embryology. 7th edition. Baltimore (MD): Williams and Wilkins; 1995. p. 1241–71.
10. Goyal RK, Padmanabhan R, Sang Q. Neural circuits in swallowing and abdominal vagal afferent-mediated lower esophageal sphincter relaxation. Am J Med 2001; 111(Suppl 8A):95S–105S.

11. Thach BT. Maturation and transformation of reflexes that protect the laryngeal airway from liquid aspiration from fetal to adult life. Am J Med 2001; 111(Suppl 8A):69S–77S.

12. Jadcherla SR, Duong HQ, Hofmann C, et al. Characteristics of upper oesophageal sphincter and oesophageal body during maturation in healthy human neonates compared with adults. Neurogastroenterol Motil 2005;17:663–70.

13. Mittal RK, Balaban DH. The esophagogastric junction. N Engl J Med 1997;336: 924–32.

14. Pena EM, Parks VN, Peng J, et al. Lower esophageal sphincter relaxation reflex kinetics: effects of peristaltic reflexes and maturation in human premature neonates. Am J Physiol Gastrointest Liver Physiol 2010;299:G1386–95.

15. Castell D, Ritcher J. The esophagus. 4th edition. Philadelphia: Lippincott Williams & Wilkins; 2004.

16. Jadcherla SR, Duong HQ, Hoffmann RG, et al. Esophageal body and upper esophageal sphincter motor responses to esophageal provocation during maturation in preterm newborns. J Pediatr 2003;143:31–8.

17. Jadcherla SR, Hoffmann RG, Shaker R. Effect of maturation of the magnitude of mechanosensitive and chemosensitive reflexes in the premature human esophagus. J Pediatr 2006;149:77–82.

18. Gupta A, Gulati P, Kim W, et al. Effect of postnatal maturation on the mechanisms of esophageal propulsion in preterm human neonates: primary and secondary peristalsis. Am J Gastroenterol 2009;104:411–9.

19. Jadcherla SR, Parks VN, Peng J, et al. Esophageal sensation in premature human neonates: temporal relationships and implications of aerodigestive reflexes and electrocortical arousals. Am J Physiol Gastrointest Liver Physiol 2012;302: G134–44.

20. Thach BT. Graded arousal responses in infants: advantages and disadvantages of a low threshold for arousal. Sleep Med 2002;3(Suppl 2):S37–40.

21. Flemstrom G, Isenberg JI. Gastroduodenal mucosal alkaline secretion and mucosal protection. News Physiol Sci 2001;16:23–8.

22. Birch JL, Newell SJ. Gastrooesophageal reflux disease in preterm infants: current management and diagnostic dilemmas. Arch Dis Child Fetal Neonatal Ed 2009; 94:F379–83.

23. Jadcherla SR, Chan CY, Moore R, et al. Impact of feeding strategies on the frequency and clearance of acid and nonacid gastroesophageal reflux events in dysphagic neonates. JPEN J Parenter Enteral Nutr 2012;36(4):449–55.

24. Jadcherla SR, Gupta A, Fernandez S, et al. Spatiotemporal characteristics of acid refluxate and relationship to symptoms in premature and term infants with chronic lung disease. Am J Gastroenterol 2008;103:720–8.

25. Jadcherla SR, Peng J, Chan CY, et al. Significance of gastroesophageal refluxate in relation to physical, chemical, and spatiotemporal characteristics in symptomatic intensive care unit neonates. Pediatr Res 2011;70:192–8.

26. Omari TI, Schwarzer A, vanWijk MP, et al. Optimisation of the reflux-symptom association statistics for use in infants being investigated by 24-hour pH impedance. J Pediatr Gastroenterol Nutr 2011;52:408–13.

27. van Wijk MP, Benninga MA, Dent J, et al. Effect of body position changes on postprandial gastroesophageal reflux and gastric emptying in the healthy premature neonate. J Pediatr 2007;151:585–90.

28. Vandenplas Y, Rudolph CD, Di Lorenzo C, et al. Pediatric gastroesophageal reflux clinical practice guidelines: joint recommendations of the North American Society for Pediatric Gastroenterology, Hepatology, and Nutrition (NASPGHAN)

and the European Society for Pediatric Gastroenterology, Hepatology, and Nutrition (ESPGHAN). J Pediatr Gastroenterol Nutr 2009;49:498–547.

29. Corvaglia L, Rotatori R, Ferlini M, et al. The effect of body positioning on gastroesophageal reflux in premature infants: evaluation by combined impedance and pH monitoring. J Pediatr 2007;151:591–6.

30. Martin RJ, Di Fiore JM, Hibbs AM. Gastroesophageal reflux in preterm infants: is positioning the answer? J Pediatr 2007;151:560–1.

31. Omari TI, Rommel N, Staunton E, et al. Paradoxical impact of body positioning on gastroesophageal reflux and gastric emptying in the premature neonate. J Pediatr 2004;145:194–200.

32. van Wijk MP, Benninga MA, Davidson GP, et al. Small volumes of feed can trigger transient lower esophageal sphincter relaxation and gastroesophageal reflux in the right lateral position in infants. J Pediatr 2010;156:744–8.

33. Vandenplas Y, De Schepper J, Verheyden S, et al. A preliminary report on the efficacy of the Multicare AR-Bed in 3-week-3-month-old infants on regurgitation, associated symptoms and acid reflux. Arch Dis Child 2010;95:26–30.

34. Committee on Fetus and Newborn, American Academy of Pediatrics. Apnea, sudden infant death syndrome, and home monitoring. Pediatrics 2003;111:914–7.

35. Moon RY. SIDS and other sleep-related infant deaths: expansion of recommendations for a safe infant sleeping environment. Pediatrics 2011;128:1030–9.

36. Oyen N, Markestad T, Skaerven R, et al. Combined effects of sleeping position and prenatal risk factors in sudden infant death syndrome: the Nordic Epidemiological SIDS Study. Pediatrics 1997;100:613–21.

37. Vandenplas Y, Sacre-Smits L. Seventeen-hour continuous esophageal pH monitoring in the newborn: evaluation of the influence of position in asymptomatic and symptomatic babies. J Pediatr Gastroenterol Nutr 1985;4:356–61.

38. Bhat RY, Rafferty GF, Hannam S, et al. Acid gastroesophageal reflux in convalescent preterm infants: effect of posture and relationship to apnea. Pediatr Res 2007;62:620–3.

39. Orenstein SR. Prone positioning in infant gastroesophageal reflux: is elevation of the head worth the trouble? J Pediatr 1990;117:184–7.

40. Skadberg BT, Morild I, Markestad T. Abandoning prone sleeping: effect on the risk of sudden infant death syndrome. J Pediatr 1998;132:340–3.

41. Franzi SJ, Martin CJ, Cox MR, et al. Response of canine lower esophageal sphincter to gastric distension. Am J Physiol 1990;259:G380–5.

42. Blackshaw LA, Staunton E, Lehmann A, et al. Inhibition of transient LES relaxations and reflux in ferrets by GABA receptor agonists. Am J Physiol 1999;277:G867–74.

43. Dent J, Dodds WJ, Friedman RH, et al. Mechanism of gastroesophageal reflux in recumbent asymptomatic human subjects. J Clin Invest 1980;65:256–67.

44. Dodds WJ, Dent J, Hogan WJ, et al. Mechanisms of gastroesophageal reflux in patients with reflux esophagitis. N Engl J Med 1982;307:1547–52.

45. Gupta A, Jadcherla SR. The relationship between somatic growth and in vivo esophageal segmental and sphincteric growth in human neonates. J Pediatr Gastroenterol Nutr 2006;43:35–41.

46. Kc P, Martin RJ. Role of central neurotransmission and chemoreception on airway control. Respir Physiol Neurobiol 2010;173:213–22.

47. Jadcherla SR, Peng J, Moore R, et al. Impact of personalized feeding program in 100 NICU infants: pathophysiology-based approach for better outcomes. J Pediatr Gastroenterol Nutr 2012;54:62–70.

48. Rudolph C, Mazur LJ, Laptak GS. Guidelines for evaluation and treatment of gastroesophageal reflux in infants and children. Recommendations of the North American Society of Pediatric Gastroenterology and Nutrition. J Pediatr Gastroenterol Nutr 2001;32(2):S1–32.

49. Blanchard C, Rothenberg ME. Basic pathogenesis of eosinophilic esophagitis. Gastrointest Endosc Clin N Am 2008;18:133–43.

50. Hommel KA, Franciosi JP, Gray WN, et al. Behavioral functioning and treatment adherence in pediatric eosinophilic gastrointestinal disorders. Pediatr Allergy Immunol 2012. [Epub ahead of print].

51. Putnam PE, Rothenberg ME. Eosinophilic esophagitis: concepts, controversies, and evidence. Curr Gastroenterol Rep 2009;11:220–5.

52. Rothenberg ME. Biology and treatment of eosinophilic esophagitis. Gastroenterology 2009;137:1238–49.

53. Hillemeier AC. Gastroesophageal reflux. Diagnostic and therapeutic approaches. Pediatr Clin North Am 1996;43:197–212.

54. Tsou VM, Bishop PR. Gastroesophageal reflux in children. Otolaryngol Clin North Am 1998;31:419–34.

55. Byars KC, Burklow KA, Ferguson K, et al. A multicomponent behavioral program for oral aversion in children dependent on gastrostomy feedings. J Pediatr Gastroenterol Nutr 2003;37:473–80.

56. Gleeson K, Eggli DF, Maxwell SL. Quantitative aspiration during sleep in normal subjects. Chest 1997;111:1266–72.

57. Orenstein SR, Hassall E. Infants and proton pump inhibitors: tribulations, no trials. J Pediatr Gastroenterol Nutr 2007;45:395–8.

58. Putnam PE. Obituary: the death of the pH probe. J Pediatr 2010;157:878–80.

59. Bredenoord AJ, Weusten BL, Timmer R, et al. Reproducibility of multichannel intraluminal electrical impedance monitoring of gastroesophageal reflux. Am J Gastroenterol 2005;100:265–9.

60. Jadcherla SR, Rudolph CD. Gastroesophageal reflux in the preterm neonate. NeoReviews 2005;6:e87–98.

61. Peter CS, Sprodowski N, Bohnhorst B, et al. Gastroesophageal reflux and apnea of prematurity: no temporal relationship. Pediatrics 2002;109:8–11.

62. Sifrim D, Castell D, Dent J, et al. Gastro-oesophageal reflux monitoring: review and consensus report on detection and definitions of acid, non-acid, and gas reflux. Gut 2004;53:1024–31.

63. Wenzl TG. Investigating esophageal reflux with the intraluminal impedance technique. J Pediatr Gastroenterol Nutr 2002;34:261–8.

64. Wenzl TG, Schenke S, Peschgens T, et al. Association of apnea and nonacid gastroesophageal reflux in infants: investigations with the intraluminal impedance technique. Pediatr Pulmonol 2001;31:144–9.

65. Jadcherla SR. Manometric evaluation of esophageal-protective reflexes in infants and children. Am J Med 2003;115(Suppl 3A):157S–60S.

66. Jadcherla SR, Gupta A, Stoner E, et al. Pharyngeal swallowing: defining pharyngeal and upper esophageal sphincter relationships in human neonates. J Pediatr 2007;151:597–603.

The Pulmonary Circulation in Neonatal Respiratory Failure

Satyan Lakshminrusimha, MD

KEYWORDS

- Pulmonary circulation • Respiratory failure • Lungs • Neonates

KEY POINTS

- Pulmonary vascular resistance increases during late gestation and decreases at birth.
- Pulmonary vascular transition at birth can be influenced by mode of delivery, asphyxia, body temperature, and oxygen concentration of the resuscitation gas.
- Neonatal hypoxemic respiratory failure (HRF) is often secondary to parenchymal lung disease, ventilation-perfusion mismatch, or extrapulmonary right-to-left shunt.
- Hypoxia causes pulmonary vasoconstriction, normoxia results in pulmonary vasodilation, but hyperoxia does not lead to additional vasodilation.
- Inhaled nitric oxide (iNO) is a specific pulmonary vasodilator and is effective in 60% to 70% of late preterm and term neonates with HRF.
- Inadequate or ill-sustained response to iNO may be secondary to poor alveolar recruitment, remodeled pulmonary vasculature, abnormalities of target enzymes, presence of reactive oxygen species, left ventricular dysfunction, or increased vasoconstrictive mediators.
- Pulmonary hypertension associated with bronchopulmonary dysplasia and congenital diaphragmatic hernia is associated with high morbidity and mortality and its management is challenging.

INTRODUCTION

The pulmonary circulation is a unique system that differs from the systemic circulation in structure, function, and regulation. For example, hypoxia causes pulmonary vasoconstriction but dilates the systemic circulation. In neonates with hypoxemic respiratory failure (HRF), circulatory changes in the lung can be primary, as in idiopathic persistent pulmonary hypertension of the newborn (PPHN), or secondary to lung disease. This article provides a brief overview of normal pulmonary circulation, changes

Conflict of interest: Dr Lakshminrusimha is a member of the speaker's bureau and a consultant for Ikaria LLC.
Division of Neonatology, Women and Children's Hospital of Buffalo, State University of New York at Buffalo, 219 Bryant Street, Buffalo, NY 14222, USA
E-mail address: slakshmi@buffalo.edu

Clin Perinatol 39 (2012) 655–683
http://dx.doi.org/10.1016/j.clp.2012.06.006
0095-5108/12/$ – see front matter © 2012 Elsevier Inc. All rights reserved.

in neonatal pulmonary circulation in common causes of neonatal HRF, and its response to therapeutic interventions in the neonatal intensive care unit (NICU).

FETAL CIRCULATION

Gas exchange is the primary function of the postnatal lung. The low-resistance, high-volume pulmonary circulation, which receives half of the combined ventricular output, is a crucial factor in achieving efficient gas exchange by the aerated lung during post-natal life. During fetal life, the placenta serves as the organ of gas exchange; placental vascular resistance is low and receives nearly half of fetal combined ventricular output. During this period, fetal pulmonary vascular resistance (PVR) is high (physiologic pulmonary hypertension), and blood flow is diverted from the pulmonary artery to the aorta and umbilical arteries toward the placenta.[1] Fetal pulmonary circulation must prepare the lungs for adequate structural growth and functional maturation in anticipation for the switch to air breathing in the postnatal period. During the normal transition at birth, PVR decreases and is associated with an increase in pulmonary blood flow. Abnormal pulmonary transition leads to sustained increase of PVR, similar to the fetal state, resulting in PPHN. Parenchymal lung diseases such as meconium aspiration syndrome can result in ventilation-perfusion (V/Q) mismatch, hypoxemia, and structural and functional changes in pulmonary circulation resulting in HRF.

Most of the knowledge of fetal pulmonary hemodynamics is derived from studies in fetal lambs. Data from fetal lambs suggest that PVR is high, with only 8% to 10% of combined ventricular output entering the lungs during fetal life.[2,3] More recently, Doppler flow studies in human fetuses have shown significantly higher flow into the left and right pulmonary arteries with 13% of combined ventricular output at 20 weeks' gestation (canalicular stage), increasing to 25% at 30 weeks (saccular stage) and 21% at 38 weeks (alveolar stage).[4] The fetal PVR is high during the canalicular stage secondary to paucity of pulmonary vascular network and reduced cross-sectional area of an immature pulmonary vascular bed (**Fig. 1**). Rasanen and colleagues[5] showed that, between 20 and 26 weeks of gestation, maternal hyperoxygenation using 60% humidified oxygen by face mask does not result in pulmonary vasodilation in human fetuses, suggesting a lack of sensitivity to oxygen in early gestation. During the early saccular stage, rapid proliferation of pulmonary vessels decreases fetal PVR. During late preterm and early term gestation (34–36 and 37–38 weeks gestational age [GA], respectively), there is a marked increase in cross-sectional area of the pulmonary vascular bed. However, pulmonary vessels become more sensitive to vaso-constrictive mediators, such as endothelin (ET) and relative hypoxemia, resulting in active pulmonary vasoconstriction and an increase in PVR.[6,7] During this period, maternal hyperoxygenation increases pulmonary blood flow in human fetuses[5] and fetal lambs.[8]

In fetal lambs, pulmonary vasodilation in response to endothelium-independent mediators, such as nitric oxide (NO), precedes responses to endothelium-dependent mediators, such as acetylcholine and oxygen. Response to NO depends on activity of its target enzyme, soluble guanylate cyclase (sGC), in the smooth muscle cell. In the ovine fetus, sGC messenger RNA levels are low during early preterm (126 days) gestation and increase during late preterm and early term gestation (137 days).[9] In rats, abundant sGC activity is present in the lung at late gestation and early newborn periods and gradually decreases in adulthood.[10] Low levels of pulmonary arterial sGC activity during late canalicular and early saccular stages of lung develop-ment are probably responsible for the poor response to iNO observed in preterm infants delivered at less than 29 weeks GA.[11]

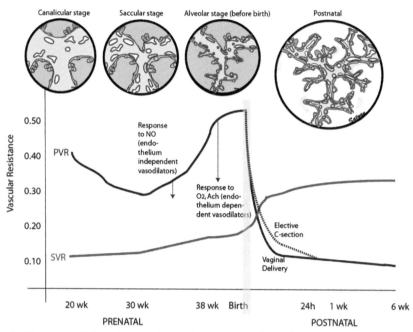

Fig. 1. Changes in PVR and systemic vascular resistance (SVR) during the last half of gestation and the postnatal period. During the canalicular phase of lung development, high PVR is caused by low density of the vasculature. In the saccular stage, broad intersaccular septae contain the double capillary network and, with increasing vascular density, PVR decreases. In the alveolar phase, despite the rapid increase in the number of small pulmonary arteries, high PVR is maintained by active vasoconstriction. Fetal pulmonary vasodilator response to endothelium-independent (direct smooth muscle relaxant) vasodilators such as NO precedes the maturation of the vasodilator response to oxygen and acetylcholine (Ach), endothelium-dependent vasodilators. After birth, lung liquid is absorbed and an air-liquid interphase is established with juxtaposition of capillaries and alveolar epithelium to promote effective gas exchange. The dashed line represents the delay in decrease of PVR observed following elective cesarean section. SVR markedly increases after occlusion of the umbilical cord and removal of the low-resistance placental circuit from the systemic circulation. (Copyright © Satyan Lakshminrusimha.)

Modulation of Fetal PVR

Conditions such as congenital diaphragmatic hernia (CDH), antenatal closure of the ductus arteriosus, and idiopathic PPHN are often associated with vascular remodeling and increased PVR during fetal life. Studies in animal models suggest that maternal therapy can alter fetal PVR. Loong and colleagues reported that antenatal administration of sildenafil improved lung structure (decreased mean linear intercept) and reduced pulmonary hypertension (decreased right ventricle/left ventricle + septum ratio) in nitrofen-induced CDH rat pups.[12] Maternal betamethasone similarly reduces oxidative stress and improves relaxation response to adenosine triphosphate (ATP) and NO donors in fetal lambs with PPHN induced by ductal ligation.[13] Antenatal tracheal occlusion in animal models of CDH reduces pulmonary circulatory impedance and pulmonary arterial remodeling.[14–17] Further translational and clinical research into reducing fetal PVR and improving lung structure and function by antenatal medical and surgical intervention is critical to reduce mortality and morbidity in CDH. Maternal medications can also increase fetal PVR and increase the risk of PPHN. Two classes of medications, antidepressants and antiinflammatory agents, have been well studied.

Selective serotonin uptake inhibitors

Maternal intake of selective serotonin uptake inhibitors (SSRIs) during the last half of pregnancy has been associated with an increased risk of PPHN.[18] Exposure of pregnant rats to fluoxetine resulted in pulmonary hypertension in rat pups (more profound in female pups) and was associated with hypoxia and increased mortality.[19,20] The mechanism by which fluoxetine induces pulmonary hypertension in newborns is unknown. It is speculated that higher drug-induced serotonin levels result in pulmonary vasoconstriction. A more recent retrospective analysis has questioned this association.[21] Obstetricians must weigh the maternal psychological benefits of antidepressant therapy during pregnancy against the risk of adverse neonatal effects.

Nonsteroidal antiinflammatory medications

Ingestion of nonsteroidal antiinflammatory drugs (NSAIDs), such as aspirin, during late gestation may be associated with in utero closure of the fetal ductus arteriosus.[22] Experimental ligation of the ductus arteriosus in lambs during fetal life is associated with pulmonary vascular remodeling and PPHN.[23] Prostaglandins maintain ductal patency in utero and are important mediators of pulmonary vasodilation in response to ventilation at birth. Pharmacologic blockade of prostaglandin production by NSAIDs can result in PPHN. Analysis of meconium from newborn infants with PPHN revealed the presence of NSAID in approximately half of the samples,[24] linking antenatal NSAID exposure to PPHN.

TRANSITION AT BIRTH

The entry of air into the alveoli with crying and breathing improves oxygenation of the pulmonary vascular bed, decreasing PVR and increasing pulmonary blood flow.[25] The increase in pulmonary blood flow raises left atrial pressures more than right atrial pressures, closing the foramen ovale. Removal of the low-resistance placental bed from the systemic circulation at birth increases systemic vascular resistance (SVR; see **Fig. 1**). As PVR decreases to less than SVR, flow reverses across the ductus. Oxygen-induced vasodilation and lung expansion decrease PVR to approximately half of SVR within a few minutes after birth. Over the first few hours after birth, the ductus arteriosus closes, largely in response to the increase in oxygen tension, and with this the normal postnatal circulatory pattern is established. The recognition of the role of NO in mediating pulmonary vascular transition at birth[26] has led to the development of inhaled NO (iNO) as a therapeutic strategy in the life-threatening clinical disorder of PPHN. A detailed review of NO and other mediators of pulmonary vascular transition at birth is presented in a previous issue.[1]

Factors Altering Pulmonary Vascular Transition at Birth

Mode of delivery

Vaginal delivery is associated with reduction in fetal PVR at birth. Delivery by elective cesarean section[27,28] delays the decrease in pulmonary arterial pressure (see **Fig. 1**), as shown by prolonged right-sided systolic time intervals, and increases the risk for PPHN.[21] Compared with matched controls, infants with PPHN are more likely to have been delivered by cesarean section.[29]

Timing of delivery

Timing of delivery influences the risk and outcome of HRF in neonates. Delivery during late preterm or early term gestation is associated with a higher risk of admission to the NICU with respiratory distress.[30] Among patients with severe HRF requiring extracorporeal membrane oxygenation (ECMO), mortality is higher among late preterm and early term infants compared with term infants.[31] However, infants with CDH without other anomalies have been observed to have reduced need for ECMO and marginally better survival when delivered early term compared with late term.[32] More recent population-based studies have not confirmed these findings.[33]

Antenatal glucocorticoids

Administration of glucocorticoids, such as betamethasone, before elective cesarean section has been shown to reduce the incidence of respiratory distress and admission to the NICU.[34,35] This regimen is being adapted in some centers in Europe.[36] Preliminary data from our laboratory suggest that antenatal betamethasone decreases PVR and increases fetal pulmonary blood flow. Recent identification of genetic variations involving corticotropin-releasing hormone in patients with PPHN, as well as the effectiveness of hydrocortisone in improving oxygenation in lambs with PPHN, suggest that glucocorticoids may have a role in prevention and management of PPHN and HRF.[37,38]

Early versus delayed cord clamping

The current neonatal resuscitation guidelines recommend delayed umbilical cord clamping for at least 1 minute for newborn infants who do not require resuscitation at birth.[39] Delayed cord clamping results in more stable blood pressures and improved iron status. Arcilla and colleagues[40] evaluated the effect of late cord clamping on pulmonary hemodynamics in newborn infants by catheterizing the pulmonary artery. The mean ratio of pulmonary artery to systemic arterial pressure decreased to 0.7 by 2 hours and to 0.5 by 4 hours following early cord clamping. Following late cord clamping, pulmonary arterial pressures were almost 90% of systemic pressures by 9 hours. The investigators speculated that increased blood volume following late cord clamping results in distension of the pulmonary capillary and venous bed, resulting in increased pulmonary arterial pressure. Polycythemia with increased viscosity may contribute to high PVR. There are no reports of an increased incidence of PPHN associated with delayed cord clamping.

Temperature

Induction of severe hypothermia in lambs between 1 and 3 days old (decreasing temperature from 40°C to 30°C) increases mean pulmonary arterial pressure from 29 to 40 mm Hg.[41] Perinatal asphyxia is a well-known predisposing factor for PPHN.[42] There was considerable concern that therapeutic hypothermia in asphyxiated infants would increase the risk of PPHN. Pooled analysis of randomized trials has not shown an increased incidence of PPHN with hypothermia in this population.[43] The type of cooling (selective head cooling vs whole body cooling) does not alter the incidence of PPHN.[44]

Asphyxia

Perinatal asphyxia interferes with the mechanisms of pulmonary transition at birth and modifies this complex adaptation impeding the decrease in PVR, and increasing the risk for PPHN.[42] Multiple mechanisms cause respiratory failure and affect pulmonary circulation in asphyxia: fetal hypoxemia, ischemia, meconium aspiration, ventricular dysfunction, and acidosis can all increase PVR.[42] Acute asphyxia is associated with reversible pulmonary vasoconstriction[45] but chronic in utero asphyxia with or without meconium aspiration may be associated with vasoconstriction and vascular remodeling.[46]

Oxygen during neonatal resuscitation

Oxygen is a potent and specific pulmonary vasodilator. The use of 100% oxygen during initial ventilation of normal lambs at birth results in a small but significant decrease in PVR during the first few minutes of life compared with 21% or 50% oxygen.[47] However, ventilation with 100% oxygen at birth impairs subsequent relaxation to iNO and acetylcholine, probably because of the formation of reactive oxygen species (ROS). Similar results were observed in lambs with pulmonary hypertension and a remodeled pulmonary vasculature.[48] In lambs with asphyxia induced by umbilical cord occlusion, PVR was lower with 100% oxygen resuscitation compared with 21% oxygen at 1 minute of age but, by 2 minutes, PVR was similar in both groups. These findings suggest that optimal ventilation (and not hyperoxygenation) is the key to reducing PVR.[49] Thirty minutes of resuscitation with 100% oxygen increased pulmonary arterial contractility and superoxide anion formation in pulmonary arteries. Using 100% oxygen therefore has transient advantages in rapidly reducing PVR but increases ROS formation, increases pulmonary arterial contractility, and impairs vasodilation to endothelium-dependent (acetylcholine) and endothelium-independent (iNO) agents. These findings support the neonatal resuscitation guidelines' recommendations to use room air for initial resuscitation of term asphyxiated newborn infants.[39]

PULMONARY CIRCULATORY CHANGES IN HRF

Fig. 2 shows the 4 different patterns of pulmonary vascular changes in neonatal HRF. PPHN is characterized by increased ratio of pulmonary vascular resistance (PVR) to SVR resulting from (1) vasoconstriction; (2) structural remodeling of the pulmonary vasculature (**Fig. 3**); (3) intravascular obstruction from increased viscosity of blood,

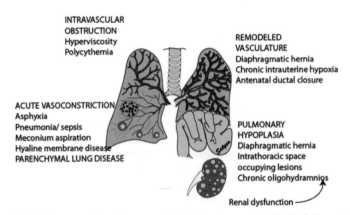

Fig. 2. Pathologic changes in pulmonary circulation in neonatal HRF follows 4 patterns. Intravascular obstruction caused by increased viscosity as seen in polycythemia in the presence of normal pulmonary vasculature can cause PPHN. Asphyxia or parenchymal lung disease can lead to alveolar hypoxia and acute pulmonary vasoconstriction. Chronic pulmonary vascular remodeling can result from chronic intrauterine hypoxia, antenatal ductal closure, or CDH. Lung hypoplasia with paucity of pulmonary vasculature accompanies CDH; intrathoracic space occupying lesions, such as adenomatoid malformations; or chronic oligohydramnios syndromes, which could be secondary to chronic leakage of amniotic fluid or fetal oliguria from renal dysfunction. (Copyright © Satyan Lakshminrusimha.)

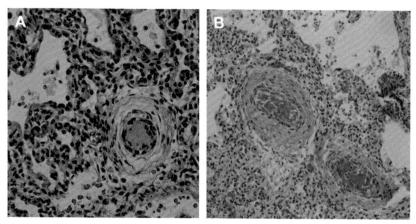

Fig. 3. Pulmonary arterial remodeling in HRF. (*A*) Preterm infant with respiratory distress syndrome and PPHN; (*B*) Term infant with asphyxia and PPHN; note the smooth muscle cell layer thickening around pulmonary arteries.

as in polycythemia; or (4) lung hypoplasia. This condition leads to right-to-left shunting of blood across the foramen ovale and ductus arteriosus, resulting in hypoxemia. Numerous disease states with diverse causes can result in a similar final pathophysiology. About 10% of cases with PPHN are idiopathic, with no associated pulmonary airspace disorder. However, PPHN is usually associated with other acute respiratory conditions, such as meconium aspiration syndrome (MAS), respiratory distress syndrome (RDS), pneumonia, or CDH. Hypoxemia in these conditions can be caused by parenchymal lung disease, surfactant deficiency (RDS) or inactivation (MAS, pneumonia), ventilation/perfusion (V/Q) mismatch, and intrapulmonary as well as extrapulmonary right-to-left shunting of blood (**Fig. 4**). In some newborns with HRF, a single mechanism predominates (eg, extrapulmonary right-to-left shunting in idiopathic PPHN). However, more commonly, several of these mechanisms contribute to hypoxemia. In MAS, obstruction of the airways by meconium results in decreasing V/Q ratios and increasing intrapulmonary right-to-left shunt. Other segments of the lungs may be overventilated relative to perfusion, causing increased physiologic dead space. The same patient may also have severe PPHN with extrapulmonary right-to-left shunting at the level of the ductus arteriosus and foramen ovale.

Pneumonia or meconium aspiration may release inflammatory mediators that induce vasoconstriction. Vasoconstrictors such as leukotrienes, platelet-activating factor, thromboxanes,[50] and ET-1[51] have been found to be increased in PPHN. Chronic intrauterine ET_A receptor blockade following antenatal ductal ligation decreases pulmonary arterial pressure in utero, decreases right ventricular hypertrophy and distal muscularization of small pulmonary arteries, and further decreases the PVR at delivery in newborn lambs with PPHN.[52] Thus ET-1 acting through ET_A receptor stimulation might contribute to the pathogenesis and pathophysiology of PPHN. Derangements in the NO pathway of vasodilation can also result in the physiologic characteristics of PPHN. Pulmonary endothelial nitric oxide synthase (eNOS) gene and protein expression and enzyme activity are decreased in fetal lambs with PPHN induced by antenatal ductal ligation.[53] In addition, the response to stimulators of eNOS is lost.[54] In these lambs with PPHN, the vascular response to NO is also diminished,[55] whereas the response to cyclic guanosine monophosphate-phosphodiesterase (cGMP) is normal. Thus, the decreased responsiveness seems to result from decreased vascular smooth

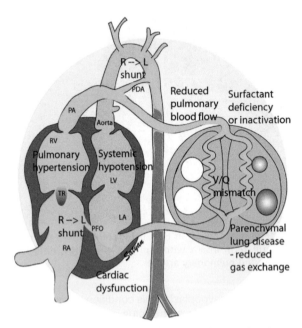

Fig. 4. Hemodynamic changes in PPHN/HRF. Surfactant deficiency (RDS) or inactivation (MAS or pneumonia) results in parenchymal lung disease and ventilation-perfusion (V/Q) mismatch. Increased PVR results in reduced pulmonary blood flow and right-to-left shunt through the PDA and/or PFO. Pulmonary hypertension, often associated with systemic hypotension, results in septal deviation to the left. Cardiac dysfunction secondary to asphyxia, sepsis, or CDH may contribute to pulmonary venous hypertension and complicate HRF. LA, left atrium; LV, left ventricle; PA, pulmonary artery; PDA, patent ductus arteriosus; PFO, patent foramen ovale; RA, right atrium; RV, right ventricle; TR, tricuspid regurgitation. (Copyright © Satyan Lakshminrusimha.)

muscle sensitivity to NO at the level of sGC. Because NO relaxes smooth muscle and inhibits vascular smooth muscle growth, diminished eNOS expression may contribute to both abnormal vasoreactivity and excessive muscularization of pulmonary vessels in PPHN.

Pulmonary hypertension sometimes occurs because of an abnormal pulmonary vascular bed despite the absence of alveolar hypoxia and hypercapnia and of lung inflammation. These infants can be grouped according to the degree of muscularization and the number of pulmonary arteries.[56] In infants with hypoplastic lungs, as in CDH and oligohydramnios sequence (sometimes secondary to fetal renal dysfunction), PPHN may arise primarily as a consequence of a decreased number of vessels, causing decreased cross-sectional area of the pulmonary vascular bed, and leading to flow restriction. Patients with alveolar capillary dysplasia may have a similar vascular hypoplasia. These cases may be complicated by increased muscularization of the vessels.

Many infants who have HRF do not have right-to-left extracardiac shunting, and may have hypoxia because of intrapulmonary shunting or cardiac dysfunction (see **Fig. 4**). Determination of the hemodynamic profile of these babies using functional echocardiography is important to make the diagnosis, initiate therapy, and follow the changes with therapy.[57] The gold standard in defining PPHN rests on the echocardiographic findings of right-to-left shunting of blood at the foramen ovale and/or the ductus arteriosus, as well as estimates of pulmonary arterial pressure using tricuspid regurgitation jet velocity. Using the modified Bernoulli equation, systolic right ventricular pressure (mm Hg) is estimated by $4v^2$ + right atrial pressure, where v is the maximal velocity of tricuspid regurgitation jet in meters per second on continuous-wave Doppler echocardiogram.[58] The velocity of tricuspid regurgitation jet may also be influenced by right ventricular dysfunction, leading to underestimation of pulmonary arterial pressure. Right ventricular dysfunction caused by excessive afterload seems to be a major risk factor for poor outcome in HRF.[42]

Doppler measurements of atrial and ductal level shunts provide essential information to optimize management of a newborn with HRF. For example, left-to-right shunting at the foramen ovale and ductus arteriosus with marked hypoxemia suggests predominant intrapulmonary shunting, and interventions should be directed at optimizing lung inflation and recruitment. Increasing mean airway pressure and administering surfactant are likely to be more effective than iNO in improving oxygenation in babies with parenchymal lung disease and left-to-right shunt at patent ductus arteriosus (PDA) and patent foramen ovale (PFO).Presence of right-to-left shunting at the ductal level and left-to-right shunting at the atrial level similarly suggests PPHN with left ventricular dysfunction with some pulmonary venous hypertension (**Table 1**). This finding may be associated with the CDH[59] and left ventricular dysfunction seen in sepsis and asphyxia.[60] If right-to-left shunting is present at ductal and atrial levels and is associated with labile hypoxemia and tricuspid regurgitation, PPHN is the most likely diagnosis. However, patients with fixed hypoxemia with right-to-left shunting at ductal and atrial levels associated with a small left atrium without tricuspid regurgitation may have anomalous pulmonary venous return (see **Table 1**).

Table 1
Differential diagnosis of hypoxemia in neonates based on the direction of shunt at atrial and ductal levels on echocardiography

Diagnosis	Ductal Shunt	Atrial Shunt	Management
Parenchymal lung disease and V/Q mismatch and intrapulmonary shunt	L → R	L → R	Lung recruitment, specific therapy (antibiotics for pneumonia) NO may be beneficial
PPHN	R → L	R → L	Oxygenation, correction of acidosis and inhaled NO
Left ventricular dysfunction (common in diaphragmatic hernia, asphyxia, and sepsis)[59,60]	R → L	L → R	Inotropes and vasodilators (Milrinone)
Tricuspid atresia/ stenosis or pulmonic atresia/stenosis	L → R	R → L	Prostaglandin E1 + surgery
Total anomalous pulmonary venous return[155]	R → L (large PA)	R → L (small LA and no tricuspid regurgitation)	Surgery

From Lakshminrusimha S, Kumar VH. Diseases of pulmonary circulation. In: Fuhrman PP, Zimmerman JJ, editors. Pediatric critical care. Mosby; 2011. p. 641; with permission.

Pulmonary Circulatory Changes in Some Specific Conditions Resulting in Neonatal Respiratory Failure

Idiopathic PPHN

Idiopathic PPHN (also known as black-lung PPHN) is characterized by increase of PVR without a primary parenchymal lung disease. Autopsy studies of fatal idiopathic PPHN show severe hypertensive structural remodeling with vessel wall thickening and smooth muscle hyperplasia. The vascular smooth muscle extends to the level of intra-acinar arteries,[61] resulting in increased PVR and failure to respond to birth-related stimuli, such as ventilation and oxygenation.[62] A well-known cause of black-lung PPHN is exposure to indomethacin during the third trimester, resulting in closure of the ductus arteriosus in utero.[24,63] A fetal lamb model of idiopathic PPHN is created by antenatal ductal ligation.[64] This model shows the clinical and histopathologic features of PPHN.[23] Abnormalities of the nitric oxide pathway (decreased eNOS,[53] decreased sGC,[55] and increased phosphodiesterase type 5 [PDE5[65]]), superoxide anion pathway (increased superoxide[66] and hydrogen peroxide[67]), and prostacyclin pathway (decreased prostacyclin synthase and prostacyclin IP receptor[68]) have been described in this model. Similar abnormalities in enzyme pathways may occur in human neonates with idiopathic PPHN.

CDH

CDH occurs in approximately 1 in 3000 births and is the most common cause of pulmonary hypoplasia in the neonate. Diaphragmatic hernia is associated with ipsilateral and contralateral lung hypoplasia, vascular paucity, and vascular remodeling. Most cases are diagnosed in the antenatal period. Initial delivery room management focuses on stabilization, gastrointestinal decompression, and immediate intubation. Bag-mask ventilation and introduction of more gas into the gastrointestinal tract should be avoided. Early corrective surgery is often associated with deterioration of respiratory function in the immediate postoperative period. There has been a paradigm shift focusing on cardiorespiratory stabilization and management of PPHN followed by surgery. There are 2 animal models of CDH: the rat model created by maternal ingestion of nitrofen, a herbicide, resulting in lung hypoplasia and a diaphragmatic defect; and a second model that is created by fetal surgery in lambs. Abnormalities in the nitric oxide synthase,[69] sGC, and PDE5 function[70] have been observed in these models. These abnormalities, associated with left ventricular hypoplasia, may contribute to poor response to iNO in CDH.

MAS

A combination of preexisting in utero hypoxia and meconium aspiration into the lungs with pulmonary hypertension often carries high morbidity. In the 1980s and 1990s, MAS was the most common cause of severe HRF and PPHN in neonates, but the incidence has decreased in recent years in the United States. A review of annual neonatal ECMO data from the Extracorporeal Life Support Organization (ELSO) registry (accessed in February 2012) shows that CDH accounts for more ECMO runs than MAS in recent years. This reduction is partly caused by reduction in postterm births in the United States in recent years, because MAS is more common in this population. Meconium aspiration with perinatal asphyxia leads to an immediate release of circulating vasoactive substances, which favor contraction and proliferation of smooth muscle fibers in the pulmonary circulation. Most cases of fatal MAS show evidence of smooth muscle hypertrophy in small pulmonary arteries.[46] In addition, a decrease in the expression of eNOS was reported in umbilical venous endothelial cells isolated from human infants with MAS.[71] In piglets, meconium instillation into the lungs increases PVR and asphyxia decreases SVR, and a combination of MAS and asphyxia worsen the ratio between PVR and SVR.[72]

Transient tachypnea of the newborn with HRF and PPHN (malignant transient tachypnea of the newborn)

Ramachandrappa and Jain[27] reviewed the pathogenesis of respiratory morbidity following elective cesarean section. Many infants with hypoxemia following elective cesarean section are considered to have transient tachypnea of the newborn and wet lung syndrome and are placed on oxygen by hood or nasal cannula without positive pressure. Absorption atelectasis results in increasing oxygen requirements and progressive respiratory failure. It is possible that formation of ROS from high alveolar Pao_2 may lead to increased pulmonary vascular reactivity and contribute to PPHN. Severe respiratory failure following elective cesarean section may occasionally require therapy with ECMO.[73]

Premature infant with bronchopulmonary dysplasia and pulmonary hypertension

Bronchopulmonary dysplasia (BPD) continues to be a major cause of morbidity and late mortality in extremely preterm infants. Pulmonary hypertension is observed in approximately 1 in 6 extremely low birth weight (ELBW) infants.[74] BPD is associated with reduced cross-sectional perfusion area with decreased arterial density and abnormal muscularization of peripheral pulmonary arteries.[75] Risk factors for developing pulmonary hypertension include low birth weight (small for GA), oligohydramnios,[76] and prolonged mechanical ventilation. A recent prospective analysis showed that the onset of pulmonary hypertension in BPD is variable and can be as late as 3 to 4 months of age.[74] A delay in diagnosis is associated with progressive pulmonary vascular disease, cor pulmonale, and high mortality. It is prudent to screen babies that are ventilated or require greater than 30% oxygen or have radiological evidence of BPD with an echocardiogram at 1 month of age and every 4 weeks until discharge to diagnose pulmonary hypertension early, leading to appropriate therapy. The optimal intervention strategies for reversing early pulmonary hypertension or treating established pulmonary hypertension are not clear. Multiple therapies, such as maintaining higher oxygen saturations, iNO, and sildenafil, are reported anecdotally to have been tried with mixed results.[77–79]

Air-leak syndromes

Air-leak syndromes such as pulmonary interstitial emphysema (PIE), pneumothorax, and pneumomediastinum are common complications of mechanical ventilation in preterm infants and are associated with respiratory failure. Among late preterm and term newborn infants, spontaneous pneumothorax is common and results in respiratory failure. Most of these infants improve spontaneously or require thoracocentesis or chest tube drainage with resolution of HRF. Smith and colleagues[80] recently reported that almost half of late preterm/term infants with spontaneous, symptomatic pneumothorax that required needle or chest tube drainage developed PPHN. Acute increases in PVR with shunting secondary to hypoxemia or acidosis or caused by the primary lung disease must be considered in the differential diagnosis of persistent HRF in infants with pneumothorax.

PULMONARY HEMODYNAMIC CHANGES CAUSED BY THERAPY

A detailed review of inhaled NO, sildenafil, milrinone, and other pulmonary vasodilator agents is provided in the March 2012 issue of *Clinics*.[81] This article focuses on the impact of various therapies in the NICU on the pulmonary circulation.

Mechanical Ventilation

Optimal lung recruitment during mechanical ventilation with appropriate use of positive end expiration pressure (PEEP) and/or mean airway pressure is a critical step during the management of HRF. When lungs are inflated at functional residual capacity (FRC), PVR is low. PVR is a combination of resistance offered by alveolar vessels and extra-alveolar vessels. When the lungs are underinflated or collapsed, the alveolar vessels are wide open but the extra-alveolar vessels are narrowed, resulting in increased PVR. When the alveoli are overinflated, the alveolar vessels are compressed, resulting in high PVR. Moreover, high PEEP or mean airway pressure may impair venous return and reduce cardiac output.[82] An optimal balance is achieved when the lung expansion is at FRC. It is important to check frequent radiographs during the acute phase of PPHN to assess optimal lung expansion.

Many clinicians use high-frequency ventilation (HFV) to manage infants with PPHN. Considering the important role of parenchymal lung disease in specific disorders resulting in PPHN, adequate lung inflation and optimal ventilation are as essential as pharmacologic vasodilator therapy. In the case of inhaled vasodilators, optimal inflation and ventilation may be necessary for drug delivery.[83] Infants with PPHN with a variety of causes have been successfully treated with HFV.[84] High-frequency oscillatory ventilation (HFOV) decreases $Paco_2$ and increases oxygenation in infants with PPHN. HFOV may improve oxygenation through safer use of higher mean airway pressures to maintain lung volume and prevent atelectasis. Two studies have evaluated the effectiveness of HFV compared with conventional ventilation in rescuing infants with respiratory failure and PPHN from potential ECMO therapy.[85,86] Neither mode of ventilation was more effective in preventing ECMO in these infants. In clinical pilot studies using iNO, a combination of HFOV and iNO resulted in the greatest improvement in oxygenation in some newborns who had severe PPHN complicated by diffuse parenchymal lung disease and underinflation.[87] A randomized controlled trial showed that treatment with HFOV and iNO was often successful in patients who failed to respond to HFOV or iNO alone in severe PPHN, and the differences in responses were related to the specific disease associated with PPHN. Infants with RDS and MAS benefit most from a combination of HFOV and iNO therapy.[88,89]

Oxygen

Oxygen is a specific and potent pulmonary vasodilator and increased oxygen tension is an important mediator of reduction in PVR at birth. Alveolar hypoxia and hypoxemia increase PVR and contribute to the pathophysiology of PPHN. Avoiding hypoxemia by mechanical ventilation with high concentrations of oxygen used to be the mainstay of PPHN management. However, exposure to hyperoxia may result in formation of oxygen free radicals and lead to lung injury. As mentioned previously, brief exposure to 100% oxygen in newborn lambs increases contractility of the pulmonary arteries[90] and formation of superoxide anions[49] and reduces response to inhaled NO.[47,48] Administration of intratracheal recombinant human superoxide dismutase (SOD; an antioxidant that breaks down superoxide anions) results in improved oxygenation in lambs with PPHN.[91,92] Based on these studies, it seems that avoiding hyperoxia is as important as avoiding hypoxia in the management of PPHN.

The optimal Pao_2 in the management of PPHN is not clear. Wung and colleagues[93] suggested that gentle ventilation with avoidance of hyperoxia and hyperventilation results in good outcomes in neonates with respiratory failure. Decreasing Pao_2 to less than 45 to 50 mm Hg results in increased PVR in newborn calves[94] and lambs.[48] In contrast, maintaining Pao_2 at greater than 70 to 80 mm Hg does not result in additional decrease in PVR in both control lambs and lambs with PPHN. Maintaining preductal oxygen saturations in the 90% to 97% range seems to be associated with low PVR in the ductal ligation model of PPHN (**Fig. 5**). In animal studies, hypoxemia results in pulmonary vasoconstriction; normoxemia reduces PVR but hyperoxemia does not result in additional pulmonary vasodilation. To date, randomized studies comparing different Pao_2 targets have not been conducted in infants with PPHN.

Acidosis/Alkalosis

Acidosis (both metabolic and respiratory) constricts the pulmonary vasculature and increases PVR, whereas alkalosis selectively decreases PVR.[94] Acidosis (pH<7.30) was associated with an exaggerated constrictor response to hypoxia. In 1978, Peckham and Fox[95] published a study of 10 infants with significant PPHN who were treated with hyperventilation and showed significant improvement. Despite the small number of infants in this report, hyperventilation soon became a common therapy in the treatment of this disease and was effectively used as a strategy to improve Pao_2.[96] In 1985, Wung and colleagues[93] challenged this practice. They managed 15 infants with severe PPHN using gentle ventilation maintaining Pao_2 between 50 and 70 mm Hg and allowing $Paco_2$ to increase as high as 60 mm Hg. All infants survived, with only 1 developing chronic lung disease, thus questioning the strategy of hyperventilation. Moreover, studies in asphyxiated lambs showed that respiratory alkalosis reduced cerebral blood flow.[97] Alkalosis achieved via ventilator-induced hypocarbia was subsequently shown to be associated with poor neurodevelopmental outcome and hearing loss.[98,99] In a retrospective review of PPHN management at National Institute of Child Health and Human Development (NICHD) centers, Walsh-Sukys and colleagues[100] reported that continuous alkali infusion was associated with increased use of ECMO and increased use of oxygen at 28 days of age. With the availability of selective pulmonary vasodilators, therapeutic alkalosis is no longer recommended in the management of PPHN. Based on animal data, avoiding acidosis (pH<7.30) may offer some protection

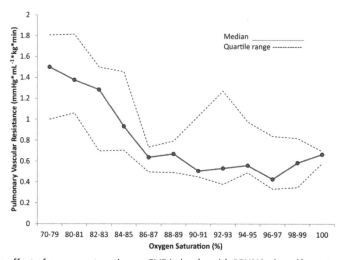

Fig. 5. The effect of oxygen saturation on PVR in lambs with PPHN induced by antenatal ductal ligation: Median (*solid line*) and 25th and 75th percentile lines (*dashed lines*) are shown in the figure. Saturation range of 90% to 97% is associated with low PVR. (*From* Lakshminrusimha S, Swartz DD, Gugino SF, et al. Oxygen concentration and pulmonary hemodynamics in newborn lambs with pulmonary hypertension. Pediatr Res 2009;66(5):542; with permission.)

against pulmonary vasoconstrictor response to hypoxia.[94] However, this effect has not been systematically evaluated in human infants with PPHN.

Surfactant

Administration of intratracheal surfactant is a common practice in the presence of RDS, pneumonia, or MAS. In surfactant-depleted piglet models, instillation of surfactant is associated with a significant reduction in systemic and pulmonary arterial pressures.[101,102] However, in human preterm infants, administration of surfactant is associated with selective reduction in pulmonary arterial pressure without any change in systemic pressure.[103] Surfactant therapy has been shown to reduce the need for ECMO in term neonates with MAS.[104–106] The effect of surfactant is probably a combination of its direct effect on compliance and recruitment and, when used in conjunction with iNO, an indirect effect through enhancing iNO delivery and V/Q matching.

iNO

The introduction of iNO, following its approval by the US Food and Drug Administration (FDA) in 1999 revolutionized the management of PPHN and HRF in the NICU. Large multicenter trials, the Neonatal Inhaled Nitric Oxide Study Group (NINOS) trial,[107] the Clinical Inhaled Nitric Oxide Research Group (CINRGI) trial,[108] and Roberts and colleagues'[109] trial, showed that iNO reduced the need for ECMO. Treatment with iNO results in improved oxygenation and reduction in oxygenation index (OI; mean airway pressure in cm H_2O × forced inspiratory oxygen [Fio_2] × $100/Pao_2$ in mm Hg) in 50% to 60% of patients over a wide range of severity of HRF.[110]

Approximately two-thirds of neonates with parenchymal lung disease, such as MAS and RDS, and HRF respond well to iNO with improved oxygenation. The percentage of responders can be further enhanced with the use of HFOV, emphasizing the importance of lung recruitment during iNO therapy.[89] A similar oxygenation response is observed in infants with idiopathic PPHN, but implementation of HFOV does not enhance this response. In contrast, HRF resulting from CDH responds poorly to both iNO and HFOV. Possible causal factors resulting in inadequate or ill-sustained response to iNO are discussed later (**Fig. 6**):

Poor alveolar recruitment

Inhaled NO has to reach its target organ, the resistance pulmonary arteriole, to induce pulmonary vasodilation. If there is parenchymal lung disease and/or atelectasis, iNO cannot reach alveoli and pulmonary vasculature. Appropriate alveolar recruitment with increased PEEP, mean airway pressure, and use of surfactant before initiation of iNO is likely to increase pulmonary vasodilation in response to iNO. Once iNO enters the pulmonary vasculature and interacts with hemoglobin in the red blood cells, methemoglobin (MHb) is formed. The increase in MHb following iNO therapy can be considered to reflect that iNO has reached the pulmonary vasculature. We have observed that MHb levels (corrected for NO dose) are significantly higher in neonates with a positive oxygenation response to iNO compared with neonates that do not respond to iNO.[83] Better alveolar recruitment with HFV and surfactant is at least partly responsible for lower ECMO/death rates following iNO therapy in recent studies (19.5%)[111] compared with the NINOS study (39%).[107]

Remodeled pulmonary vasculature

Chronic intrauterine pulmonary hypertension, such as is seen in CDH, and antenatal closure of the ductus arteriosus can result in thickening of the smooth muscle layer and adventitia with distal extension of musculature to normally nonmuscular arterioles. Remodeled vasculature tends to be associated with a fixed component of

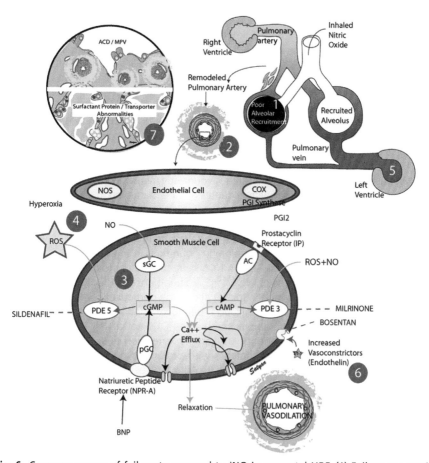

Fig. 6. Common causes of failure to respond to iNO in neonatal HRF. (1) Failure to recruit alveoli before iNO administration prevents delivery of NO to its target organ, the resistance level pulmonary artery. (2) Remodeled pulmonary artery may have a fixed component of pulmonary vasoconstriction and not respond to vasodilators. (3) Enzyme abnormalities such as decreased sGC activity or increased PDE5 activity can decrease cGMP formation. (4) Increased formation of ROS such as superoxide anions can inactivate NO and stimulate PDE5. (5) Left ventricular failure results in pulmonary venous hypertension, and use of NO in this situation may worsen pulmonary edema and oxygenation. (6) High concentrations of vasoconstrictors, such as ET, may counteract the vasodilation induced by iNO. (7) Rare abnormalities such as alveolar capillary dysplasia with misaligned pulmonary veins (ACD/ MPV) and surfactant protein-B deficiency or ATP binding cassette A3 (ABCA3) deficiency. AC, adenylate cyclase; BNP, B-type natriuretic peptide; COX, cyclooxygenase; NO, nitric oxide; NOS, nitric oxide synthase; PDE, phosphodiesterase; pGC, particulate guanylate cyclase; PGI, prostacyclin; ROS, reactive oxygen species; sGC, soluble guanylate cyclase. (Copyright © Satyan Lakshminrusimha.)

vasoconstriction and does not respond well to exogenous vasodilators. Endothelial dysfunction results in poor response to endothelium-dependent vasodilators, such as oxygen and acetylcholine. These abnormal vasodilator responses secondary to impaired sGC activity are well described in animal models of neonatal pulmonary hypertension[55] and diaphragmatic hernia.[70]

Abnormalities of target enzymes

Nitric oxide stimulates sGC in the pulmonary arterial smooth muscle cell (PASMC) to produce cGMP. sGC is a heme-containing enzyme and can be inactivated by a variety of conditions. Animal models of PPHN have decreased sGC activity reducing cGMP production and relaxation to NO donors.[55] More recently, specific activators of sGC have been shown to relax PASMC and may be potentially more effectively than iNO.[112,113] An increase in PDE5 activity results in catabolism of cGMP and limitation of NO-induced vasodilation. Ventilation with high concentrations of inspired oxygen and exposure to ROS stimulates PDE5 activity[114] and decreases cGMP levels. Inhibition of PDE5 with the use of sildenafil has been an effective strategy in the treatment of PPHN.[115,116] Sildenafil, the first PDE5 inhibitor to be approved by the FDA for treatment of pulmonary hypertension in adults, is currently available for both oral and intravenous administration. Therapy with sildenafil has been studied in the acute phase of PPHN and in patients with chronic pulmonary hypertension. Sildenafil is currently not approved for use in neonates but has been used off label in the following circumstances: (1) management of PPHN in the acute phase in situations in which iNO and ECMO are not available,[115] as in developing countries. In a recent pharmacokinetic study, intravenous sildenafil was shown to be effective in improving oxygenation as a primary agent (without the use of iNO).[116] (2) To augment the effect of iNO in patients with partial or ill-sustained response to iNO. It may be particularly effective in patients following prolonged hyperoxic ventilation because ventilation with high oxygen concentrations and superoxide anions stimulates PDE5 activity.[114] (3) To reduce the severity of, or to prevent rebound, pulmonary hypertension observed after weaning iNO.[117] (4) Chronic oral therapy in infants with prolonged pulmonary hypertension, as in that associated with BPD[118] or CDH. (5) Antenatal use of sildenafil was recently shown to decrease pulmonary hypertension in nitrofen-induced CDH in rat pups; there are no human studies to show the effect of antenatal sildenafil on fetal PVR. The primary concern with the use of intravenous or oral vasodilators, such as sildenafil, is the potential for a decrease in SVR with worsening of right-to-left shunt. The dose of sildenafil should be carefully adjusted to achieve pulmonary vasodilation without significant systemic vasodilation. The optimal dose of sildenafil in term neonates has been evaluated in a recent pharmacokinetic study.[119] A slow load of 0.4 mg/kg over 3 hours results in early buildup of therapeutic plasma levels without significant reduction in systemic blood pressure. The dose of continuous infusion is 1.6 mg/kg/d. This intravenous dose (approximately 2 mg/kg/d) corresponds with the recommended oral dose of 4 to 8 mg/kg/d, assuming that oral bioavailability of sildenafil in neonates is similar to that in adults (40%).[120–122] Hepatic immaturity or dysfunction and severe renal impairment can prolong the half-life of sildenafil[121] and potentially increase in the risk of systemic hypotension.

ROS

The primary determinant of the biologic half-life of endogenous NO is the local concentration of superoxide anions. The reaction between NO and superoxide anion yields toxic peroxynitrite with a second-order rate constant near the diffusion-controlled limit (K constant = $6.7 \pm 0.9 \times 10^9$ M^{-1} s^{-1}). This reaction constitutes an important sink for superoxide anions because it is about twice as fast as the maximum velocity of superoxide dismutase.[123] In addition to direct inactivation of NO, ROS can decrease eNOS activity and sGC activity, and increase PDE5 activity, resulting in decreased cGMP levels. Increased ROS can be secondary to (1) ventilation or exposure to high oxygen[49]; (2) poor antioxidant defense mechanisms such as superoxide dismutase, catalase, and glutathione peroxidase levels[124]; and (3) increased production of superoxide anions from increased activity of enzymes such as nicotinamide adenine dinucleotide phosphate hydrogen (NADPH) oxidase (Nox).[66] The effect of prior oxygen exposure (in the form of OI) on response to iNO has been evaluated. Konduri and colleagues[125] randomized near-term and term infants with HRF into early initiation of iNO (when OI is ≥15 but <25) or standard initiation (OI ≥25). There was no difference in the incidence of death (early iNO, 6.7% vs standard, 9.4%), ECMO (10.7% vs 12.1%), or death and ECMO combined (16.7% vs 19.5%). However, control infants receiving standard iNO deteriorated to OI greater than 40 more often than the early iNO group (14% vs 7%, $P = .056$). Based on this study, starting iNO at an OI less than 25 does not reduce the need for ECMO but may prevent progression of HRF and decrease exposure to high levels of oxygen in some neonates with HRF. Data from multiple trials of iNO in HRF are shown in **Fig. 7**. Based on these results, it seems that OI at initiation of iNO roughly corresponds with the frequency of ECMO/death in that cohort. The case series of gentle ventilation and iNO use from Columbia-Presbyterian hospital[126] with lower target Pao_2 and permissive hypercapnia was associated with a lower frequency of ECMO/death (28%) despite a high mean OI at initiation of iNO (46.8 ± 24.5). This association suggests that targeting lower Pao_2 and limiting Fio_2 (and possibly ROS generation) and barotrauma improves outcomes in PPHN.

Left ventricular dysfunction

Patients with HRF and PPHN typically have a right-to-left shunt at the level of ductus arteriosus and foramen ovale. In the presence of left ventricular dysfunction and/or hypoplasia, left atrial pressures are increased, resulting in a left-to-right shunt at the foramen ovale (see **Table 1**). Increased left atrial pressure results in pulmonary venous hypertension. Administration of iNO to a patient with pulmonary venous hypertension can result in potential flooding of the pulmonary capillary bed and worsening of pulmonary edema, resulting in clinical deterioration.[59] Left ventricular hypoplasia associated

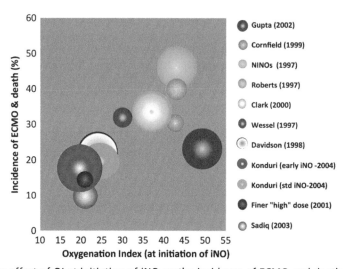

Fig. 7. The effect of OI at initiation of iNO on the incidence of ECMO and death in various trials: the size of the bubble is based on the number of infants enrolled in the iNO arm in that trial. The OI at initiation corresponds approximately with the incidence of ECMO or death. A case series from Columbia-Presbyterian Hospital using gentle ventilation is associated with lower incidence of ECMO/death despite high OI at initiation of iNO,[126] suggesting that prior exposure to oxygen is a more important factor than precise OI at initiation of iNO.

with CDH[127,128] may contribute to pulmonary venous hypertension and could be a potential explanation for impaired response to iNO in these patients.[129] It has been suggested that an inodilator such as milrinone may be more effective than iNO in improving left ventricular function and reducing pulmonary venous hypertension.

Two case series report the effectiveness of milrinone in improving oxygenation in iNO-resistant PPHN.[130,131] Unlike iNO, which acts through cGMP, milrinone inhibits phosphodiesterase 3A (PDE3A) enzyme in PASMCs and increases the level of a different second messenger, cAMP, resulting in pulmonary vasodilation. Pulmonary vasodilation in response to milrinone is proportional to PDE3A activity in PASMCs. Exposure to NO donors increases PDE3A expression in rat PASMCs.[132] Ventilation of newborn lambs with oxygen and iNO increases PDE3A activity in resistance level pulmonary arteries compared with ventilation with oxygen alone.[133] Pulmonary arterial rings isolated from lambs ventilated with iNO relax significantly better to milrinone compared with lambs ventilated with oxygen only. These studies suggest that exposure to iNO increases PDE3A activity and that milrinone may be uniquely effective in promoting pulmonary vasodilation and improving oxygenation in iNO-resistant PPHN,[130,131] in addition to its cardiac inotropic effect.

Increased vasoconstrictor mediators

ET-1 is produced by the endothelium and exerts its powerful vasoconstrictor effect by acting on ET-A receptors on vascular smooth muscle cells.[134] Increased levels of plasma immunoreactive ET-1 levels have been reported in neonates with PPHN, and these levels correlate with the severity of disease.[135,136] Bosentan, an ET receptor antagonist, has been used in PPHN.[137,138] Mohamed and colleagues[137] recently reported a prospective randomized trial of bosentan versus placebo in PPHN. Oral bosentan (1 mg/kg twice a day) resulted in a significant improvement in OI compared with placebo. Close monitoring of liver function is important during bosentan therapy.

Rare causes of PPHN/HRF in term neonates

In some patients with PPHN/HRF resistant to all treatments including ECMO, lung biopsy may be required to confirm the diagnosis.[139] Patients with alveolar capillary dysplasia and misalignment of pulmonary veins (ACD/MPV) typically present with HRF and PPHN shortly after birth. Lung histology shows simplification of alveolar architecture, widened and poorly developed septa, with a paucity of capillaries. Small pulmonary arteries are muscularized, accompanied by pulmonary veins within the same connective tissue sheath (see **Fig. 6**). Patients with surfactant protein-B (SPB) deficiency and ATP binding cassette A3 (ABCA3) transporter deficiencies present with intractable HRF. Infants with prolonged, severe HRF/PPHN out of proportion to their lung disease may require a lung biopsy or targeted genetic evaluation for definitive diagnosis.

Inotropes

PPHN is a syndrome associated with an increased PVR/SVR ratio. Systemic hypotension is a common feature of patients with PPHN and can be multifactorial. Common causes include (1) direct effect of the primary underlying disease such as sepsis or pneumonia, (2) myocardial dysfunction secondary to asphyxia or sepsis,[60] (3) septal deviation to the left impinging on left ventricular end-diastolic volume and outflow tract, (4) ventilator therapies such as increased mean airway pressure reducing venous return,[82] and (5) decreased pulmonary venous return caused by increased PVR reduces left ventricular preload.

It is a common practice in the NICU to obtain an echocardiogram to estimate systolic pulmonary arterial pressure and to increase systemic systolic pressure with an infusion of inotropes such as dopamine. Dopamine is a nonselective vasoconstrictor and can increase systemic arterial pressure as well as pulmonary arterial pressure in newborn goats[140] and preterm human infants with PDA. Initiation of norepinephrine infusion (0.5–1 μg/kg/min) increased mean systemic arterial pressure from 39 ± 4 to 49 ± 4 mm Hg and increased mean pulmonary arterial pressure from 33 ± 4 to 42 ± 5 mm Hg, decreased pulmonary/systemic pressure ratio, and improved oxygenation in late preterm and term infants with PPHN.[141] The investigators report echocardiographic findings that suggest increased pulmonary blood flow and speculate that norepinephrine may mediate an α2 receptor–mediated pulmonary vasodilation.

We recently evaluated the effect of dopamine on systemic arterial pressure and pulmonary arterial pressure in newborn lambs with PPHN induced by antenatal ductal ligation[64] and their control twins. Control lambs without PPHN have significantly higher systemic blood pressure compared with pulmonary arterial pressure (**Fig. 8**). Administration of dopamine selectively increases systemic arterial pressure at a lower dose without significantly increasing pulmonary arterial pressure, and increases pulmonary blood flow in control lambs with normal pulmonary vasculature. In PPHN lambs with remodeled pulmonary arteries, pulmonary arterial pressure is at systemic levels and is more sensitive to vasoconstrictor effects of dopamine. Dopamine did not increase pulmonary blood flow in lambs with PPHN. These findings emphasize the need for frequent echocardiograms to evaluate pulmonary arterial pressure in patients with PPHN on high doses of dopamine and norepinephrine.

Partial Liquid Ventilation

Partial liquid ventilation (PLV) with perfluorocarbons has been studied in HRF in animal models[142,143] and human infants.[144] PLV has been shown to improve gas exchange and improve spatial distribution of pulmonary blood flow in models of lung injury.[145] However, PLV does not prevent hypoxic pulmonary vasoconstriction in the absence of parenchymal lung injury.[146] A combination of iNO and PLV improved oxygenation in a lamb model of CDH[147] but did not decrease PVR in a piglet model of MAS[142] with conventional ventilation. The use of high-frequency PLV results in a significant

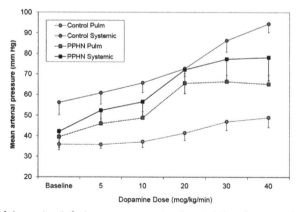

Fig. 8. Effect of dopamine infusion on mean systemic arterial and mean pulmonary arterial pressure in normal newborn lambs and lambs with PPHN induced by antenatal ductal ligation. In newborn lambs with normal pulmonary vasculature, systemic blood pressure is significantly higher than pulmonary arterial pressure and increases relatively selectively in response to low doses of dopamine. In PPHN, systemic and pulmonary blood pressures are similar and increase in parallel in response to dopamine.

decrease in PVR and an improvement in pulmonary blood flow in a preterm lamb model of RDS.[148] It is likely that PLV improves alveolar recruitment, compliance, and gas exchange, and its effect on pulmonary hemodynamics is secondary to these changes.

ECMO

ECMO refers to a life support technique designed to enhance gas exchange and provide pulmonary and/or cardiac support in severe HRF. ECMO requires diversion of blood from a major systemic vessel through a gas exchange device (membrane oxygenator) and back to a major vessel. The venoarterial approach (VA) has served as the primary mode of cannulation for both cardiac and respiratory failure in neonates and uses a central vein (usually jugular) for drainage and an artery (usually carotid) for return. As blood is diverted from the pulmonary circuit, immediate decompression of the right ventricle occurs in VA-ECMO. Venovenous (VV) cannulation is appropriate for patients with severe respiratory failure who do not require cardiac support and uses a major vein for blood drainage and a vein for return of oxygenated blood to the right heart.[149,150] Pulmonary and right ventricular hemodynamics are not altered, although the blood entering the pulmonary artery has substantially higher Po_2. The impact of such increased oxygen tension in the pulmonary circulation on PVR is not known. The presence of pulsatile flow in VV ECMO is associated with better cerebral hemodynamics but this could be a reflection of patient selection bias.[151] Overall, no major differences have been reported in respiratory outcome between VA and VV ECMO.[152,153]

SUMMARY

Increased understanding of the pathophysiologic changes in the pulmonary circulation in neonatal HRF and PPHN in the last 2 decades has led to a substantial decrease in the number of neonatal respiratory patients requiring ECMO. Further clinical research into pulmonary vasodilator therapy has become more challenging because of a decreased number of patients and widespread availability of iNO, resulting in difficult study recruitment. Two unmet challenges remain in pulmonary circulatory disorders: CDH and premature infants with BPD and pulmonary hypertension.[154] Multicenter trials to evaluate and develop appropriate strategies to ameliorate pulmonary vascular disease in these conditions are warranted.

ACKNOWLEDGMENTS

I thank Drs Bobby Mathew, Veena Manja, and Corinne Leach for their critical review of this article.

REFERENCES

1. Lakshminrusimha S, Steinhorn RH. Pulmonary vascular biology during neonatal transition. Clin Perinatol 1999;26(3):601–19.
2. Dawes GS. Pulmonary circulation in the foetus and new-born. Br Med Bull 1966; 22(1):61–5.
3. Ardran G, Dawes GS, Prichard MM, et al. The effect of ventilation of the foetal lungs upon the pulmonary circulation. J Physiol 1952;118(1):12–22.
4. Rasanen J, Wood DC, Weiner S, et al. Role of the pulmonary circulation in the distribution of human fetal cardiac output during the second half of pregnancy. Circulation 1996;94(5):1068–73.

5. Rasanen J, Wood DC, Debbs RH, et al. Reactivity of the human fetal pulmonary circulation to maternal hyperoxygenation increases during the second half of pregnancy: a randomized study. Circulation 1998;97(3):257–62.
6. Heymann MA, Lewis AB, Rudolph AM. Pulmonary vascular responses during advancing gestation in fetal lambs in utero. Chest 1977;71(Suppl 2):270–1.
7. Lewis AB, Heymann MA, Rudolph AM. Gestational changes in pulmonary vascular responses in fetal lambs in utero. Circ Res 1976;39(4):536–41.
8. Accurso FJ, Alpert B, Wilkening RB, et al. Time-dependent response of fetal pulmonary blood flow to an increase in fetal oxygen tension. Respir Physiol 1986;63(1):43–52.
9. Mensah E, Morin FC 3rd, Russell JA, et al. Soluble guanylate cyclase mRNA expression change during ovine lung development. Pediatr Res 1998;43:290.
10. Bloch KD, Filippov G, Sanchez LS, et al. Pulmonary soluble guanylate cyclase, a nitric oxide receptor, is increased during the perinatal period. Am J Physiol 1997;272(3 Pt 1):L400–6.
11. Kumar VH, Hutchison AA, Lakshminrusimha S, et al. Characteristics of pulmonary hypertension in preterm neonates. J Perinatol 2007;27(4):214–9.
12. Luong C, Rey-Perra J, Vadivel A, et al. Antenatal sildenafil treatment attenuates pulmonary hypertension in experimental congenital diaphragmatic hernia. Circulation 2011;123(19):2120–31.
13. Chandrasekar I, Eis A, Konduri GG. Betamethasone attenuates oxidant stress in endothelial cells from fetal lambs with persistent pulmonary hypertension. Pediatr Res 2008;63(1):67–72.
14. Cruz-Martinez R, Moreno-Alvarez O, Prat J, et al. Lung tissue blood perfusion changes induced by in utero tracheal occlusion in a rabbit model of congenital diaphragmatic hernia. Fetal Diagn Ther 2009;26(3):137–42.
15. Jelin E, Lee H. Tracheal occlusion for fetal congenital diaphragmatic hernia: the US experience. Clin Perinatol 2009;36(2):349–61, ix.
16. Bratu I, Flageole H, Laberge JM, et al. Pulmonary structural maturation and pulmonary artery remodeling after reversible fetal ovine tracheal occlusion in diaphragmatic hernia. J Pediatr Surg 2001;36(5):739–44.
17. Luks FI, Wild YK, Piasecki GJ, et al. Short-term tracheal occlusion corrects pulmonary vascular anomalies in the fetal lamb with diaphragmatic hernia. Surgery 2000;128(2):266–72.
18. Chambers CD, Hernandez-Diaz S, Van Marter LJ, et al. Selective serotonin-reuptake inhibitors and risk of persistent pulmonary hypertension of the newborn. N Engl J Med 2006;354(6):579–87.
19. Belik J. Fetal and neonatal effects of maternal drug treatment for depression. Semin Perinatol 2008;32(5):350–4.
20. Fornaro E, Li D, Pan J, et al. Prenatal exposure to fluoxetine induces fetal pulmonary hypertension in the rat. Am J Respir Crit Care Med 2007;176(10):1035–40.
21. Wilson KL, Zelig CM, Harvey JP, et al. Persistent pulmonary hypertension of the newborn is associated with mode of delivery and not with maternal use of selective serotonin reuptake inhibitors. Am J Perinatol 2011;28(1):19–24.
22. Talati AJ, Salim MA, Korones SB. Persistent pulmonary hypertension after maternal naproxen ingestion in a term newborn: a case report. Am J Perinatol 2000;17(2):69–71.
23. Wild LM, Nickerson PA, Morin FC 3rd. Ligating the ductus arteriosus before birth remodels the pulmonary vasculature of the lamb. Pediatr Res 1989;25(3):251–7.

24. Alano MA, Ngougmna E, Ostrea EM Jr, et al. Analysis of nonsteroidal antiinflammatory drugs in meconium and its relation to persistent pulmonary hypertension of the newborn. Pediatrics 2001;107(3):519–23.

25. Teitel DF, Iwamoto HS, Rudolph AM. Changes in the pulmonary circulation during birth-related events. Pediatr Res 1990;27(4 Pt 1):372–8.

26. Abman SH, Chatfield BA, Hall SL, et al. Role of endothelium-derived relaxing factor during transition of pulmonary circulation at birth. Am J Physiol 1990; 259(6 Pt 2):H1921–7.

27. Ramachandrappa A, Jain L. Elective cesarean section: its impact on neonatal respiratory outcome. Clin Perinatol 2008;35(2):373–93, vii.

28. Sulyok E, Csaba IF. Elective repeat cesarean delivery and persistent pulmonary hypertension of the newborn. Am J Obstet Gynecol 1986;155(3):687–8.

29. Hernandez-Diaz S, Van Marter LJ, Werler MM, et al. Risk factors for persistent pulmonary hypertension of the newborn. Pediatrics 2007;120(2):e272–82.

30. Ramachandrappa A, Jain L. Health issues of the late preterm infant. Pediatr Clin North Am 2009;56(3):565–77, Table of Contents.

31. Ramachandrappa A, Rosenberg ES, Wagoner S, et al. Morbidity and mortality in late preterm infants with severe hypoxic respiratory failure on extra-corporeal membrane oxygenation. J Pediatr 2011;159(2):192–8.e3.

32. Stevens TP, van Wijngaarden E, Ackerman KG, et al. Timing of delivery and survival rates for infants with prenatal diagnoses of congenital diaphragmatic hernia. Pediatrics 2009;123(2):494–502.

33. Hutcheon JA, Butler B, Lisonkova S, et al. Timing of delivery for pregnancies with congenital diaphragmatic hernia. BJOG 2010;117(13):1658–62.

34. Sotiriadis A, Makrydimas G, Papatheodorou S, et al. Corticosteroids for preventing neonatal respiratory morbidity after elective caesarean section at term. Cochrane Database Syst Rev 2009;(4):CD006614.

35. Stutchfield P, Whitaker R, Russell I. Antenatal betamethasone and incidence of neonatal respiratory distress after elective caesarean section: pragmatic randomised trial. BMJ 2005;331(7518):662.

36. Guilherme R, Rotten D. Betamethasone before elective caesarean section at term: a survey of practice in France. Eur J Obstet Gynecol Reprod Biol 2010; 150(1):104.

37. Byers HM, Dagle JM, Klein JM, et al. Variations in CRHR1 are associated with persistent pulmonary hypertension of the newborn. Pediatr Res 2012;71(2): 162–7.

38. Perez M, Lakshminrusimha S, Wedgwood S, et al. Hydrocortisone normalizes oxygenation and cGMP regulation in lambs with persistent pulmonary hypertension of the newborn. Am J Physiol Lung Cell Mol Physiol 2012;302(6): L595–603.

39. Perlman JM, Wyllie J, Kattwinkel J, et al. Part 11: Neonatal resuscitation: 2010 International Consensus on cardiopulmonary resuscitation and emergency cardiovascular care science with treatment recommendations. Circulation 2010;122(16 Suppl 2):S516–38.

40. Arcilla RA, Oh W, Lind J, et al. Pulmonary arterial pressures of newborn infants born with early and late clamping of the cord. Acta Paediatr Scand 1966;55(3): 305–15.

41. Toubas PL, Hof RP, Heymann MA, et al. Effects of hypothermia and rewarming on the neonatal circulation. Arch Fr Pediatr 1978;35(Suppl 10):84–92.

42. Lapointe A, Barrington KJ. Pulmonary hypertension and the asphyxiated newborn. J Pediatr 2011;158(Suppl 2):e19–24.

43. Thoresen M. Hypothermia after perinatal asphyxia: selection for treatment and cooling protocol. J Pediatr 2011;158(Suppl 2):e45–9.
44. Sarkar S, Barks JD, Bhagat I, et al. Pulmonary dysfunction and therapeutic hypothermia in asphyxiated newborns: whole body versus selective head cooling. Am J Perinatol 2009;26(4):265–70.
45. Cornish JD, Dreyer GL, Snyder GE, et al. Failure of acute perinatal asphyxia or meconium aspiration to produce persistent pulmonary hypertension in a neonatal baboon model. Am J Obstet Gynecol 1994;171(1):43–9.
46. Murphy JD, Vawter GF, Reid LM. Pulmonary vascular disease in fatal meconium aspiration. J Pediatr 1984;104(5):758–62.
47. Lakshminrusimha S, Russell JA, Steinhorn RH, et al. Pulmonary hemodynamics in neonatal lambs resuscitated with 21%, 50%, and 100% oxygen. Pediatr Res 2007;62(3):313–8.
48. Lakshminrusimha S, Swartz DD, Gugino SF, et al. Oxygen concentration and pulmonary hemodynamics in newborn lambs with pulmonary hypertension. Pediatr Res 2009;66(5):539–44.
49. Lakshminrusimha S, Steinhorn RH, Wedgwood S, et al. Pulmonary hemodynamics and vascular reactivity in asphyxiated term lambs resuscitated with 21% and 100% oxygen. J Appl Physiol 2011;111(5):1441–7.
50. Dobyns EL, Wescott JY, Kennaugh JM, et al. Eicosanoids decrease with successful extracorporeal membrane oxygenation therapy in neonatal pulmonary hypertension. Am J Respir Crit Care Med 1994;149(4 Pt 1):873–80.
51. Langleben D, DeMarchie M, Laporta D, et al. Endothelin-1 in acute lung injury and the adult respiratory distress syndrome. Am Rev Respir Dis 1993;148(6 Pt 1): 1646–50.
52. Ivy DD, Parker TA, Ziegler JW, et al. Prolonged endothelin A receptor blockade attenuates chronic pulmonary hypertension in the ovine fetus. J Clin Invest 1997;99(6):1179–86.
53. Shaul PW, Yuhanna IS, German Z, et al. Pulmonary endothelial NO synthase gene expression is decreased in fetal lambs with pulmonary hypertension. Am J Physiol 1997;272(5 Pt 1):L1005–12.
54. McQueston JA, Kinsella JP, Ivy DD, et al. Chronic pulmonary hypertension in utero impairs endothelium-dependent vasodilation. Am J Physiol 1995;268(1 Pt 2): H288–94.
55. Steinhorn RH, Russell JA, Morin FC 3rd. Disruption of cGMP production in pulmonary arteries isolated from fetal lambs with pulmonary hypertension. Am J Physiol 1995;268(4 Pt 2):H1483–9.
56. Geggel RL, Reid LM. The structural basis of PPHN. Clin Perinatol 1984;11(3): 525–49.
57. El-Khuffash AF, McNamara PJ. Neonatologist-performed functional echocardiography in the neonatal intensive care unit. Semin Fetal Neonatal Med 2011; 16(1):50–60.
58. Yock PG, Popp RL. Noninvasive estimation of right ventricular systolic pressure by Doppler ultrasound in patients with tricuspid regurgitation. Circulation 1984; 70(4):657–62.
59. Kinsella JP. Inhaled nitric oxide in the term newborn. Early Hum Dev 2008; 84(11):709–16.
60. Sehgal A, Athikarisamy SE, Adamopoulos M. Global myocardial function is compromised in infants with pulmonary hypertension. Acta Paediatr 2012;101(4):410–3.
61. Murphy JD, Rabinovitch M, Goldstein JD, et al. The structural basis of persistent pulmonary hypertension of the newborn infant. J Pediatr 1981;98(6):962–7.

62. Allen K, Haworth SG. Human postnatal pulmonary arterial remodeling. Ultrastructural studies of smooth muscle cell and connective tissue maturation. Lab Invest 1988;59(5):702–9.

63. Manchester D, Margolis HS, Sheldon RE. Possible association between maternal indomethacin therapy and primary pulmonary hypertension of the newborn. Am J Obstet Gynecol 1976;126(4):467–9.

64. Morin FC 3rd. Ligating the ductus arteriosus before birth causes persistent pulmonary hypertension in the newborn lamb. Pediatr Res 1989;25(3):245–50.

65. Hanson KA, Ziegler JW, Rybalkin SD, et al. Chronic pulmonary hypertension increases fetal lung cGMP phosphodiesterase activity. Am J Physiol 1998; 275(5 Pt 1):L931–41.

66. Brennan LA, Steinhorn RH, Wedgwood S, et al. Increased superoxide generation is associated with pulmonary hypertension in fetal lambs: a role for NADPH oxidase. Circ Res 2003;92(6):683–91.

67. Wedgwood S, Steinhorn RH, Bunderson M, et al. Increased hydrogen peroxide downregulates soluble guanylate cyclase in the lungs of lambs with persistent pulmonary hypertension of the newborn. Am J Physiol Lung Cell Mol Physiol 2005;289(4):L660–6.

68. Lakshminrusimha S, Porta NF, Farrow KN, et al. Milrinone enhances relaxation to prostacyclin and iloprost in pulmonary arteries isolated from lambs with persistent pulmonary hypertension of the newborn. Pediatr Crit Care Med 2009;10(1): 106–12.

69. Karamanoukian HL, Peay T, Love JE, et al. Decreased pulmonary nitric oxide synthase activity in the rat model of congenital diaphragmatic hernia. J Pediatr Surg 1996;31(8):1016–9.

70. de Buys Roessingh A, Fouquet V, Aigrain Y, et al. Nitric oxide activity through guanylate cyclase and phosphodiesterase modulation is impaired in fetal lambs with congenital diaphragmatic hernia. J Pediatr Surg 2011;46(8):1516–22.

71. Villanueva ME, Zaher FM, Svinarich DM, et al. Decreased gene expression of endothelial nitric oxide synthase in newborns with persistent pulmonary hypertension. Pediatr Res 1998;44(3):338–43.

72. Aaltonen M, Soukka H, Halkola L, et al. Asphyxia aggravates systemic hypotension but not pulmonary hypertension in piglets with meconium aspiration. Pediatr Res 2003;53(3):473–8.

73. Keszler M, Carbone MT, Cox C, et al. Severe respiratory failure after elective repeat cesarean delivery: a potentially preventable condition leading to extracorporeal membrane oxygenation. Pediatrics 1992;89(4 Pt 1):670–2.

74. Bhat R, Salas AA, Foster C, et al. Prospective analysis of pulmonary hypertension in extremely low birth weight infants. Pediatrics 2012;129(3):e682–9.

75. Gorenflo M, Vogel M, Obladen M. Pulmonary vascular changes in bronchopulmonary dysplasia: a clinicopathologic correlation in short- and long-term survivors. Pediatr Pathol 1991;11(6):851–66.

76. Kim DH, Kim HS, Choi CW, et al. Risk factors for pulmonary artery hypertension in preterm infants with moderate or severe bronchopulmonary dysplasia. Neonatology 2012;101(1):40–6.

77. Nyp M, Sandritter T, Poppinga N, et al. Sildenafil citrate, bronchopulmonary dysplasia and disordered pulmonary gas exchange: any benefits? J Perinatol 2012;32(1):64–9.

78. Banks BA, Seri I, Ischiropoulos H, et al. Changes in oxygenation with inhaled nitric oxide in severe bronchopulmonary dysplasia. Pediatrics 1999;103(3): 610–8.

79. Mourani PM, Ivy DD, Gao D, et al. Pulmonary vascular effects of inhaled nitric oxide and oxygen tension in bronchopulmonary dysplasia. Am J Respir Crit Care Med 2004;170(9):1006–13.

80. Smith J, Schumacher RE, Donn SM, et al. Clinical course of symptomatic spontaneous pneumothorax in term and late preterm newborns: report from a large cohort. Am J Perinatol 2011;28(2):163–8.

81. Porta NF, Steinhorn RH. Pulmonary vasodilator therapy in the NICU: inhaled nitric oxide, sildenafil, and other pulmonary vasodilating agents. Clin Perinatol 2012;39(1):149–64.

82. Linde LM, Simmons DH, Ellman EL. Pulmonary hemodynamics during positive-pressure breathing. J Appl Physiol 1961;16:644–6.

83. Pabalan MJ, Nayak SP, Ryan RM, et al. Methemoglobin to cumulative nitric oxide ratio and response to inhaled nitric oxide in PPHN. J Perinatol 2009; 29(10):698–701.

84. Carlo WA, Beoglos A, Chatburn RL, et al. High-frequency jet ventilation in neonatal pulmonary hypertension. Am J Dis Child 1989;143(2):233–8.

85. Clark RH, Yoder BA, Sell MS. Prospective, randomized comparison of high-frequency oscillation and conventional ventilation in candidates for extracorporeal membrane oxygenation. Journal of Pediatrics 1994;124(3):447–54.

86. Engle WA, Yoder MC, Andreoli SP, et al. Controlled prospective randomized comparison of high-frequency jet ventilation and conventional ventilation in neonates with respiratory failure and persistent pulmonary hypertension. J Perinatol 1997;17(1):3–9.

87. Kinsella JP, Abman SH. Clinical approaches to the use of high-frequency oscillatory ventilation in neonatal respiratory failure. J Perinatol 1996;16(2 Pt 2 Su):S52–5.

88. Kinsella JP, Abman SH. High-frequency oscillatory ventilation augments the response to inhaled nitric oxide in persistent pulmonary hypertension of the newborn: Nitric Oxide Study Group. Chest 1998;114(Suppl 1):100S.

89. Kinsella JP, Truog WE, Walsh WF, et al. Randomized, multicenter trial of inhaled nitric oxide and high-frequency oscillatory ventilation in severe, persistent pulmonary hypertension of the newborn. J Pediatr 1997;131(1 Pt 1):55–62.

90. Lakshminrusimha S, Russell JA, Steinhorn RH, et al. Pulmonary arterial contractility in neonatal lambs increases with 100% oxygen resuscitation. Pediatr Res 2006;59(1):137–41.

91. Lakshminrusimha S, Russell JA, Wedgwood S, et al. Superoxide dismutase improves oxygenation and reduces oxidation in neonatal pulmonary hypertension. Am J Respir Crit Care Med 2006;174(12):1370–7.

92. Steinhorn RH, Albert G, Swartz DD, et al. Recombinant human superoxide dismutase enhances the effect of inhaled nitric oxide in persistent pulmonary hypertension. Am J Respir Crit Care Med 2001;164(5):834–9.

93. Wung JT, James LS, Kilchevsky E, et al. Management of infants with severe respiratory failure and persistence of the fetal circulation, without hyperventilation. Pediatrics 1985;76(4):488–94.

94. Rudolph AM, Yuan S. Response of the pulmonary vasculature to hypoxia and H+ ion concentration changes. J Clin Invest 1966;45(3):399–411.

95. Peckham GJ, Fox WW. Physiologic factors affecting pulmonary artery pressure in infants with persistent pulmonary hypertension. J Pediatr 1978;93(6):1005–10.

96. Fox WW, Duara S. Persistent pulmonary hypertension in the neonate: diagnosis and management. J Pediatr 1983;103(4):505–14.

97. Rosenberg AA. Response of the cerebral circulation to hypocarbia in postasphyxia newborn lambs. Pediatr Res 1992;32(5):537–41.

98. Bifano EM, Pfannenstiel A. Duration of hyperventilation and outcome in infants with persistent pulmonary hypertension. Pediatrics 1988;81(5):657–61.

99. Hendricks-Munoz KD, Walton JP. Hearing loss in infants with persistent fetal circulation. Pediatrics 1988;81(5):650–6.

100. Walsh-Sukys MC, Tyson JE, Wright LL, et al. Persistent pulmonary hypertension of the newborn in the era before nitric oxide: practice variation and outcomes. Pediatrics 2000;105(1 Pt 1):14–20.

101. Yu XQ, Feet BA, Moen A, et al. Nitric oxide contributes to surfactant-induced vasodilation in surfactant-depleted newborn piglets. Pediatr Res 1997;42(2): 151–6.

102. Moen A, Yu XQ, Rootwelt T, et al. Acute effects on systemic and pulmonary hemodynamics of intratracheal instillation of porcine surfactant or saline in surfactant-depleted newborn piglets. Pediatr Res 1997;41(4 Pt 1):486–92.

103. Kaapa P, Seppanen M, Kero P, et al. Pulmonary hemodynamics after synthetic surfactant replacement in neonatal respiratory distress syndrome. J Pediatr 1993;123(1):115–9.

104. Soll RF, Dargaville P. Surfactant for meconium aspiration syndrome in full term infants. Cochrane Database Syst Rev 2000;(2):CD002054.

105. Lotze A, Mitchell BR, Bulas DI, et al. Multicenter study of surfactant (beractant) use in the treatment of term infants with severe respiratory failure. Survanta in Term Infants Study Group. J Pediatr 1998;132(1):40–7.

106. Findlay RD, Taeusch HW, Walther FJ. Surfactant replacement therapy for meconium aspiration syndrome. Pediatrics 1996;97(1):48–52.

107. Inhaled nitric oxide in full-term and nearly full-term infants with hypoxic respiratory failure. The Neonatal Inhaled Nitric Oxide Study Group. N Engl J Med 1997; 336(9):597–604.

108. Clark RH, Kueser TJ, Walker MW, et al. Low-dose nitric oxide therapy for persistent pulmonary hypertension of the newborn. Clinical Inhaled Nitric Oxide Research Group. N Engl J Med 2000;342(7):469–74.

109. Roberts JD Jr, Fineman JR, Morin FC 3rd, et al. Inhaled nitric oxide and persistent pulmonary hypertension of the newborn. The Inhaled Nitric Oxide Study Group. N Engl J Med 1997;336(9):605–10.

110. Golombek SG, Young JN. Efficacy of inhaled nitric oxide for hypoxic respiratory failure in term and late preterm infants by baseline severity of illness: a pooled analysis of three clinical trials. Clin Ther 2010;32(5):939–48.

111. Konduri GG. New approaches for persistent pulmonary hypertension of newborn. Clin Perinatol 2004;31(3):591–611.

112. Deruelle P, Balasubramaniam V, Kunig AM, et al. BAY 41-2272, a direct activator of soluble guanylate cyclase, reduces right ventricular hypertrophy and prevents pulmonary vascular remodeling during chronic hypoxia in neonatal rats. Biol Neonate 2006;90(2):135–44.

113. Deruelle P, Grover TR, Storme L, et al. Effects of BAY 41-2272, a soluble guanylate cyclase activator, on pulmonary vascular reactivity in the ovine fetus. Am J Physiol Lung Cell Mol Physiol 2005;288(4):L727–33.

114. Farrow KN, Groh BS, Schumacker PT, et al. Hyperoxia increases phosphodiesterase 5 expression and activity in ovine fetal pulmonary artery smooth muscle cells. Circ Res 2008;102(2):226–33.

115. Baquero H, Soliz A, Neira F, et al. Oral sildenafil in infants with persistent pulmonary hypertension of the newborn: a pilot randomized blinded study. Pediatrics 2006;117(4):1077–83.

116. Steinhorn RH, Kinsella JP, Pierce C, et al. Intravenous sildenafil in the treatment of neonates with persistent pulmonary hypertension. J Pediatr 2009;155(6): 841–847.e1.

117. Atz AM, Wessel DL. Sildenafil ameliorates effects of inhaled nitric oxide withdrawal. Anesthesiology 1999;91(1):307–10.

118. Farrow KN, Steinhorn RH. Sildenafil therapy for bronchopulmonary dysplasia: not quite yet. J Perinatol 2012;32(1):1–3.

119. Mukherjee A, Dombi T, Wittke B, et al. Population pharmacokinetics of sildenafil in term neonates: evidence of rapid maturation of metabolic clearance in the early postnatal period. Clin Pharmacol Ther 2009;85(1):56–63.

120. Muirhead GJ, Rance DJ, Walker DK, et al. Comparative human pharmacokinetics and metabolism of single-dose oral and intravenous sildenafil. Br J Clin Pharmacol 2002;53(Suppl 1):13S–20S.

121. Muirhead GJ, Wilner K, Colburn W, et al. The effects of age and renal and hepatic impairment on the pharmacokinetics of sildenafil. Br J Clin Pharmacol 2002;53(Suppl 1):21S–30S.

122. Nichols DJ, Muirhead GJ, Harness JA. Pharmacokinetics of sildenafil after single oral doses in healthy male subjects: absolute bioavailability, food effects and dose proportionality. Br J Clin Pharmacol 2002;53(Suppl 1):5S–12S.

123. Huie RE, Padmaja S. The reaction of NO with superoxide. Free Radic Res Commun 1993;18(4):195–9.

124. Auten RL, Davis JM. Oxygen toxicity and reactive oxygen species: the devil is in the details. Pediatr Res 2009;66(2):121–7.

125. Konduri GG, Kim UO. Advances in the diagnosis and management of persistent pulmonary hypertension of the newborn. Pediatr Clin North Am 2009;56(3): 579–600.

126. Gupta A, Rastogi S, Sahni R, et al. Inhaled nitric oxide and gentle ventilation in the treatment of pulmonary hypertension of the newborn–a single-center, 5-year experience. J Perinatol 2002;22(6):435–41.

127. Schwartz SM, Vermilion RP, Hirschl RB. Evaluation of left ventricular mass in children with left-sided congenital diaphragmatic hernia. J Pediatr 1994;125(3):447–51.

128. Siebert JR, Haas JE, Beckwith JB. Left ventricular hypoplasia in congenital diaphragmatic hernia. J Pediatr Surg 1984;19(5):567–71.

129. Inhaled nitric oxide and hypoxic respiratory failure in infants with congenital diaphragmatic hernia. The Neonatal Inhaled Nitric Oxide Study Group (NINOS). Pediatrics 1997;99(6):838–45.

130. Bassler D, Choong K, McNamara P, et al. Neonatal persistent pulmonary hypertension treated with milrinone: four case reports. Biol Neonate 2006;89(1):1–5.

131. McNamara PJ, Laique F, Muang- S, et al. Milrinone improves oxygenation in neonates with severe persistent pulmonary hypertension of the newborn. J Crit Care 2006;21(2):217–22.

132. Busch CJ, Graveline AR, Jiramongkolchai K, et al. Phosphodiesterase 3A expression is modulated by nitric oxide in rat pulmonary artery smooth muscle cells. J Physiol Pharmacol 2010;61(6):663–9.

133. Chen B, Lakshminrusimha S, Czech L, et al. Regulation of phosphodiesterase 3 in the pulmonary arteries during the perinatal period in sheep. Pediatr Res 2009; 66(6):682–7.

134. Steinhorn RH, Millard SL, Morin FC 3rd. Persistent pulmonary hypertension of the newborn. Role of nitric oxide and endothelin in pathophysiology and treatment. Clin Perinatol 1995;22(2):405–28.

135. Kumar P, Kazzi NJ, Shankaran S. Plasma immunoreactive endothelin-1 concentrations in infants with persistent pulmonary hypertension of the newborn. Am J Perinatol 1996;13(6):335–41.

136. Rosenberg AA, Kennaugh J, Koppenhafer SL, et al. Elevated immunoreactive endothelin-1 levels in newborn infants with persistent pulmonary hypertension. J Pediatr 1993;123(1):109–14.

137. Mohamed WA, Ismail M. A randomized, double-blind, placebo-controlled, prospective study of bosentan for the treatment of persistent pulmonary hypertension of the newborn. J Perinatol 2011. [Epub ahead of print].

138. Nakwan N, Choksuchat D, Saksawad R, et al. Successful treatment of persistent pulmonary hypertension of the newborn with bosentan. Acta Paediatr 2009; 98(10):1683–5.

139. Inwald D, Brown K, Gensini F, et al. Open lung biopsy in neonatal and paediatric patients referred for extracorporeal membrane oxygenation (ECMO). Thorax 2004;59(4):328–33.

140. Sakamoto H, Takenoshita M, Asakura Y, et al. Comparison of circulatory effects between arginine vasopressin (AVP) and dopamine in conscious newborn goats. J Vet Med Sci 1996;58(6):511–4.

141. Tourneux P, Rakza T, Bouissou A, et al. Pulmonary circulatory effects of norepinephrine in newborn infants with persistent pulmonary hypertension. J Pediatr 2008;153(3):345–9.

142. Barrington KJ, Singh AJ, Etches PC, et al. Partial liquid ventilation with and without inhaled nitric oxide in a newborn piglet model of meconium aspiration. Am J Respir Crit Care Med 1999;160(6):1922–7.

143. Shaffer TH, Lowe CA, Bhutani VK, et al. Liquid ventilation: effects on pulmonary function in distressed meconium-stained lambs. Pediatr Res 1984;18(1):47–52.

144. Leach CL, Greenspan JS, Rubenstein SD, et al. Partial liquid ventilation with perflubron in premature infants with severe respiratory distress syndrome. The LiquiVent Study Group. N Engl J Med 1996;335(11):761–7.

145. Enrione MA, Papo MC, Leach CL, et al. Regional pulmonary blood flow during partial liquid ventilation in normal and acute oleic acid-induced lung-injured piglets. Crit Care Med 1999;27(12):2716–23.

146. Lueders M, Weiswasser J, Aly H, et al. Changes in pulmonary vascular resistance in response to partial liquid ventilation. J Pediatr Surg 1998;33(1):85–90.

147. Wilcox DT, Glick PL, Karamanoukian HL, et al. Partial liquid ventilation and nitric oxide in congenital diaphragmatic hernia. J Pediatr Surg 1997;32(8):1211–5.

148. Sukumar M, Bommaraju M, Fisher JE, et al. High-frequency partial liquid ventilation in respiratory distress syndrome: hemodynamics and gas exchange. J Appl Physiol 1998;84(1):327–34.

149. Klein MD, Andrews AF, Wesley JR, et al. Venovenous perfusion in ECMO for newborn respiratory insufficiency. A clinical comparison with venoarterial perfusion. Ann Surg 1985;201(4):520–6.

150. Andrews AF, Klein MD, Toomasian JM, et al. Venovenous extracorporeal membrane oxygenation in neonates with respiratory failure. J Pediatr Surg 1983;18(4):339–46.

151. Fukuda S, Aoyama M, Yamada Y, et al. Comparison of venoarterial versus venovenous access in the cerebral circulation of newborns undergoing extracorporeal membrane oxygenation. Pediatr Surg Int 1999;15(2):78–84.

152. Knight GR, Dudell GG, Evans ML, et al. A comparison of venovenous and venoarterial extracorporeal membrane oxygenation in the treatment of neonatal respiratory failure. Crit Care Med 1996;24(10):1678–83.

153. Anderson HL 3rd, Snedecor SM, Otsu T, et al. Multicenter comparison of conventional venoarterial access versus venovenous double-lumen catheter access in newborn infants undergoing extracorporeal membrane oxygenation. J Pediatr Surg 1993;28(4):530–4 [discussion 534–5].
154. Aschner JL, Fike CD. New developments in the pathogenesis and management of neonatal pulmonary hypertension. In: Bancalari E, editor. The newborn lung. Philadelphia: Saunders Elsevier; 2008. p. 241–99.
155. Lakshminrusimha S, Wynn RJ, Youssfi M, et al. Use of CT angiography in the diagnosis of total anomalous venous return. J Perinatol 2009;29(6):458–61.

Novel Methods for Assessment of Right Heart Structure and Function in Pulmonary Hypertension

Gautam K. Singh, MD[a,*], Philip T. Levy, MD[a],
Mark R. Holland, PhD[b], Aaron Hamvas, MD[a]

KEYWORDS

- Pulmonary hypertension • Right ventricle • Heart function • Echocardiography
- Magnetic resonance imaging

KEY POINTS

- Long-term increases in pulmonary vascular resistance (PVR) and pulmonary arterial pressure (PAP) resulting from structural alterations and abnormal vasoreactivity of the pulmonary vasculature may lead to changes in geometry, structure, and function of the right ventricle (RV), a process known as cardiac remodeling. The remodeling is orchestrated by modulation of the myofiber architecture and distribution and ventricle-specific anisotropy in the contractile pattern.
- Many conditions in infants and children such as persistent fetal circulation, primary pulmonary parenchymal and vascular diseases, and structural malformation of heart and lungs can result in PH that may lead to RV remodeling from increased afterload and neurohormonal changes. The clinical course of the disease and prognosis in PH are mainly determined by the dysfunction of the target organ, the RV.
- Conventional methods of assessment of RV structure and function are often qualitative and do not provide sensitive markers of RV remodeling for prognostic information.
- Advances in cardiac imaging of the RV, including ultrasonic tissue characterization by integrated backscatter imaging, tissue Doppler imaging, speckle tracking echocardiography, and flow dynamics, have provided the capability to obtain quantitative information that often precedes the qualitative information provided by conventional methods.
- This article reviews the clinical conditions that result in PH and discusses the novel and emerging methods for the assessment of right heart structure and function in PH in infants and children.

Disclosures: None.
[a] Department of Pediatrics, Washington University School of Medicine, St Louis, MO, USA;
[b] Department of Physics, Washington University, St Louis, MO, USA
* Corresponding author. One Children's place, Campus Box 8116-NWT, St Louis, MO 63132.
E-mail address: singh_g@kids.wustl.edu

Pulmonary hypertension (PH) is defined by an increased pulmonary arterial pressure (PAP) (mean pulmonary arterial pressure >25 mm Hg). However, the clinical course of the disease and prognosis in PH are mainly determined by the dysfunction of the target organ, the right ventricle (RV).[1] Long-term increases in pulmonary vascular resistance (PVR) and PAP resulting from structural alterations and abnormal vasoreactivity of the pulmonary vasculature may lead to changes in geometry, structure, and function of the RV,[2,3] a process known as cardiac remodeling.[4] The RV remodeling is dictated by many factors including the severity of RV afterload caused by increased PVR, the duration of the PH, neurohormonal activation, and altered gene expression.[5] The remodeling is orchestrated by modulation of the myofiber architecture and distribution and ventricle-specific anisotropy in the contractile pattern, particularly if these events occur during myocardial maturation.[6,7] Conventional methods, such as two-dimensional (2D) and Doppler echocardiography, are frequently inaccurate in estimating PAP,[8,9] their assessment of RV structure and function are often qualitative, and they are not sufficiently sensitive markers of the changes in myofiber architecture and RV contractile function[10] to provide robust prognostic information. Advances in cardiac imaging of the RV, including ultrasonic tissue characterization by integrated backscatter imaging (IBI), tissue Doppler imaging (TDI), speckle tracking echocardiography (STE), and flow dynamics, provide quantitative information that often precedes conventional qualitative echocardiographic indicators of structural and functional changes in the RV. This article reviews the clinical conditions that result in PH and discusses the novel and emerging methods for the assessment of right heart structure and function in PH in infants and children.

CONDITIONS THAT RESULT IN PH
Fetal Circulation

In the fetus, PVR is increased and is maintained by a combination of a low oxygen environment, suppression of mediators of vasodilation, and production of mediators of vasoconstriction.[11–13] As a result, only approximately 10% of the cardiac output circulates through the lungs. At birth, PVR rapidly decreases in response to lung expansion and oxygen exposure and then gradually declines toward adult levels over the next several months. Many developmental, intrauterine, or postnatal factors may prevent this natural decline and influence the effective pulmonary circulation. These factors may be intrinsic to the pulmonary vasculature per se or in the structural development of the lung, or may be secondary to pulmonary or cardiac disorders (the more common of these conditions are listed in **Table 1**).

Primary Pulmonary Parenchymal Disease

Failure of normal decrease in PVR at or shortly after birth is most commonly associated with diffuse pulmonary parenchymal disease, such as hyaline membrane disease or sepsis/pneumonia. In this case, hypoxic vasoconstriction to optimize ventilation-perfusion matching results in generalized pulmonary vasoconstriction and a secondary increase in PVR and PH. This mechanism is also likely to be operative in the PH associated with inherited deficiencies in surfactant protein B or the ATP-binding cassette member A3 (ABCA3).[14–17]

Primary Pulmonary Vascular Disease

Persistent increase of PVR after birth in the absence of pulmonary parenchymal disease results in the syndrome of idiopathic persistent PH of the newborn (PPHN). Insight into this phenomenon comes primarily from autopsy findings that the development of the

Table 1 Mechanisms of newborn PH			
Primary Pulmonary Parenchymal Disease	**Primary Pulmonary Vascular Disease**	**Structural Malformations of the Lung**	**Structural Malformation of the Heart/Great Vessels**
Hyaline membrane disease	Idiopathic PPHN	Congenital diaphragmatic hernia	Premature closure of the ductus arteriosus
Pneumonia/sepsis	ACD-MPV	Pulmonary hypoplasia	Pulmonary venous obstruction: TAPVR, HLHS
Meconium aspiration	Meconium aspiration	BPD	Persistent left to right shunts with pulmonary overcirculation

Abbreviations: ACD-MPV, alveolar-capillary dysplasia with misalignment of the pulmonary veins; BPD, bronchopulmonary dysplasia; HLHS, hypoplastic left heart syndrome with a restrictive foramen ovale; PPHN, persistent PH of the newborn; TAPVR, total anomalous pulmonary venous return.

pulmonary vasculature is significantly advanced with muscular thickening of the arterial walls and extension of the musculature to intra-acinar arteries.[18] Although the cause is unknown, animal models of ligation of the fetal ductus arteriosus or intrauterine hypoxia from umbilical cord or uterine artery occlusion mimic the clinical findings.

PH has been associated with use of selective serotonin reuptake inhibitors (SSRI) for the treatment of depression during pregnancy. Serotonin causes pulmonary vaso-constriction, and chronic use of SSRIs is postulated to contribute to sustained high levels of serotonin and prevention of the postnatal decrease in PVR.[19]

Severe hypoxemic respiratory failure and PH from birth may result from alveolar-capillary dysplasia with misalignment of the pulmonary veins (ACD-MPV). Newborns with this disorder come to attention by virtue of the severity and refractory nature of the hypoxia (with normal ability to ventilate). Often these children are placed on extra-corporeal membrane oxygenation before the diagnosis becomes more apparent. Diagnosis can only be made by examination of lung tissue by biopsy or at autopsy. Loss-of-function mutations or deletions of 1 allele of the gene encoding the forkhead box transcription factor *FOXF1* have been identified as a cause of ACD-MPV in approximately 25% of cases.[20] ACD-MPV is usually fatal during the neonatal period but there is a spectrum of severity of the disease, with reports of some children pre-senting beyond the neonatal period.[21]

Although difficult to categorize in this classification scheme, infants undergoing therapeutic hypothermia for treatment of neonatal encephalopathy often show echo-cardiographic evidence of increased PVR and PH, which can significantly complicate their management. Several mechanisms likely contribute to this decreased pulmonary blood flow, including the perinatal factors that resulted in the encephalopathy to begin with, decreased cardiac output from myocardial injury, and the hypothermia inducing pulmonary vasoconstriction.[22] This condition often reverses with warming.

Several mechanisms contribute to the PH associated with meconium aspiration. First, it is a parenchymal disease with impaired oxygen diffusion between the alveolar space and the capillary bed and resultant hypoxic vasoconstriction.[23] Second, in infants with prolonged intrauterine stress, the pulmonary vasculature resembles that seen in PPHN with muscular thickening of the pulmonary arteries, and thus there is a component of primary vascular disease as well.

Structural Malformations of the Lung

Because the pulmonary vasculature and airways develop in parallel, factors that inhibit growth of the lung in utero result in PH because of diminished vascular surface area. Most notable is the lung hypoplasia associated with congenital diaphragmatic hernia (CDH), which is commonly attributed to a mass effect from herniated abdominal contents, although some animal models as well as clinical experience suggest a more global disruption of lung airspace and vascular development in which there seems to be discordance between the clinically assessed lung volume and the gas exchanging capacity. Conditions associated with low amniotic fluid volume, such as prolonged rupture of membranes at critical stages of fetal lung development or urinary tract or renal malformations, in which urine production or excretion is disrupted, also result in pulmonary hypoplasia that can be associated with PH.

Bronchopulmonary dysplasia (BPD) is a form of structural malformation of the lung that results from arrest of vascular and airway development that develops after premature birth. The interaction of multiple factors, including intrauterine and postnatal inflammation, oxidant stress, and genetic factors, contribute to structural airway simplification, decreased vascular surface area, and increased PVR.[24–26] PH develops over time and significantly increases mortality.

Structural Malformation of the Heart

Cardiovascular malformations in which there is an obstruction to pulmonary venous return or pulmonary overcirculation are less common, but nonetheless are associated with significant neonatal mortality. Intrauterine pulmonary venous obstruction associated with anomalous pulmonary venous return or left-sided outflow obstruction with a restrictive foramen ovale results in pulmonary venous hypertension, and intrauterine constriction of the ductus arteriosus results in pulmonary overcirculation and vascular remodeling. Cardiac lesions that result in long-standing pulmonary overcirculation as PVR decreases postnatally, such as ventricular or atrial septal defects, persistently patent ductus arteriosus, ultimately result in PH if the primary defect is untreated.

In all these disease states, the right heart is affected, although the left heart may also be affected to some degree. A sensitive and objective assessment of early alterations and progression of changes in the structure and function of the RV may provide insight into the prognosis of the PH even before or during the course of an intervention. Quantitative evaluation by newer modalities may define the dysfunction of RV and left ventricle (LV) and may thus predict the course of the disease.

ASSESSMENT OF RIGHT VENTRICULAR STRUCTURE
Ultrasonic Myocardial Tissue Characterization of the RV

Right ventricular myoarchitecture can be quantitatively evaluated by ultrasonic tissue characterization. There is a close relationship between measured ultrasonic parameters (attenuation, backscatter, speed of sound) and the inherent properties of myocardial tissue. Both the biochemical properties (different types and concentrations of proteins present that result in specific intracellular and extracellular viscoelastic properties) and the geometric properties (organization of myoskeleton) of the myocardium combine to produce the observed ultrasonic parameters.[27–30] Studies have shown regional dependence of backscattered ultrasound on intrinsic myofiber organization,[31] and an increase in both the measured ultrasonic attenuation[32–34] and backscatter[27,33,35–37] correlates well with increased collagen concentration. The measurement of the systematic variation of backscattered ultrasonic energy from the myocardium over the heart cycle (ie, the cyclic variation of myocardial backscatter) can characterize myocardial intrinsic properties in several cardiac disorders, including PH.[38–46]

Quantification of the cyclic variation of backscatter from the myocardium

The quantification of the cyclic variation of backscatter from the myocardium is a method that compares the level of backscatter during systole with that during diastole and is easy to implement clinically. The echocardiographic imaging system is configured first to provide a linear relationship between the measured backscattered ultrasound intensity and grayscale value,[47] so images of the standard echocardiographic views[48] of a subject can be obtained. The cyclic variation is measured and data are expressed in terms of the magnitude and normalized time delay (**Fig. 1**).[47,49,50] In practice, an automated algorithm is often used to determine the magnitude and time delay values.[50]

Clinical application of ultrasonic myocardial tissue characterization

Studies have shown that ultrasonic tissue characterization has the ability to differentiate normal from abnormal myocardium in the RV.[47–53] In patients with an intracardiac shunt leading to RV overload, integrated backscatter ultrasonography revealed interstitial and replacement fibrosis in the RV myocardium, which was consistent with histologic analysis, despite preserved systolic function in the early stages.[47] Pacileo and colleagues[48] used tissue characterization measurements to detect differences in myocardial functional and textural properties in the presence of pressure and/or volume RV overload. An association between the levels of cellular adhesion

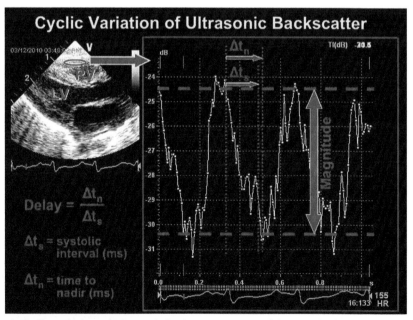

Fig. 1. Cyclic variation of ultrasonic backscatter expressed in magnitude and normalized time delay of the backscatter energy. The magnitude of cyclic variation is defined as the difference in backscatter between the average peak and average nadir values. The normalized time delay of cyclic variation is expressed in terms of a dimensionless ratio, obtained by dividing the time interval from end-diastole to the nadir of the mean backscatter trace (Δt_n) by the systolic interval (Δt_s).

molecules, deterioration of diastolic function of the RV, and altered myocardial ultrasonic properties were found in patients with Behçet disease, which may lead to PH.[53]

ASSESSMENT OF RIGHT VENTRICULAR FUNCTION
Strain Imaging

Helical myocardial fiber arrangement orchestrates changes in the geometry and dimensions of the ventricular wall in 3 dimensions during phases of the cardiac cycle. Strain measures the percentage change in myocardial deformation, whereas its time derivative, strain rate, defines the rate of deformation of myocardium over time. Strain rate is a load-independent global measure of ventricular systolic function and correlates closely with myocardial contractility.[54] RV myocardial strain in 2 dimensions can be measured by a novel echocardiographic method that determines myocardial deformation from continuous frame-by-frame tracking of the speckle pattern in images.[55,56] The speckle pattern within B-mode images of myocardium represent natural acoustic markers, which are considered to be stable between consecutive image frames; hence, a change in the pattern's position follows tissue motion.[56,57] STE is angle independent, can track in 2 and 3 dimensions, and therefore can assess the magnitude and timing of regional and global RV deformation in the longitudinal, radial, and circumferential directions. For the RV, longitudinal and radial strain and strain rate are typically assessed in practice (**Fig. 2**), although circumferential strain can also be assessed. Optimum quality images with frame rates between 60 and 90 frames/s during image acquisition are necessary prerequisites for reproducibility and reliability of the data.[58]

2D strain estimated by STE has been applied to assess RV function in adult patients with PH.[59] RV strain and strain rate showed a close relationship with invasive pulmonary hemodynamics (PVR, mean PAP, and cardiac output), exercise capacity, and independently predicted functional classes in 1 study.[60] In other studies, 2D strain and strain rate changed in proportion to the degree of increase in PAP in patients with idiopathic PH[61] and was further changed in those with concomitant RV failure.[62] It even proved sensitive enough to detect early alterations of RV function in patients with systemic sclerosis and pulmonary fibrosis but normal PAP.[63] Assessment of RV longitudinal systolic strain and strain rate by STE has been reported to independently predict future right-sided heart failure, clinical deterioration, and mortality in adult patients with PH.[64] RV longitudinal systolic strain has also been shown to discriminate RV response to pressure overload in different conditions including PH. The nature and degree of RV response to pressure overload provide a better assessment of survival profile[65] and prognosis in patients with PH.[60]

In a prospective pilot study in extremely low gestational age neonates (ELGANs) (born at 27 ± 2 weeks, n = 13) to discern the predictive and tracking sensitivity, we compared longitudinal global strain of the RV at 32 ± 1 weeks postconceptional age between ELGANs who did and did not require respiratory support at 36 ± 1 weeks postconceptional age (supplemental flow via nasal cannula, continuous positive airway pressure, or mechanical ventilation, the National Institutes of Health consensus definition of moderate and severe bronchopulmonary dysplasia).[66,67] ELGANs requiring respiratory support at 36 weeks postconceptional age had lower RV longitudinal global strain at both 32 weeks ($P<.003$) and 36 weeks ($P<.05$) than those not requiring respiratory support at 36 weeks postconceptional age (**Fig. 3**A). RV free wall global longitudinal strain of $-16.7\% \pm 1.5\%$ (significantly less than normal) at 32 weeks predicted with a sensitivity of 76% and specificity of 79% those ELGANs who either developed or continued to have the need for respiratory support at 36

A

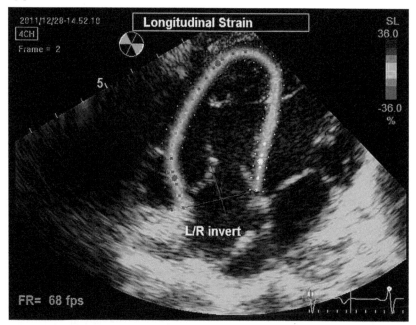

B

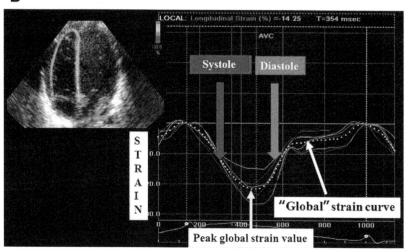

Fig. 2. Strain imaging of the RV in an extremely low gestational age neonate with broncho-pulmonary dysplasia and increased pulmonary pressure using speckle tracking echocardiography (A). The segmental strain is graphically presented by different color codes and curves and global longitudinal strain by dotted curve with its peak as peak systolic longitudinal strain (B). The segmental strains are not synchronous and peak global longitudinal strain is decreased (−21%, normal >−23%). AVC, aortic valve closure; FR, frame rate.

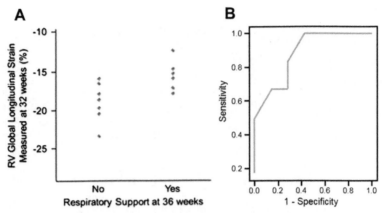

Fig. 3. (*A*) Significant difference in right ventricular global longitudinal strains at 32 weeks postconceptional age between groups of ELGANs requiring respiratory support versus not requiring respiratory support at 36 weeks postconceptional age. (*B*) Receiver operative curve depicting sensitivity and specificity of right ventricular global strain of −16.7% at 32 weeks postconceptional age in predicting the need for respiratory support at 36 weeks postconceptional age.

weeks (see **Fig. 3**B).[68,69] The data suggest that RV global longitudinal strain in ELGAN may serve as a marker that can identify and track cardiopulmonary alterations in the clinical setting of bronchopulmonary dysplasia.

Strength and weakness
STE is angle independent, has a high signal/noise ratio, and can provide regional as well as a global function assessment. However, the global RV strain is derived only from a single view, making it not a truly global assessment of RV function. Furthermore, different speckle tracking algorithms are used by the currently available imaging platforms, which may result in different normal values and ranges.[70]

Tissue Doppler Imaging
Because longitudinally oriented myofibers are the dominant architectural element of the RV, measurements of longitudinal velocity of myocardial segments during specific phases of the same cardiac cycle provide direct assessment of regional myocardial function. TDI is used to measure the velocity of the myocardial tissue. Myocardial velocities can be measured using pulsed tissue Doppler and color-coded tissue Doppler at the tricuspid annulus as well as segments of the RV free wall. This velocity has been termed the RV S′ for systolic excursion velocity, e′ for the early diastolic excursion, and a′ for the late diastolic excursion (**Fig. 4**). The basal segments must be aligned parallel to the insonifying ultrasonic beam for the accurate measurements of the velocities. Assessment of the mid and apical RV segmental velocities may be less reliable because of the difficulty in aligning these segments parallel to the insonifying beam. Tissue Doppler–based indexes of myocardial velocities are less flow dependent than conventional tricuspid flow Doppler and are a preload-independent means of evaluating ventricular diastolic function.[71]

RV myocardial performance index
RV myocardial performance index (RVMPI), or the Tei index, is a measure of the relationship of the work performance between the ejection and nonejection cycle of the heart. It provides a quantitative index of RV systolic and diastolic function, which is

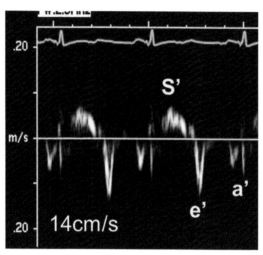

Fig. 4. TDI of myocardial velocity at the tricuspid level of the right ventricular free wall in a normal neonate.

derived from the ratio of the sum of isovolumic contraction time (IVCT) and isovolumic relaxation time (IVRT) to the ejection time. These time intervals are measured using TDI or standard pulsed Doppler (**Fig. 5**). TDI offers the quantitative assessment of the RV function during 1 cardiac cycle, whereas the standard pulsed Doppler method uses measurements from different cardiac cycles and, therefore, may be affected by heart rate variability.

The RVMPI has shown significant correlation with RV ejection fraction (EF) by nuclear ventriculography and is reported to be less affected by heart rate, loading conditions, or the presence and the severity of tricuspid regurgitation.[72,73] Tei and colleagues[74] showed abnormal RVMPIs in patients with primary PH compared with age-matched controls. Another study showed that the index correlated with symptoms and that values more than 0.83 predicted poor survivals.[75]

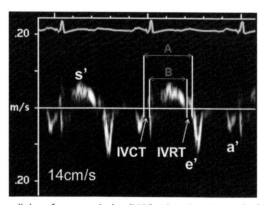

Fig. 5. TDI of myocardial performance index (MPI) using time interval of different phases of the cardiac cycle. Myocardial velocities were measured at the tricuspid level of the right ventricular free wall in a normal neonate. ET, ejection time; IVCT, isovolumic contraction time; IVRT, isovolumic relaxation time. MPI is the ratio (IVCT + IVRT)/ET. A, time interval includes sum of IVCT, IVRT, and ET; B, ejection time.

Myocardial isovolumic acceleration

Myocardial isovolumic acceleration (IVA) is a TDI-derived parameter that has been reported to measure RV contractility and, therefore, to be less affected by preload or afterload.[76] It is calculated by dividing the maximal isovolumic myocardial velocity by the time to peak velocity. It has been reported as a sensitive contractility index of RV[77] but its discriminatory power and reproducibility in the evaluation of RV performance in infants with PH warrant further study.

Strength and weakness

TDI can be incorporated in clinical practice without difficulty. It is not greatly affected by the RV geometry and flow dynamics. It is a reproducible technique with good discriminatory ability to detect normal versus abnormal RV function. However, TDI is angle dependent and is affected by regional tethering and translational and tractional motions of the ventricle. Therefore, it is considered to be a less sensitive measure of RV myocardial function than RV strain and strain rate. Further, it assumes that the function of a single segment represents the function of the entire RV ventricle, which may not be true in conditions in which regions of RV are differentially affected, such as RV infarction or pulmonary embolism. The MPI in RV may be limited by the short isovolumic periods in the normal RV and the pseudonormalization of the index when right atrial pressure is increased, resulting in shortening of the IVRT.[78]

Thus, RVMPI is a simple and quick measure that can be used in patients with PH to assess the RV function. Furthermore, RVMPI can provide insight into the evolving relationship between the pulmonary vasculature and the RV and may be used when evaluating the global function of the RV to assess patients at risk for PH.

THREE-DIMENSIONAL ECHOCARDIOGRAPHY/MAGNETIC RESONANCE IMAGING: STUDY OF RIGHT VENTRICULAR VOLUMES

The RV volume and EF constitute indications for both surgical and catheter-based intervention for lesions causing RV dilation and deterioration of RV function including pulmonary regurgitation caused by structural heart defects compounded by PH. The RV-EF, like the LV-EF, can be an indicator of prognosis besides that of diagnosis of RV function.[79] However, because of the tripartite anatomy of the RV and its complex geometry seen in patients with PH, formulae using 2D analyses for volume quantification and EF calculation for LV cannot be applied to RV. The new modality of third-generation three-dimensional echocardiography (3DE) now offers the ability to measure RV volume and EF in real time.[80] Simultaneous acquisition of large, sequential, multiplane volumetric data sets of the RV allows offline four-dimensional analysis (3 dimensions+ time), which provides RV volumes, EF, and mass. The RV volume and EF measured by 3DE compared well with those measured by cardiac magnetic resonance imaging in studies in patients with PH[81] and in children.[82] It is now proposed that RV volume and EF measured by 3DE should be used to assess remodeling and treatment effects of PH.[83] Further studies are needed to validate the prognostic and monitoring abilities of 3DE for RV volume, EF, and remodeling in infants with PH.

EMERGING METHODS: ECHOCARDIOGRAPHIC ASSESSMENT OF FLOW CHARACTERISTICS

Evaluation of ventricular function mostly focuses on wall motion–related indices. However, the flow dynamics of blood inside the heart and blood vessels influence the tissue perfusion of the end-organs. The heart is a dynamic organ that functions according to the principles of fluid dynamics. The structural form and mechanical function of the normal heart create time-varying and spatially complex flow patterns that are optimal for minimizing the energy required for normal function. Flow is immediately affected by changes in cardiac function and adaptation. Heart diseases and vascular alterations, including those caused by PH, have the potential of adversely altering these energy-efficient flow patterns. Therefore, analyzing the spatial and temporal distribution of blood flow in the heart and blood vessels may provide early diagnostic and prognostic information.

Although Doppler-based methods for characterizing cardiac hemodynamics represent a critical component of clinical evaluation, inherent limitations of conventional Doppler-based measurements (ie, the dependence of Doppler measurements on the direction of flow relative to the insonifying beam direction) do not permit a complete assessment of complex cardiovascular flow characteristics over the heart cycle. The development and implementation of new approaches that permit more detailed measurements of flow characteristics within the cardiovascular system will enhance understanding of cardiopulmonary diseases including PH and their impact on overall cardiac function.

The medical literature[84] reviewing the advances made in these emerging methods points to the use of conventional color Doppler flow measurements in conjunction with additional information to obtain a more complete characterization of blood flow properties. These methods include crossed-beam approaches that use multiple transmitting and receiving transducers,[85] vector flow mapping that combines the measured blood velocity along the ultrasonic beam axis with estimated orthogonal velocities obtained from the application of fundamental fluid dynamic principles,[86] and methods that combine color Doppler measurements along with endocardial wall motion measurements and fundamental physical principles.[87] Methods that use measurements of blood speckle patterns are also being developed.[88]

The widespread use of ultrasound contrast agents permits the visualization of blood flow in the chambers of the heart and vessels. Echocardiography-based particle image velocimetry (Echo-PIV) is a new method for quantifying blood flow dynamics.[89–95] The Echo-PIV method uses pairs of sequential image frames for calculating the direction and magnitude of contrast-enhanced blood flow. Tracking the displacement of contrast patterns in the second image, relative to the position of the patterns in the first image, provides a measure of the motion of blood. This Echo-PIV–derived blood flow information can be exported and used for further analyses and quantification of flow characteristics over the cardiac cycle.

Although these emerging methods for assessing cardiac chamber blood flow have primarily been used to characterize flow in the LV, they are equally applicable for characterization of flow within the RV. It is anticipated that these methods may provide a means for recognizing early changes in flow dynamics that occur before the onset of clinical manifestations of cardiac dysfunction. Such early changes may provide markers for screening and for discerning therapeutic effectiveness, which is not discernible by current diagnostic modalities.

REFERENCES

1. D'Alonzo GE, Barst RJ, Ayres SM, et al. Survival in patients with primary pulmonary hypertension. Results from a national prospective registry. Ann Intern Med 1991;115:343–9.
2. Haddad F, Doyle R, Murphy DJ, et al. Right ventricular function in cardiovascular disease, part II: pathophysiology, clinical importance, and management of right ventricular failure. Circulation 2008;117:1717–31.

3. Bogaard HJ, Natarajan R, Henderson SC, et al. Chronic pulmonary artery pressure elevation is insufficient to explain right heart failure. Circulation 2009;120: 1951–60.

4. Cohn JN, Ferrari R, Sharpe N. Cardiac remodeling–concepts and clinical implications: a consensus paper from an international forum on cardiac remodeling. Behalf of an International Forum on Cardiac Remodeling. J Am Coll Cardiol 2000;35:569–82.

5. Voelkel NF, Quaife RA, Leinwand LA, et al. Right ventricular function and failure: report of a National Heart, Lung, and Blood Institute Working Group on Cellular and Molecular Mechanisms of Right Heart Failure. Circulation 2006;114:1883–91.

6. Sedmera D, Hu N, Weiss KM, et al. Cellular changes in experimental left heart hypoplasia. Anat Rec 2002;267:137–45.

7. Tobita K, Garrison JB, Liu LJ, et al. Three-dimensional myofiber architecture of the embryonic left ventricle during normal development and altered mechanical loads. Anat Rec A Discov Mol Cell Evol Biol 2005;283:193–201.

8. Fisher MR, Forfia PR, Chamera E, et al. Accuracy of Doppler echocardiography in the hemodynamic assessment of pulmonary hypertension. Am J Respir Crit Care Med 2009;179:615–21.

9. Rich JD, Shah SJ, Swamy RS, et al. Inaccuracy of Doppler echocardiographic estimates of pulmonary artery pressures in patients with pulmonary hypertension: implications for clinical practice. Chest 2011;139:988–93.

10. Giusca S, Dambrauskaite V, Scheurwegs C, et al. Deformation imaging describes right ventricular function better than longitudinal displacement of the tricuspid ring. Heart 2010;96:281–8.

11. Hyvelin J-M, Howell K, Nichol A, et al. Inhibition of rho-kinase attenuates hypoxia-induced angiogenesis in the pulmonary circulation. Circ Res 2005;97:185–91.

12. Ivy DD, Kinsella JP, Abman SH. Endothelin blockade augments pulmonary vasodilation in the ovine fetus. J Appl Physiol 1996;81:2481–7.

13. Gao Y, Raj JU. Regulation of the pulmonary circulation in the fetus and newborn. Physiol Rev 2010;90:1291–335.

14. Brasch F, Schimanski S, Muhlfeld C, et al. Alteration of the pulmonary surfactant system in full-term infants with hereditary ABCA3 deficiency. Am J Respir Crit Care Med 2006;174:571–80.

15. Shulenin S, Nogee L, Annilo T, et al. ABCA3 gene mutations in newborns with fatal surfactant deficiency. N Engl J Med 2004;350:1296–303.

16. Somaschini M, Wert S, Mangili G, et al. Hereditary surfactant protein B deficiency resulting from a novel mutation. Intensive Care Med 2000;26:97–100.

17. Tredano M, van Elburg RM, Kaspers AG, et al. 1549c'GAA (121ins2) and 457delC heterozygosity in severe congenital lung disease and surfactant protein B (SP-B) deficiency. Hum Mutat 1999;14:502–9.

18. Murphy JD, Rabinovitch M, Goldstein JD, et al. The structural basis of persistent pulmonary hypertension of the newborn infant. J Pediatr 1981;98:962–7.

19. Delaney C, Gien J, Grover TR, et al. Pulmonary vascular effects of serotonin and selective serotonin reuptake inhibitors in the late-gestation ovine fetus. Am J Physiol Lung Cell Mol Physiol 2011;301:L937–44.

20. Stankiewicz P, Sen P, Bhatt SS, et al. Genomic and genic deletions of the FOX gene cluster on 16q24.1 and inactivating mutations of FOXF1 cause alveolar capillary dysplasia and other malformations. Am J Hum Genet 2009;84:780–91.

21. Ahmed S, Ackerman V, Faught P, et al. Profound hypoxemia and pulmonary hypertension in a 7-month-old infant: late presentation of alveolar capillary dysplasia. Pediatr Crit Care Med 2008;9:e43–6.

22. Sarkar S, Barks JD, Bhagat I, et al. Pulmonary dysfunction and therapeutic hypothermia in asphyxiated newborns: whole body versus selective head cooling. Am J Perinatol 2009;26:265–70.

23. Ban R, Ogihara T, Mori Y, et al. Meconium aspiration delays normal decline of pulmonary vascular resistance shortly after birth through lung parenchymal injury. Neonatology 2011;99:272–9.

24. Baraldi E, Filippone M. Chronic lung disease after premature birth. N Engl J Med 2007;357:1946–55.

25. Jobe AH, Bancalari E. Bronchopulmonary dysplasia. Am J Respir Crit Care Med 2001;163:1723–9.

26. Stenmark KR, Abman SH. Lung vascular development: implications for the pathogenesis of bronchopulmonary dysplasia. Annu Rev Physiol 2005;67:623–61.

27. Hall CS, Scott MJ, Lanza GM, et al. The extracellular matrix is an important source of ultrasound backscatter from myocardium. J Acoust Soc Am 2000;107:612–9.

28. O'Brien WD Jr, Sagar KB, Warltier DC, et al. Acoustic propagation properties of normal, stunned, and infarcted myocardium: morphological and biochemical determinants. Circulation 1995;91:154–60.

29. Rose JH, Kaufmann MR, Wickline SA, et al. A proposed microscopic elastic wave theory for ultrasonic backscatter from myocardial tissue. J Acoust Soc Am 1995;97:656–68.

30. Wickline SA, Thomas LJ 3rd, Miller JG, et al. A relationship between ultrasonic integrated backscatter and myocardial contractile function. J Clin Invest 1985;76:2151–60.

31. Holland MR, Wilkenshoff UM, Finch-Johnston AE, et al. Effects of myocardial fiber orientation in echocardiography: quantitative measurements and computer simulation of the regional dependence of backscattered ultrasound in the parasternal short-axis view. J Am Soc Echocardiogr 1998;11:929–37.

32. Hall CS, Dent CL, Scott MJ, et al. High-frequency ultrasound detection of the temporal evolution of protein cross linking in myocardial tissue. IEEE Trans Ultrason Ferroelectr Freq Control 2000;47:1051–8.

33. Mimbs JW, O'Donnell M, Bauwens D, et al. The dependence of ultrasonic attenuation and backscatter on collagen content in dog and rabbit hearts. Circ Res 1980;47:49–58.

34. O'Donnell M, Mimbs JW, Miller JG. The relationship between collagen and ultrasonic attenuation in myocardial tissue. J Acoust Soc Am 1979;65:512–7.

35. Hoyt RM, Skorton DJ, Collins SM, et al. Ultrasonic backscatter and collagen in normal ventricular myocardium. Circulation 1984;69:775–82.

36. O'Donnell M, Mimbs JW, Miller JG. The relationship between collagen and ultrasonic backscatter in myocardial tissue. J Acoust Soc Am 1981;69:580–8.

37. Pohlhammer J, O'Brien WD Jr. Dependence of the ultrasonic scatter coefficient on collagen concentration in mammalian tissues. J Acoust Soc Am 1981;69:283–5.

38. Coucelo J, Joaquim N, Carreira G, et al. The cyclic variation of the 2-dimensional echocardiographic densitometry spectrum as a function of the phase of the cardiac cycle. Experimental work and its clinical application in arterial hypertension. Rev Port Cardiol 1997;16:63–7 [in Portuguese].

39. Di Bello V, Pedrinelli R, Bertini A, et al. Cyclic variation of the myocardial integrated backscatter signal in hypertensive cardiopathy: a preliminary study. Coron Artery Dis 2001;12:267–75.

40. Di Bello V, Pedrinelli R, Bianchi M, et al. Ultrasonic myocardial texture in hypertensive mild-to-moderate left ventricular hypertrophy: a videodensitometric study. Am J Hypertens 1998;11:155–64.

41. Di Bello V, Pedrinelli R, Giorgi D, et al. Ultrasonic myocardial texture versus Doppler analysis in hypertensive heart: a preliminary study. Hypertension 1999; 33:66–73.
42. Di Bello V, Pedrinelli R, Giorgi D, et al. Ultrasonic videodensitometric analysis of two different models of left ventricular hypertrophy. Athlete's heart and hypertension. Hypertension 1997;29:937–44.
43. Di Bello V, Pedrinelli R, Giorgi D, et al. Ultrasonic myocardial textural parameters and midwall left ventricular mechanics in essential arterial hypertension. J Hum Hypertens 2000;14:9–16.
44. Maceira AM, Barba J, Beloqui O, et al. Ultrasonic backscatter and diastolic function in hypertensive patients. Hypertension 2002;40:239–43.
45. Maceira AM, Barba J, Varo N, et al. Ultrasonic backscatter and serum marker of cardiac fibrosis in hypertensives. Hypertension 2002;39:923–8.
46. Sutton MSJ, Plappert T. Myocardial texture in hypertrophic remodeling: new insight into ventricular load and function? J Hum Hypertens 2000;14:7–8.
47. Hopkins WE, Waggoner AD, Gussak H. Quantitative ultrasonic tissue characterization of myocardium in cyanotic adults with an unrepaired congenital heart defect. Am J Cardiol 1994;74:930–4.
48. Pacileo G, Limongelli G, Verrengia M, et al. Backscatter evaluation of myocardial functional and textural findings in children with right ventricular pressure and/or volume overload. Am J Cardiol 2004;93:594–7.
49. Waggoner AD, Perez JE, Miller JG, et al. Differentiation of normal and ischemic right ventricular myocardium with quantitative two-dimensional integrated backscatter imaging. Ultrasound Med Biol 1992;18:249–53.
50. Yildirim N, Saricam E, Ozbakir C, et al. Assessment of the relationship between functional capacity and right ventricular ultrasound tissue characterization by integrated backscatter in patients with isolated mitral stenosis. Int Heart J 2007;48:87–96.
51. Pacileo G, Limongelli G, Verrengia M, et al. Impact of pulmonary regurgitation and age at surgical repair on textural and functional right ventricular myocardial properties in patients with tetralogy of Fallot. Ital Heart J 2005;6:745–50.
52. Pacileo G, Calabro P, Limongelli G, et al. Feasibility and usefulness of right ventricular ultrasonic tissue characterization with integrated backscatter in patients with unsuccessfully operatively "repaired" tetralogy of Fallot. Am J Cardiol 2002;90:669–71.
53. Yildirim N, Tekin NS, Tekin IO, et al. Myocardial functional and textural findings of the right and left ventricles and their association with cellular adhesion molecules in Behçet's disease. Echocardiography 2007;24:702–11.
54. Jamal F, Bergerot C, Argaud L, et al. Longitudinal strain quantitates regional right ventricular contractile function. Am J Physiol Heart Circ Physiol 2003;285:H2842–7.
55. Amundsen BH, Helle-Valle T, Edvardsen T, et al. Noninvasive myocardial strain measurement by speckle tracking echocardiography: validation against sonomicrometry and tagged magnetic resonance imaging. J Am Coll Cardiol 2006;47:789–93.
56. Korinek J, Wang J, Sengupta PP, et al. Two-dimensional strain–a Doppler-independent ultrasound method for quantitation of regional deformation: validation in vitro and in vivo. J Am Soc Echocardiogr 2005;18:1247–53.
57. Leitman M, Lysyansky P, Sidenko S, et al. Two-dimensional strain–a novel software for real-time quantitative echocardiographic assessment of myocardial function. J Am Soc Echocardiogr 2004;17:1021–9.
58. Singh GK, Cupps B, Pasque M, et al. Accuracy and reproducibility of strain by speckle tracking in pediatric subjects with normal heart and single ventricular

physiology: a two-dimensional speckle-tracking echocardiography and magnetic resonance imaging correlative study. J Am Soc Echocardiogr 2010;23:1143–52.

59. Chow PC, Liang XC, Cheung EW, et al. New two-dimensional global longitudinal strain and strain rate imaging for assessment of systemic right ventricular function. Heart 2008;94:855–9.

60. Filusch A, Mereles D, Gruenig E, et al. Strain and strain rate echocardiography for evaluation of right ventricular dysfunction in patients with idiopathic pulmonary arterial hypertension. Clin Res Cardiol 2010;99:491–8.

61. Pirat B, McCulloch ML, Zoghbi WA. Evaluation of global and regional right ventricular systolic function in patients with pulmonary hypertension using a novel speckle tracking method. Am J Cardiol 2006;98:699–704.

62. Simon MA, Rajagopalan N, Mathier MA, et al. Tissue Doppler imaging of right ventricular decompensation in pulmonary hypertension. Congest Heart Fail 2009;15:271–6.

63. Matias C, Isla LP, Vasconcelos M, et al. Speckle-tracking-derived strain and strain-rate analysis: a technique for the evaluation of early alterations in right ventricle systolic function in patients with systemic sclerosis and normal pulmonary artery pressure. J Cardiovasc Med (Hagerstown) 2009;10:129–34.

64. Sachdev A, Villarraga HR, Frantz RP, et al. Right ventricular strain for prediction of survival in patients with pulmonary arterial hypertension. Chest 2011;139: 1299–309.

65. Jurcut R, Giusca S, Ticulescu R, et al. Different patterns of adaptation of the right ventricle to pressure overload: a comparison between pulmonary hypertension and pulmonary stenosis. J Am Soc Echocardiogr 2011;24:1109–17.

66. Ambalavanan N, Walsh M, Bobashev G, et al. Intercenter differences in bronchopulmonary dysplasia or death among very low birth weight infants. Pediatrics 2011;127:e106–16.

67. Network VO. 2007 Very low birth weight database summary. 2008.

68. Levy PT, Holland MR, Singh GK, et al. Echocardiogaphic tissue characterization measurements of the right ventricle discriminate the need for respiratory support in premature infants. J Ultrasound Med 2012;31:S70.

69. Levy PT, Holland MR, Singh GK, et al. Novel echocardiographic measures of right ventricular performance discriminate need for respiratory support in premature infants. E-PAS2012:3853.687 (Abstract).

70. Kaul S, Miller JG, Grayburn PA, et al. A suggested roadmap for cardiovascular ultrasound research for the future. J Am Soc Echocardiogr 2011;24:455–64.

71. Sohn DW, Chai IH, Lee DJ, et al. Assessment of mitral annulus velocity by Doppler tissue imaging in the evaluation of left ventricular diastolic function. J Am Coll Cardiol 1997;30:474–80.

72. Dyer KL, Pauliks LB, Das B, et al. Use of myocardial performance index in pediatric patients with idiopathic pulmonary arterial hypertension. J Am Soc Echocardiogr 2006;19:21–7.

73. Karnati PK, El-Hajjar M, Torosoff M, et al. Myocardial performance index correlates with right ventricular ejection fraction measured by nuclear ventriculography. Echocardiography 2008;25:381–5.

74. Tei C, Dujardin KS, Hodge DO, et al. Doppler echocardiographic index for assessment of global right ventricular function. J Am Soc Echocardiogr 1996;9: 838–47.

75. Yeo TC, Dujardin KS, Tei C, et al. Value of a Doppler-derived index combining systolic and diastolic time intervals in predicting outcome in primary pulmonary hypertension. Am J Cardiol 1998;81:1157–61.

76. Vogel M, Schmidt MR, Kristiansen SB, et al. Validation of myocardial acceleration during isovolumic contraction as a novel noninvasive index of right ventricular contractility: comparison with ventricular pressure-volume relations in an animal model. Circulation 2002;105:1693–9.

77. Vogel M, Derrick G, White PA, et al. Systemic ventricular function in patients with transposition of the great arteries after atrial repair: a tissue Doppler and conductance catheter study. J Am Coll Cardiol 2004;43:100–6.

78. Yoshifuku S, Otsuji Y, Takasaki K, et al. Pseudonormalized Doppler total ejection isovolume (Tei) index in patients with right ventricular acute myocardial infarction. Am J Cardiol 2003;91:527–31.

79. van Wolferen SA, Marcus JT, Boonstra A, et al. Prognostic value of right ventricular mass, volume, and function in idiopathic pulmonary arterial hypertension. Eur Heart J 2007;28:1250–7.

80. Angelini ED, Homma S, Pearson G, et al. Segmentation of real-time three-dimensional ultrasound for quantification of ventricular function: a clinical study on right and left ventricles. Ultrasound Med Biol 2005;31:1143–58.

81. Grapsa J, O'Regan DP, Pavlopoulos H, et al. Right ventricular remodelling in pulmonary arterial hypertension with three-dimensional echocardiography: comparison with cardiac magnetic resonance imaging. Eur J Echocardiogr 2010;11:64–73.

82. Lu X, Nadvoretskiy V, Bu L, et al. Accuracy and reproducibility of real-time three-dimensional echocardiography for assessment of right ventricular volumes and ejection fraction in children. J Am Soc Echocardiogr 2008;21:84–9.

83. Badano LP, Ginghina C, Easaw J, et al. Right ventricle in pulmonary arterial hypertension: haemodynamics, structural changes, imaging, and proposal of a study protocol aimed to assess remodelling and treatment effects. Eur J Echocardiogr 2010;11:27–37.

84. Sengupta PP, Pedrizzetti G, Kilner PJ, et al. Emerging trends in CV flow visualization. JACC Cardiovasc Imaging 2012;5:305–16.

85. Dunmire B, Beach KW, Labs K, et al. Cross-beam vector Doppler ultrasound for angle-independent velocity measurements. Ultrasound Med Biol 2000;26:1213–35.

86. Uejima T, Koike A, Sawada H, et al. A new echocardiographic method for identifying vortex flow in the left ventricle: numerical validation. Ultrasound Med Biol 2010;36:772–88.

87. Garcia D, Del Alamo JC, Tanne D, et al. Two-dimensional intraventricular flow mapping by digital processing conventional color-Doppler echocardiography images. IEEE Trans Med Imaging 2010;29:1701–13.

88. Lovstakken L, Bjaerum S, Martens D, et al. Blood flow imaging–a new real-time, 2-D flow imaging technique. IEEE Trans Ultrason Ferroelectr Freq Control 2006;53:289–99.

89. Kim HB, Hertzberg JR, Shandas R. Echo PIV for flow field measurements in vivo. Biomed Sci Instrum 2004;40:357–63.

90. Hong GR, Pedrizzetti G, Tonti G, et al. Characterization and quantification of vortex flow in the human left ventricle by contrast echocardiography using vector particle image velocimetry. JACC Cardiovasc Imaging 2008;1:705–17.

91. Zhang F, Lanning C, Mazzaro L, et al. In vitro and preliminary in vivo validation of echo particle image velocimetry in carotid vascular imaging. Ultrasound Med Biol 2011;37:450–64.

92. Kheradvar A, Houle H, Pedrizzetti G, et al. Echocardiographic particle image velocimetry: a novel technique for quantification of left ventricular blood vorticity pattern. J Am Soc Echocardiogr 2010;23:86–94.

93. Sengupta PP, Khandheria BK, Korinek J, et al. Left ventricular isovolumic flow sequence during sinus and paced rhythms: new insights from use of high-resolution Doppler and ultrasonic digital particle imaging velocimetry. J Am Coll Cardiol 2007;49:899–908.
94. Faludi R, Szulik M, D'Hooge J, et al. Left ventricular flow patterns in healthy subjects and patients with prosthetic mitral valves: an in vivo study using echocardiographic particle image velocimetry. J Thorac Cardiovasc Surg 2010;139: 1501–10.
95. Sengupta PP, Burke R, Khandheria BK, et al. Following the flow in chambers. Heart Fail Clin 2008;4:325–32.

Cell-Based Strategies to Reconstitute Lung Function in Infants with Severe Bronchopulmonary Dysplasia

Megan O'Reilly, PhD[a], Bernard Thébaud, MSc, MD, PhD[a,b,c],*

KEYWORDS

- Premature birth • Bronchopulmonary dysplasia • Oxygen • Lung injury • Stem cells
- Regeneration • Cell therapy

KEY POINTS

- Various types of stem/progenitor cells have shown potential promise in preventing and/or repairing neonatal lung injury.
- Mesenchymal stem cells derived from both bone marrow and umbilical cord blood are being popularly studied and appear to function in a paracrine manner rather than through cell engraftment.
- Further knowledge and understanding in this novel and exciting area of research is necessary before safe clinical translation of cell-based therapies is warranted.
- Strong emphasis must be placed on developing and standardizing techniques for stem/progenitor cell definition, isolation, expansion, and therapeutic administration.
- Experimental studies also need to focus on the long-term outcomes of such therapies.
- By identifying the most appropriate "reparative cell(s)" and its source, combined with understanding alternative mechanisms of action beyond cell replacement, we can advance in the quest of providing therapeutic strategies to prevent/repair neonatal lung injury.

INTRODUCTION

Advances in perinatal care have led to improved survival following very preterm birth, with infants born as early as 23 to 24 weeks of gestation now being capable of survival. However, with this shift in the limit of viability toward a lower gestational age, the task of protecting the more immature lung from injury becomes increasingly challenging.

[a] Department of Pediatrics, Women and Children Health Research Institute, University of Alberta, 87 Avenue, T6G 1C9, Edmonton, Alberta, Canada; [b] Department of Pediatrics, Cardiovascular Research Center, University of Alberta, 87 Avenue, T6G 2S2, Edmonton, Alberta, Canada; [c] Department of Physiology, University of Alberta, 87 Avenue, T6G 2H7, Edmonton, Alberta, Canada
* Corresponding author. University of Alberta, 3020 Katz Centre, Edmonton, Alberta T6G 2S2, Canada.
E-mail address: bthebaud@ualberta.ca

Clin Perinatol 39 (2012) 703–725
http://dx.doi.org/10.1016/j.clp.2012.06.009
0095-5108/12/$ – see front matter © 2012 Elsevier Inc. All rights reserved.

Extreme prematurity is one of the major risk factors for the development of chronic lung disease of prematurity or bronchopulmonary dysplasia (BPD).[1] Preterm infants born between 24 and 28 weeks of gestation (ie, extremely preterm) have an immature pulmonary surfactant system, immature airway and vascular architecture, and an underdeveloped surface area for gas exchange (**Fig. 1**).[2] Many very preterm infants require prolonged respiratory support to ensure survival, which further increases their risk of developing BPD.

Recent evidence suggests that BPD may have long-term respiratory complications that reach beyond childhood. Numerous follow-up studies indicate that children and young adults who were born very preterm are at an increased risk of respiratory symptoms, poor lung function, and lower exercise capacity[3-7] this is especially apparent in infants who have developed BPD. More alarmingly, isolated case studies are surfacing of irreversible arrested alveolar development at adult age in former premature infants with BPD,[8,9] mirroring results from experimental models of BPD.[10]

Progress toward decreasing the incidence/severity of BPD over the next few years using currently available techniques and strategies is likely (ie, optimization of antenatal management combined with surfactant and early noninvasive ventilatory support targeting lower oxygen saturations).[11] However, further understanding of the mechanisms involved in lung development, injury, and repair are necessary to advance toward preventing lung injury and/or promoting lung development/regeneration in prematurely born infants. Exciting discoveries in stem cell biology in recent years may offer new insight into the pathogenesis of BPD and, more importantly, open new therapeutic avenues.

BASIC CONCEPTS OF STEM CELL BIOLOGY

Stem cells are primitive cells capable of extensive self-renewal with the potential to give rise to multiple differentiated cellular phenotypes.[12] These cells are not only critical for organogenesis and growth during the early stages of development but also contribute to organ repair and regeneration throughout life.

Developmental Potency of Stem Cells

The concept of developmental potency refers to the range of possible fates open to cells during differentiation. Stem cells exhibit varying differentiation potencies, and

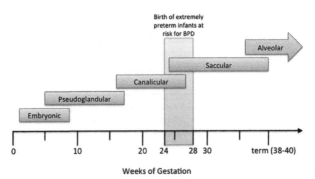

Fig. 1. Stages and gestational ages of normal lung development and preterm infants at risk of BPD. Schematic depicting stages of lung development in the human: embryonic (1–7 weeks), pseudoglandular (~5–16/17 weeks), canalicular (~16/17–24/26 weeks), saccular (~24–38 weeks), and alveolar (~36 weeks to postnatal) stages. Preterm infants at risk of developing BPD are born during the late canalicular to early saccular phase of lung development.

are typically categorized into embryonic and somatic stem cells. Embryonic stem cells (ESCs) are derived from the early blastocyst and represent the most potent of stem cells owing to their pluripotency (ie, ability to differentiate into cell types derived from all 3 germinal lineages: endoderm, mesoderm, or ectoderm) and their ability for indefinite self-renewal. By contrast, somatic stem cells (also termed adult stem cells [ASCs]) are cells that have assumed increasing degrees of fate restriction and are either multipotent (ie, can differentiate into a limited range of cell types) or unipotent (ie, can generate only one cell type).[13] Residual pools of such multipotent or unipotent stem cells are hypothesized to reside in almost all adult organs, and have the ability to contribute to tissue repair and regeneration via repopulation during growth, injury, or disease.

Classical Versus Nonclassical Stem Cell Hierarchies

While stem cells are essential for growth and development, residual pools of ASCs are considered important for tissue repair and maintenance through adulthood. Highly proliferative tissues, such as the intestinal epithelium or the hematopoietic compartment of the bone marrow, depend on a pool of ASCs that are organized in a "classical hierarchy" to maintain homeostasis.[14] By contrast, anatomically complex tissues that turn over more slowly (ie, brain, heart, lung, and kidney) do not appear to support a classical stem cell hierarchy. Such tissues are thought to be maintained by stem/progenitor cell populations that are organized in a nonclassical hierarchy and are recruited in a facultative manner for regeneration following injury.

In the lung, several local epithelial cell types function both as differentiated functional cells and as transit-amplifying progenitors that proliferate in response to airway or alveolar injuries.[15] Recent research suggests that the adult lung harbors rare populations of multipotent epithelial stem cells that are regulated by specific microenvironmental cellular niches, and are putatively recruited to repopulate the damaged epithelium.[16–19] With new insights into stem cell biology, other types of resident lung stem/progenitor cells have also been described over the past 5 years.

RESIDENT LUNG STEM/PROGENITOR CELLS

Lungs are complex organs constituted by more than 40 cell types derived from all 3 germ layers.[20] Normal lung morphogenesis involves spatiotemporally coordinated interactions between the stem/progenitor cells of different cellular compartments, which are later recapitulated during lung regeneration and repair following injury.[21] At present, the localization and properties of lung stem/progenitor cell niches and the type of cells within each niche are of major interest, yet also present controversy. Complexity of the lung architecture combined with an extensive diversity of cell types and niches has hindered the identification of true lung stem/progenitor cells. Because of the exceptionally low rate of epithelial cell turnover in the steady-state adult lung, the use of injury models has become necessary in unveiling the identity, fate, and specificity of resident lung stem/progenitor cells that contribute to homeostatic maintenance in the lung.[22] In doing so, it has been observed that relatively differentiated airway and alveolar epithelial cell types are capable of proliferating in response to epithelial injury.[15] This observation has drawn the focus of lung stem/progenitor cell research into identifying and defining those epithelial cell subpopulations that appear to contribute to postinjury regeneration.[15] Indeed, putative populations of such endogenous progenitor cells within the adult lung have been located in the basal layer of the proximal conducting airways (trachea and major bronchi) and more distally (bronchioles and alveolar ducts) within or near neuroendocrine bodies (NEBs), in the bronchoalveolar duct junction (BADJ), and the alveolar surface.[23] A representative list of putative endogenous lung epithelial stem/progenitor cells is summarized in **Table 1**. While stem/progenitor cells in the proximal airways have been explored more extensively, the study of distal stem/progenitor cells remains more controversial.

Proximal Airway Stem/Progenitor Cells

Airway submucosal glands (SMGs) and SMG ducts are major secretory structures situated below the epithelium of the proximal trachea.[24] Studies have indicated that SMGs may serve as a protective niche for adult epithelial stem/progenitor cells of the proximal airways.[25,26] Using a model of epithelial damage induced by intratracheal detergent or SO_2 inhalation, Borthwick and colleagues[25] identified a population of 5-bromo-2′-deoxyuridine label–retaining cells that were localized to the gland ducts of the upper trachea and were able to reconstitute a surface-like tracheal epithelium. In support of these findings, SMG duct cells ($K5^+$, $K14^+$) survive severe hypoxic-ischemic injury and contain stem/progenitor cell populations for regenerating the pseudostratified surface epithelium, SMGs, and SMG ducts.[26]

An additional niche of stem/progenitor cells in the proximal airway is the K14-expressing tracheobronchial basal cells, which have been shown to repopulate the denuded airway epithelium, including columnar secretory and ciliated cells, following naphthalene-induced epithelial ablation.[27] This finding indicates that the K14-expressing basal cells are implicated as a stem/progenitor cell for this airway location. The potential contribution of these cells to the repair of the distal lung remains unknown.

Distal Lung Epithelial Stem/Progenitor Cells

With transition from the proximal to distal airways, it can be seen that the notion of multiple niches supporting different populations and their progenitors within the lung is evident. This idea is supported by studies using naphthalene to deplete the airways of Clara cells, revealing a subset of Clara cells that are $CCSP^+$, yet naphthalene resistant. These cells, termed variant Clara ($Clara^V$) cells, exhibit stem cell characteristics, including ability to efflux Hoechst dye and Sca-1 expression, and have been located either within NEBs or at the bronchoalveolar duct junctions (BADJs).[28,29] More recently, Volckaert and colleagues[30] also proposed that parabronchial smooth muscle cells (PSMCs) constitute a stem/progenitor cell niche for the $Clara^V$ cells. Activation of the $Clara^V$ cell for epithelial repair following naphthalene injury was shown to be dependent on the paracrine signaling of fibroblast growth factor 10 from the PSMC niche.[30]

Recently, multipotent stem cells in the distal lung capable of differentiating into epithelial cells specific to the bronchioles and the alveoli have been identified. Kim and colleagues[17] demonstrated the existence of dual-lineage bronchoalveolar stem cells (BASCs) at the BADJ that express both bronchiolar ($CCSP^+$) and alveolar ($SP-C^+$) markers, which proliferate in response to airway and alveolar injury. However, based on the techniques used, there has been some ambiguity regarding the lineage potential[23,31] and contribution of these cells to alveolar repair.[32] McQualter and colleagues[18] used a multiparameter cell separation strategy and an organotypic in vitro clonogenic assay to detect and characterize a rare population of multipotent adult lung epithelial stem cells that give rise to airway and alveolar epithelial lineages in vitro. More recently, p63-expressing cells in the bronchiolar epithelium have been

Table 1
A selective list of candidate endogenous lung stem/progenitor cells in the rodent lung

Anatomic Location	Candidate Stem/Progenitor Cell	Attributed Differentiated Phenotype	Niche	Defining Characteristics	References
Proximal trachea	SMG duct cells	Tracheal epithelial cells, SMGs, SMG ducts	SMGs	Express cytokeratin-14 and -5; survives and repopulates tracheal epithelium following hypoxic-ischemic injury; BrdU labeling–retained cells following i.t. detergent or SO_2-mediated epithelial injury	25,26
Distal trachea and bronchi	Basal cells	Tracheobronchial epithelial cells	Intercartilaginous zone	Cytokeratin-14-expressing multipotent progenitor cells capable of restoring differentiated tracheal epithelium following naphthalene injury; associated with innervated NEBs	27
Bronchioles	Clara^V cells	Distal airway epithelium	BADJs, NEBs, and PSMCs	Express CCSP; survives and repopulates distal airway epithelium following naphthalene injury; dependent on paracrine signaling of Fgf10	29,30
Bronchioles and alveoli	BASCs	Bronchoalveolar epithelial cells	BADJs	Resistant to naphthalene injury and proliferate in response; coexpress CCSP and SP-C	17
	Pulmonary Oct-4$^+$ stem/progenitor cells	Alveolar type-I and -II pneumocytes	BADJs	Oct4$^+$, SSEA-1$^+$, Sca-1$^+$, cytokeratin-7$^+$ cells; serially passaged, differentiate terminally into type-II and -I pneumocytes; susceptible to SARS-CoV infection	78
	Multipotent lung epithelial progenitors	Airway and alveolar epithelium	Intrapulmonary airways and alveoli (not localized)	EpCAMhi, CD49f$^+$, CD104$^+$, CD24lo, Sca-1$^-$, CD45$^-$, CD31$^-$ lung epithelial colony-forming units, form colonies in Matrigel; serially passaged and retain multipotent potential	18
Alveoli	Alveolar type-II pneumocytes	Alveolar type-I pneumocytes	Alveolar surface	All alveolar type-II pneumocytes	34
	A subset of alveolar type-II pneumocytes	Alveolar type-I and mature type-II pneumocytes	Alveolar surface	E-cadherin negative subset of alveolar type-II cells, proliferative, high telomerase activity, resistant to oxygen-induced injury	37

Abbreviations: BADJ, bronchoalveolar duct junction; BASC, bronchoalveolar stem cell; BrdU, 5-bromo-2'-deoxyuridine; CCSP, Clara cell secretory protein; Clara^V, variant Clara; EpCAMhi, epithelial cell adhesion molecule Fgf10, fibroblast growth factor 10; NEBs, neuroendocrine bodies; Oct-4, octamer-binding transcription factor 4; PSMC, parabronchial smooth muscle cell; Sca-1, stem cell antigen 1; SMG, submucosal gland; SP-C, surfactant protein C; SSEA-1, stage-specific embryonic antigen-1; SARS-CoV, severe acute respiratory syndrome coronavirus.

shown to undergo rapid proliferation after H1N1 influenza virus infection and to radiate to interbronchiolar regions of alveolar ablation. These cells assemble into Krt5[+] pods and initiate expression of markers typical of alveoli. Gene-expression profiles of these pods suggest that they are intermediates in the reconstitution of the alveolar-capillary network.[33] The presence of such putative endogenous alveolar stem cell populations provides fresh hope of target-directed, regenerative therapies for alveolar diseases.

Cuboidal type-II pneumocytes have long been considered as progenitors of the alveolar epithelium, based on their capacity to replenish themselves and generate terminally differentiated type I pneumocytes.[34,35] Since then, type-II pneumocytes have been speculated to contain a subpopulation of progenitors cells that can undergo reactivation into a progenitor-like state in response to injury cues. Using an acute model of oxygen-induced injury, Driscoll and colleagues[36] demonstrated the existence of a telomerase-positive subpopulation within the general type-II cell population during the recovery phase. These findings were further strengthened by a later study in which Reddy and colleagues[37] classified type-II cells into E-cadherin–positive and -negative fractions, and showed heightened telomerase activity and injury resistance in the latter subset.

Lung Mesenchymal Stem Cells

Additional lung cell types, including airway smooth muscle, fibroblasts, and the vasculature, are derived from the mesoderm. Interactions between the epithelial cells, mesenchymal microenvironment (including extracellular matrix proteins and growth factors), and the adjacent pulmonary vasculature regulate the structural and functional maturation of the developing lung.[21] Current knowledge of lung mesenchymal precursors is limited; however, there is evidence that small populations of resident lung cells expressing certain phenotypic characteristics of mesenchymal cells with progenitor capacity exist within the lung.

Resident lung "side population" (SP) cells, which appear to have both mesenchymal and epithelial potential, have been isolated based on their capacity to efflux Hoechst dye.[38–40] These SP cells have been shown to be present at all levels of the airway tree, and regardless of which lung compartment they were derived from, exhibited a relatively uniform phenotype.[40] Although it has been demonstrated that these SP cells are a source of adult lung mesenchymal stem cells (MSCs),[39] the role of SP cells in endogenous lung repair is not completely understood.

Furthermore, McQualter and colleagues[41] described a population of endogenous fibroblastic progenitor cells with clonogenic potential in the adult lung, which are predominantly representative of mesenchymal cell lineages. The cell fraction defined by McQualter and colleagues[18] was of similar cell phenotype (CD45[-], CD31[-], Sca-1[+], CD43[+]) to the cell fraction defined as BASCs; however, they coexpressed immunophenotypic markers definitive of lung fibroblastic rather than epithelial cells.[41] These findings highlight the need for alternative, specific markers to enable precise identification of endogenous stem/progenitor cell subpopulations within the lung.

Following the discovery of the plasticity characteristics of ASCs that allow them to cross lineage barriers and adopt functional phenotypes of other tissues, much interest has been diverted to understanding their role in repair and maintenance of the lungs.[42] Experimental evidence indicates that the injured lung stimulates the release and preferential homing of MSCs, a population of ASCs derived from the bone marrow.[43,44] However, the mechanism by which exogenous progenitors, such as bone marrow MSCs, assume lung phenotype remains unclear, as does its clinical significance.[45,46]

Lung Endothelial Progenitor Cells

Endothelial progenitor cells (EPCs), a population of vascular precursor cells, have also recently received attention in the context of lung development and regeneration. Indeed, given the importance of lung angiogenesis and vascular growth factors during lung growth and repair, vascular progenitor cells are appealing candidate cells likely to be involved in the same mechanisms.[47] However, assessment of the contribution of endogenous lung EPCs in lung vascular repair and lung regeneration and remodeling is impeded by their rarity, lack of distinguishing markers, and the inability to discriminate circulating EPCs and tissue EPCs.[22] Alvarez and colleagues[48] demonstrated that the lung microvasculature is enriched with a population of EPCs, termed resident microvascular endothelial progenitor cells, which were shown to be highly proliferative and capable of renewing the entire hierarchy of endothelial cell growth potentials. It has been demonstrated that both circulating and resident lung EPCs are likely to contribute to endothelial cell regeneration and repair in the lung.[49,50]

The recent surge in our knowledge of stem cell biology and the availability of advanced research tools in this field has motivated researchers in exploring the role of lung stem cells in the pathogenesis of lung diseases. Indeed, several major lung diseases likely involve dysregulation in the numbers and/or the function of resident lung stem/progenitor cells.[46] For instance, depletion or functional impairment of alveolar epithelial and/or EPCs could putatively underlie the pathogenesis of alveolar growth arrest or destruction observed in BPD and emphysema, respectively. In such a scenario, augmentation of stem cells is an appealing strategy to minimize lung injury, promote repair, or possibly regenerate lost tissue.

LUNG STEM/PROGENITOR CELLS: IMPLICATIONS FOR THE PATHOGENESIS OF BPD

Recent animal and human studies suggest that damage or depletion of epithelial and/or vascular stem/progenitor cells in the developing lung likely contributes to the pathogenesis of BPD.

Perturbation of Distal Lung Epithelial and Mesenchymal Stem Cells

Exposure of neonatal rodents to high levels of oxygen is extensively used as an injury model to investigate experimental BPD. Irwin and colleagues[51] showed a reduction in the number and endothelial differentiation potential of multipotent lung SP cells. Observations from the authors' own laboratory in an oxygen-challenged neonatal rat model of BPD have also shown decreased numbers of circulating and resident MSCs in the lungs.[52] This finding highlights the potential of stem cell supplementation for the prevention or repair of neonatal lung injury. Accordingly, systemic treatment of neonatal hyperoxia–exposed mice with MSCs significantly increases the number of BASCs compared with untreated controls. In addition, treatment of BASCs with MSC-derived conditioned media (CdM) in culture stimulated BASC growth efficiency, indicating a direct effect of MSCs on BASCs.[53]

In contrast to the aforementioned reports of depleted numbers of stem/progenitor cells, Popova and colleagues[54] demonstrated that the presence of MSCs in tracheal aspirates of preterm infants indicated an increased risk for developing BPD. Those cells isolated from the tracheal aspirates expressed the markers STRO-1, CD73, CD90, CD105, CD166, CCR2b, CD13, propyl-4-hydroxylase, and α-smooth muscle actin, and were negative for CD11b, CD31, CD34, and CD45.[55] Furthermore, these cells were shown to acquire a myofibroblast phenotype, which suggest that they could contribute to the profibrotic changes and arrested alveolarization in BPD.[56] However, in contrast to tracheal aspirate MSCs, human bone marrow–derived MSCs did not undergo myofibroblastic differentiation in response to transforming growth factor β1, suggesting distinct properties between these 2 populations of MSCs.[56] Indeed, it is possible that these reported resident lung MSCs are perturbed in BPD, as their cell phenotype is not analogous to the endogenous MSCs described by McQualter and colleagues[41] in the absence of lung injury. Therefore, with the growing interest in harnessing the therapeutic effects of stem progenitor cells for neonatal lung injury, it is necessary to perform further thorough investigations to understand the behavior of MSCs from different populations (ie, lung, umbilical cord blood [UCB], bone marrow) in the presence and absence of lung injury, and how this could affect potential cell-based therapies for BPD.[57]

Perturbation of Lung and Circulating EPCs

Neonatal mice with oxygen-induced chronic lung injury have depleted numbers of putative lung-resident EPCs ($CD45^-/Sca-1^+/CD133^+/VEGFR-2^+$).[50] Baker and colleagues[58] demonstrated that UCB of preterm infants yielded a higher amount of endothelial colony-forming cells (ECFCs; a specific subset of EPCs) than from UCB of term infants. Preterm ECFCs had an increased susceptibility to in vitro oxygen exposure than term ECFCs.[58] Borghesi and colleagues[59] reported that the number of ECFCs was lower in UCB of preterm infants who subsequently developed BPD, compared with preterm infants who did not develop BPD. In contrast to the findings of Borghesi and colleagues,[59] Paviotti and colleagues[60] recently reported no association between the number of EPCs at birth and the subsequent development of BPD. The apparent discordance between studies reporting EPCs in preterm infants highlights the importance of appropriately defining an EPC and establishing criteria similar to the "minimal criteria" for characterizing MSCs.[61] Furthermore, assessing EPC function may be more revealing than assessing EPC number.

These observations suggest that the capacity of resident stem cell populations to undergo self-renewal and regeneration can be limited, because of the natural effect of increasing age and/or the presence of disease. This situation forms the rationale for the therapeutic potential of stem cell–based therapies, either through stimulation of endogenous stem cell pools or their therapeutic replacement with exogenous-derived stem cells. Such cell-replacement therapies already show promise in debilitating childhood and adult disorders.[62–64] In the laboratory, stem cell–based strategies have shown therapeutic benefit in experimental models of lung disease.

THERAPEUTIC POTENTIAL OF STEM CELLS TO PREVENT OR REPAIR THE DAMAGED LUNG

Numerous studies in experimental animal models provide compelling evidence for the beneficial effects of stem cell therapy approaches for a wide variety of adult lung diseases (**Table 2**), including acute lung injury/acute respiratory distress syndrome, pulmonary hypertension, asthma, and chronic obstructive pulmonary disease (including emphysema).[65–67]

Of the many different stem/progenitor cell therapies that have been used in experimental models, MSCs appear to be the most extensively examined cell type. MSCs can be sourced from the bone marrow, UCB, Wharton jelly, the placenta, and adipose tissue.[68] As outlined in **Table 2** benefits of MSC therapy in experimental adult lung diseases include, but are not limited to, improvements in alveolar, airway, and vascular structure; attenuation of lung inflammation; decreased pulmonary fibrosis; reduced pulmonary edema, hemorrhage, and alveolar and endothelial permeability; and

Table 2
Studies testing the therapeutic effect of stem/progenitor cells in experimental adult lung disease models

Experimental Model	Therapeutic Cell of Product	Outcomes	Suggested Mechanisms	References
Bleomycin Lung Injury/Acute Respiratory Distress Syndrome				
Bleomycin-induced (i.t.)	Human ESC-derived cells with AT2 epithelial phenotype (i.t.)	Improved body weight and survival Improved arterial oxygen saturation Decreased collagen deposition	Engraftment and AT1 differentiation Paracrine mechanisms	79
	Bone marrow–derived MSCs (i.v.)	Reduced fibrosis and inflammation	IL-1 receptor antagonism Decrease in NO metabolites, proinflammatory, and angiogenic cytokines	44,80,81
	hUC Wharton jelly–derived MSCs (i.v.)	Reduced fibrosis	Decreased TGF-β and TIMP activity Increased MMP-2 activity	82
	Bone marrow–derived HSCs ± KGF overexpression (i.v.)	Reduced fibrosis	KGF-induced endogenous AT2 cell proliferation	83
Bleomycin-induced (i.n.)	hAECs (i.p.)	Reduced fibrosis and collagen deposition Improved lung function Modulated inflammatory response	Anti-inflammatory effects	84
Escherichia coli endotoxin-induced (i.p.)	Bone marrow–derived MSCs (i.v.; i.t.)	Improved survival Decreased systemic and local inflammation	Cell-cell interactions Paracrine mechanisms Decreased proinflammatory and increased anti-inflammatory cytokines Antioxidant mechanisms	85–87
E coli endotoxin-induced (i.t.)	iPS cells and CdM (i.v.)	Attenuated lung injury Reduced inflammation Reduced MPO and NF-κB activity Improved Pao₂ and lung function	Paracrine mechanisms Regulation of neutrophil activity Attenuating inflammatory cascade Immunomodulatory effects	88
	Bone marrow–derived MSCs overexpressing Ang-1 (i.v.; i.t.)	Decreased inflammation Decreased alveolar permeability	Decreased inflammatory cytokines Ang-1–mediated effects	89,90
	hUCB-derived MSCs (i.t.)	Increased survival Attenuated lung injury Reduced inflammation Increased MPO activity Inhibited bacterial growth	Down-modulating inflammatory process Enhancing bacterial clearance	91

(continued on next page)

Table 2
(continued)

Experimental Model	Therapeutic Cell of Product	Outcomes	Suggested Mechanisms	References
LPS-induced (i.t.)	Human orbital fat–derived stem/stromal cells (i.v.)	Decreased systemic and local inflammation Decreased alveolar and endothelial permeability	Inhibition of macrophage and neutrophil-associated inflammatory responses	92
	EPCs (i.v.)	Improved Pao_2 and SaO_2 Preservation of alveolocapillary permeability	Paracrine mechanisms Anti-inflammatory effects	93
	hUCB-derived MSCs (i.t.)	Reduced interstitial edema, hyaline membrane formation, hemorrhage Increased survival Reduced edema, hemorrhage, alveolar and endothelial permeability Reduced inflammation	Paracrine mechanisms Anti-inflammatory effects	94
LPS-induced (i.v.)	EPCs (i.v.)	Reduced pulmonary edema, inflammation, hemorrhage, and hyaline membrane formation Decreased adhesion molecule expression Reduced endothelial and epithelial cell apoptosis	Engraftment of EPCs Re-endothelialization Downregulation of adhesion molecules Alleviation of inflammatory response Apoptosis prevention	95
Ventilator-induced	Bone marrow–derived MSCs and CdM (i.v.)	Improved lung function Modulated inflammation Restored lung structure	Paracrine mechanisms	96
Pulmonary Hypertension				
Monocrotaline-induced	Bone marrow–derived MSCs ± eNOS overexpression (i.v.; i.t.)	Improved survival Improved RV pressure overload and function Improved lung structure	eNOS-mediated vasodilation VEGF-mediated enhanced microvasculature	97–100
	Bone marrow–derived EPCs (i.v.)	Restored pulmonary hemodynamics Increased microvascular perfusion Improved cardiac function	Paracrine effects	101
	Peripheral blood–derived EPCs (i.t.)	Improved vasculature thickness and lung neovascularization	eNOS-mediated vascular growth	102

Asthma/Allergic Airway Inflammation

Ovalbumin-induced (i.p. and i.t.; nebulized)	Adipose tissue–derived MSCs (i.v.)	Decreased local and systemic allergic response	Decreased Th2 activity	103,104
	Bone marrow–derived MSCs (i.v.)	Reduced airway hyperresponsiveness and remodeling; Reduced serum NO levels; Reduced inflammatory cell infiltration and mast cell degranulation	Immunomodulatory effects; Anti-inflammatory effects	105,106
	BMC-CdM	Prevented airway inflammation; Reduced airway remodeling; Prevented airway hyperresponsiveness	Paracrine mechanisms; Anti-inflammatory effects of adipokine, APN	107
Ragweed-induced (i.p.)	Bone marrow–derived MSCs (i.v.)	Decreased asthma-specific allergic response	TGF-β production; Regulatory T-cell recruitment	108

Chronic Obstructive Pulmonary Disease/Emphysema

Cigarette smoke–induced	Bone marrow–derived MSCs, CdM, and BMCs (i.v.)	Restoration of alveolar structure; Increased pulmonary vascularity; Alleviation of pulmonary hypertension (by BMCs)	Paracrine mechanisms; Recruitment of BMCs by donor cells	109
Papain-induced	Bone marrow–derived MSCs (i.v.)	Improved alveolar structure	Engraftment and AT2 differentiation; Reduced alveolar epithelial apoptosis	110
Elastase-induced (i.t.)	Adipose tissue–derived MSCs (i.v. or cultured on PGA and transplanted after LVRS)	Restored gas exchange; Improved exercise tolerance	Growth factor release (HGF, VEGF)	111,112
	Bone marrow–derived MSCs (i.t.)	Preservation of alveolar structure; Reduced inflammation; Upregulated growth factors; Improved survival; Attenuated alveolar damage	Paracrine mechanisms; HGF, EGF, and secretory leukocyte protease inhibitor secretion	113
	Lung resident multilineage progenitors Sca1+CD45− CD31− (i.t.)		Immunomodulatory effects; Paracrine mechanisms	114

Abbreviations: Ang-1, angiopoietin-1; APN, adiponectin; AT1, alveolar epithelial type 1; AT2, alveolar epithelial type 2; BMC, bone marrow–derived cells; CdM, conditioned media; EGF, epidermal growth factor; eNOS, endothelial nitric oxide synthase; EPC, endothelial progenitor cell; HGF, hepatocyte growth factor; HSC, hematopoietic stem cell; hAEC, human amnion epithelial cell; hUC, human umbilical cord; hUCB, human umbilical cord blood; IL, interleukin; i.n., intranasal; i.p., intraperitoneal; iPS, induced pluripotent stem; i.t., intratracheal; i.v., intravenous; KGF, keratinocyte growth factor; LPS, lipopolysaccharide; LVRS, lung volume reduction surgery; MMP-2, matrix metalloproteinase 2; MPO, myeloperoxidase; MSC, mesenchymal stem cell; NF-κB, nuclear factor kappa light-chain enhancer of activated B cells; NO, nitric oxide; Pao₂, partial pressure of oxygen in arterial blood; PGA, polyglycolic acid; RV, right ventricle; Sao₂, oxygen saturation; TGF-β, transforming growth factor β; Th2, helper T cell type 2; TIMP, tissue inhibitor of metalloproteinase; VEGF, vascular endothelial growth factor.

restoration of lung function and exercise capacity. Of importance, the beneficial therapeutic actions of MSCs appear to be mediated through paracrine mechanisms and immunomodulatory effects, rather than cell engraftment and direct actions in the lungs.[69]

The use of MSCs and other types of stem/progenitor cells are also being increasingly examined in experimental models of neonatal lung disease, in particular BPD. Given the perturbations of resident lung stem cells in BPD, the ideal therapeutic approach would involve replenishing the lung with healthy multipotent stem/progenitor cells that repopulate, repair, and regenerate the injured, developing lung. Indeed, several recent studies have demonstrated promising outcomes using different stem/progenitor cell types in animal models of BPD (**Fig. 2, Table 3**).

Mesenchymal Stem Cell Therapy in Experimental BPD

Administration of bone marrow–derived MSCs, either intratracheally, intravenously, or intraperitoneally, have ameliorated numerous aspects of neonatal lung injury, as evident by mitigation of lung inflammation, prevention of lung vascular damage and alveolar growth arrest, inhibition of lung fibrosis, and improvement in exercise tolerance (**Fig. 3**).[52,53,70,71] Low engraftment and differentiation of these MSCs into the injured neonatal lung suggest that the potential mechanisms through which MSCs exert their actions are paracrine mediated. These speculations are supported by in vitro and in vivo studies demonstrating that administration of CdM from MSCs has the ability to protect alveolar epithelial and lung microvascular endothelial cells from oxidative stress, prevent oxygen-induced alveolar growth arrest, and stimulate a subset of stem/progenitor cells, namely BASCs, to aid in lung repair.[52,53,70] Furthermore, the therapeutic benefits of MSC-CdM may surpass those of MSCs, with in vivo

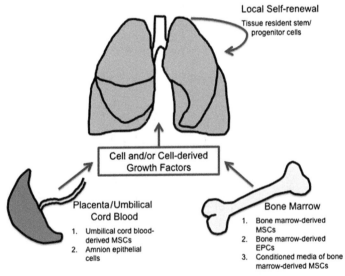

Fig. 2. Current sources of stem/progenitor cells for lung regeneration in experimental models of neonatal lung injury. Several studies have demonstrated the effects of stem/progenitor cells and stem/progenitor cell-derived growth factors (ie, conditioned media) to promote lung regeneration following neonatal lung injury in animal models of BPD. These cells were sourced from the bone marrow, umbilical cord blood, and placenta amnion.

Table 3
Studies testing the therapeutic effect of stem/progenitor cells in experimental models of neonatal chronic lung disease

Experimental Model	Therapeutic Cell or Product	Outcomes	Suggested Mechanism	References
Hyperoxia-induced lung injury (mice, rats)	Bone marrow–derived MSCs (i.t.)	Improved survival	Engraftment as AT2 Paracrine mechanisms	52
	Bone marrow–derived MSCs or CdM (i.v.)	Improved alveolar structure/prevented alveolar arrest Prevented vascular growth arrest Improved exercise capacity Reduced pulmonary hypertension	Paracrine mechanisms Immunomodulatory effects	70
	Bone marrow–derived MSCs or CdM (i.v.)	Improved alveolar structure/prevented alveolar arrest Attenuated inflammation Prevented vascular growth arrest Prevented pulmonary hypertension Increased number of BASCs	Stimulation of BASCs Paracrine mechanisms	53
	Bone marrow–derived MSCs (i.p.)	Improved survival Improved alveolar structure/prevented alveolar arrest Attenuated inflammation Inhibited lung fibrosis	Engraftment as AT2 Reduction in ECM remodeling and fibrosis gene expression (TGF-β1, collagen 1α, TIMP-1) Anti-inflammatory effects	71
	hUCB-derived MSCs (i.t.)	Improved survival and growth restriction Improved alveolar structure Attenuated lung fibrosis, inflammation, and ROS activity	Paracrine anti-inflammatory, antifibrotic, and antioxidative effects	72,73
	BMDACs (i.v.)	Improved alveolar structure Improved vascular growth	Paracrine mechanisms	74
LPS-induced (i.a.) lung injury (sheep)	hAECs (i.t.; i.v.)	Improved alveolar structure Increased surfactant protein expression Attenuated inflammation	Immunomodulatory effects	75

Abbreviations: AT2, alveolar epithelial type 2; BASC, bronchoalveolar stem cell; BMDAC, bone marrow–derived angiogenic cell; CdM, conditioned media; ECM, extracellular matrix; hAEC, human amnion epithelial cell; hUCB, human umbilical cord blood; i.a., intra-amniotic; i.p., intraperitoneal; i.t., intratracheal; i.v., intravenous; LPS, lipopolysaccharide; MSC, mesenchymal stem cell; ROS, reactive oxygen species; TGF-β1, transforming growth factor β1; TIMP-1, tissue inhibitor of metalloproteinase 1.

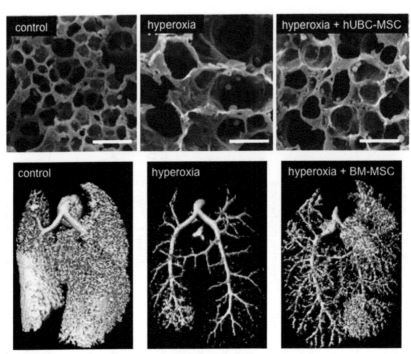

Fig. 3. Therapeutic effects of bone marrow–derived MSCs and human umbilical cord (hUBC) blood-derived MSCs in experimental oxygen-induced BPD. Intratracheal delivery of MSCs derived from hUBC and from bone marrow (BM) improves hyperoxia-induced alveolar and lung vascular growth in neonatal rats, as demonstrated by electron microscopy (*top panels*) and micro–computed tomography (*bottom panels*) of the alveolar structure and pulmonary vasculature, respectively. (*Adapted from* Chang YS, Oh W, Choi SJ, et al. Human umbilical cord blood-derived mesenchymal stem cells attenuate hyperoxia-induced lung injury in neonatal rats. Cell Transplant 2009;18:869–86; with permission; and van Haaften T, Byrne R, Bonnet S, et al. Airway delivery of mesenchymal stem cells prevents arrested alveolar growth in neonatal lung injury in rats. Am J Respir Crit Care Med 2009;180:1131–42; with permission.)

findings indicating a more profound therapeutic effect of MSC-CdM in preventing and repairing lung injury than that of MSCs.[70]

UCB also represents an appealing source of MSCs for therapeutic use in the newborn because of its clinically relevant, easily accessible, ethically viable, and readily available source of stem/progenitor cells. Chang and colleagues[72,73] demonstrated that MSCs obtained from human UCB prevent hyperoxia-induced alveolar growth arrest and alleviate fibrotic changes in the neonatal rat lung (see **Fig. 3**). Chang and colleagues[73] also show that the route of administration may alter the outcome, with intratracheal transplantation resulting in a more prominent attenuation of hyperoxia-induced lung injury than intraperitoneal transplantation. Furthermore, Chang and colleagues[72] recently demonstrated the dose-dependent effects of human UCB-derived MSCs in the oxygen-challenged neonatal rat lung. This study indicated that intratracheal delivery of a minimum of 5×10^4 cells is required to exhibit efficient anti-inflammatory, antifibrotic, and antioxidant effects following hyperoxia-induced lung injury in neonatal rats.[72] In light of these findings, further studies determining the optimal dose of MSCs for potential clinical benefit in human neonates are anticipated.

Endothelial Progenitor Cell Therapy in Experimental BPD

The therapeutic potential of EPCs in neonatal lung injury has been effectively demonstrated in an oxygen-induced BPD mouse model.[74] Treatment of neonatal mice exposed to hyperoxia with intravenously administered bone marrow–derived angiogenic cells (a population of bone marrow myeloid-like precursor cells) showed restoration of the alveolar structure and vessel density to that of control (room air–exposed) levels.[74]

Amnion Epithelial Cell Therapy in Experimental BPD

The therapeutic potential of human amnion epithelial cells (hAECs) has recently been investigated in a sheep model of neonatal lung injury, induced by lipopolysaccharide (LPS) administration in fetal sheep.[75] Because hAECs are sourced from placentae, which are normally discarded after birth, they present an easily accessible and ethically viable candidate for cell therapy. Administration of hAECs to fetal sheep exposed to LPS attenuated inflammation-induced changes in lung function and structure, and reduced pulmonary inflammation.[75] Of particular interest is the ability of hAECs to significantly increase the expression levels of SP-A and SP-C. The low engraftment into the lungs indicates that these hAECs act via immune modulation rather than cell engraftment and differentiation. More detailed assessment of the therapeutic potential of these cells in other models of neonatal lung injury will be of interest.

In summary, findings from several exciting studies indicate that a variety of stem/progenitor cells can prevent and/or regenerate neonatal lung injury in experimental models. Additional studies in different animal models of BPD are necessary to broaden the current knowledge and understanding of the therapeutic potential of stem/progenitor cells. In doing so, further evidence for creating a strong rationale for transitioning this potential breakthrough into clinic can be generated.

REMAINING CHALLENGES

Although stem/progenitor cell therapies present potential promise in preventing and/or repairing lung injury, many gaps in our knowledge and understanding of stem cell biology in health and disease are yet to be filled (**Box 1**). In part, it is important to more precisely define putative reparative cells. One of the obstacles is the lack of biomarkers available for the characterization of candidate stem/progenitor cells in different species[22] and the inability to easily study these cells in vivo.

Current studies elegantly detail the short-term effects of stem/progenitor cell therapies in animal models of neonatal lung injury.[52,53,70–75] However, few of these studies have reported the long-term outcomes (ie, in mid-adult or aged lung) of such stem/progenitor cell therapies,[52,71] which is a vital and clinically important area of research that needs to be understood to warrant safe clinical translation.

In addition, it would be valuable to understand the effects of such stem/progenitor cell therapies in other animal models of neonatal lung injury closely mimicking the clinical setting (ie, ventilator-induced, fetal/neonatal inflammation-induced), rather than the frequently used hyperoxia-induced model; indeed, this is already being used by some.[75]

Current studies highlight the beneficial effects of stem/progenitor cell therapy on attenuating structural and/or molecular alterations to the injured developing lung, yet the effects on lung function are infrequently reported.[52] This aspect of experimental studies requires further investigation and thorough documentation, because

---

Box 1
Future directions and questions for the use of stem/progenitor cells in neonatal lung injury

Determine Optimal Stem Cell-Based Strategy for Lung Diseases

- What is the best reparative cell to treat a given lung disease?
  - ESCs, MSCs, EPCs, amniotic fluid stem cells, amnion epithelial cells
- What is the appropriate strategy for cell-based therapies?
  - Administration of exogenous stem cells: stem cells, stem cell–derived CdM, CdM-derived factors
  - Protection of endogenous lung progenitor cells
- What is the best mode of delivery of stem cells for lung diseases?
  - Intravenous
  - Intratracheal

Long-Term Outcomes of Cell Therapy in BPD Models

- Can stem/progenitor cell therapies permanently prevent/repair neonatal lung injury, or will continuous treatment be required for life?
- Would additional later in life "insults" reduce the protective effects of stem/progenitor cell therapies?
  - Lung infection
  - Smoking
- What are the effects of stem/progenitor cell therapies on short-term and long-term lung function outcomes?
  - Baseline lung function
  - Challenged lung function: exercise-induced, asthma/allergy-induced
  - Age-induced decline in lung function
- What are the potential adverse effects of stem cell–based therapies?
  - Tumor formation
  - Ectopic tissue formation
  - Immune rejection of the transplanted stem cells

Cell Therapy in Other Experimental Models of BPD

- What are the effects of stem/progenitor cell therapies in other relevant animal models of neonatal lung injury?
  - Type of lung injury: ventilator-induced, inflammation/infection-induced
  - Type of animal model: rodent, sheep, baboon

---

the overall aim of treating neonatal lung injury with stem/progenitor cells is to reduce and/or prevent lung dysfunction.

SUMMARY

Half a century since the landmark discovery of stem cells by the Canadian researchers Till and McCulloch in 1961,[76] their therapeutic potential in regenerative medicine is now being harnessed for treatment of neonatal lung injury, almost half a century since Northway and colleagues[77] described BPD. Various types of stem/progenitor cells have shown benefit in experimental models of neonatal lung injury, with MSCs derived from both bone marrow and UCB being popularly studied, as well as CdM from these cells. However, before safe clinical translation of cell-based therapies is warranted, we must broaden our knowledge and understanding in this novel and exciting area of research. Strong emphasis must be placed on developing and standardizing techniques for stem/progenitor cell definition, isolation, expansion, and therapeutic administration. Experimental studies also need to focus on the long-term outcomes of such therapies. By identifying the most appropriate reparative cell(s) and its source, combined with understanding alternative mechanisms of action beyond cell replacement and assessing the short-term and long-term efficacy and safety, we can advance in the quest of providing therapeutic strategies to prevent and repair neonatal lung injury.

REFERENCES

1. Henderson-Smart DJ, Hutchinson JL, Donoghue DA, et al. Prenatal predictors of chronic lung disease in very preterm infants. Arch Dis Child Fetal Neonatal Ed 2006;91:F40–5.
2. Kinsella JP, Greenough A, Abman SH. Bronchopulmonary dysplasia. Lancet 2006;367:1421–31.
3. Brostrom EB, Thunqvist P, Adenfelt G, et al. Obstructive lung disease in children with mild to severe BPD. Respir Med 2010;104:362–70.
4. Doyle LW, Faber B, Callanan C, et al. Bronchopulmonary dysplasia in very low birth weight subjects and lung function in late adolescence. Pediatrics 2006; 118:108–13.
5. Filippone M, Bonetto G, Corradi M, et al. Evidence of unexpected oxidative stress in airways of adolescents born very preterm. Eur Respir J 2012. [Epub ahead of print].
6. Narang I, Rosenthal M, Cremonesini D, et al. Longitudinal evaluation of airway function 21 years after preterm birth. Am J Respir Crit Care Med 2008;178: 74–80.
7. Smith LJ, van Asperen PP, McKay KO, et al. Reduced exercise capacity in children born very preterm. Pediatrics 2008;122:e287–93.
8. Cutz E, Chiasson D. Chronic lung disease after premature birth. N Engl J Med 2008;358:743–5 [author reply: 745–6].
9. Wong PM, Lees AN, Louw J, et al. Emphysema in young adult survivors of moderate-to-severe bronchopulmonary dysplasia. Eur Respir J 2008;32: 321–8.
10. Yee M, Chess PR, McGrath-Morrow SA, et al. Neonatal oxygen adversely affects lung function in adult mice without altering surfactant composition or activity. Am J Physiol Lung Cell Mol Physiol 2009;297:L641–9.
11. Jobe AH. The new bronchopulmonary dysplasia. Curr Opin Pediatr 2011;23: 167–72.
12. Blau HM, Brazelton TR, Weimann JM. The evolving concept of a stem cell: entity or function? Cell 2001;105:829–41.
13. Stevenson K, McGlynn L, Shiels PG. Stem cells: outstanding potential and outstanding questions. Scott Med J 2009;54:35–7.
14. Stripp BR. Hierarchical organization of lung progenitor cells: is there an adult lung tissue stem cell? Proc Am Thorac Soc 2008;5:695–8.
15. Rawlins EL, Hogan BL. Epithelial stem cells of the lung: privileged few or opportunities for many? Development 2006;133:2455–65.

16. Giangreco A, Reynolds SD, Stripp BR. Terminal bronchioles harbor a unique airway stem cell population that localizes to the bronchoalveolar duct junction. Am J Pathol 2002;161:173–82.

17. Kim CF, Jackson EL, Woolfenden AE, et al. Identification of bronchoalveolar stem cells in normal lung and lung cancer. Cell 2005;121:823–35.

18. McQualter JL, Yuen K, Williams B, et al. Evidence of an epithelial stem/progenitor cell hierarchy in the adult mouse lung. Proc Natl Acad Sci U S A 2010;107:1414–9.

19. Rawlins EL, Clark CP, Xue Y, et al. The Id2+ distal tip lung epithelium contains individual multipotent embryonic progenitor cells. Development 2009;136:3741–5.

20. Kim CF. Paving the road for lung stem cell biology: bronchoalveolar stem cells and other putative distal lung stem cells. Am J Physiol Lung Cell Mol Physiol 2007;293:L1092–8.

21. Shi W, Xu J, Warburton D. Development, repair and fibrosis: what is common and why it matters. Respirology 2009;14:656–65.

22. McQualter JL, Bertoncello I. Concise review: deconstructing the lung to reveal its regenerative potential. Stem Cells 2012;30(5):811–6.

23. Bertoncello I, McQualter JL. Endogenous lung stem cells: what is their potential for use in regenerative medicine? Expert Rev Respir Med 2010;4:349–62.

24. Liu X, Engelhardt JF. The glandular stem/progenitor cell niche in airway development and repair. Proc Am Thorac Soc 2008;5:682–8.

25. Borthwick DW, Shahbazian M, Krantz QT, et al. Evidence for stem-cell niches in the tracheal epithelium. Am J Respir Cell Mol Biol 2001;24:662–70.

26. Hegab AE, Ha VL, Gilbert JL, et al. Novel stem/progenitor cell population from murine tracheal submucosal gland ducts with multipotent regenerative potential. Stem Cells 2011;29:1283–93.

27. Hong KU, Reynolds SD, Watkins S, et al. Basal cells are a multipotent progenitor capable of renewing the bronchial epithelium. Am J Pathol 2004;164:577–88.

28. Giangreco A, Shen H, Reynolds SD, et al. Molecular phenotype of airway side population cells. Am J Physiol Lung Cell Mol Physiol 2004;286:L624–30.

29. Hong KU, Reynolds SD, Giangreco A, et al. Clara cell secretory protein-expressing cells of the airway neuroepithelial body microenvironment include a label-retaining subset and are critical for epithelial renewal after progenitor cell depletion. Am J Respir Cell Mol Biol 2001;24:671–81.

30. Volckaert T, Dill E, Campbell A, et al. Parabronchial smooth muscle constitutes an airway epithelial stem cell niche in the mouse lung after injury. J Clin Invest 2011;121:4409–19.

31. Snyder JC, Teisanu RM, Stripp BR. Endogenous lung stem cells and contribution to disease. J Pathol 2009;217:254–64.

32. Rawlins EL, Okubo T, Xue Y, et al. The role of Scgb1a1+ Clara cells in the long-term maintenance and repair of lung airway, but not alveolar, epithelium. Cell Stem Cell 2009;4:525–34.

33. Kumar PA, Hu Y, Yamamoto Y, et al. Distal airway stem cells yield alveoli in vitro and during lung regeneration following H1N1 influenza infection. Cell 2011;147:525–38.

34. Adamson IY, Bowden DH. The type 2 cell as progenitor of alveolar epithelial regeneration. A cytodynamic study in mice after exposure to oxygen. Lab Invest 1974;30:35–42.

35. Brody JS, Williams MC. Pulmonary alveolar epithelial cell differentiation. Annu Rev Physiol 1992;54:351–71.

36. Driscoll B, Buckley S, Bui KC, et al. Telomerase in alveolar epithelial development and repair. Am J Physiol Lung Cell Mol Physiol 2000;279:L1191–8.
37. Reddy R, Buckley S, Doerken M, et al. Isolation of a putative progenitor subpopulation of alveolar epithelial type 2 cells. Am J Physiol Lung Cell Mol Physiol 2004;286:L658–67.
38. Majka SM, Beutz MA, Hagen M, et al. Identification of novel resident pulmonary stem cells: form and function of the lung side population. Stem Cells 2005;23:1073–81.
39. Martin J, Helm K, Ruegg P, et al. Adult lung side population cells have mesenchymal stem cell potential. Cytotherapy 2008;10:140–51.
40. Reynolds SD, Shen H, Reynolds PR, et al. Molecular and functional properties of lung SP cells. Am J Physiol Lung Cell Mol Physiol 2007;292:L972–83.
41. McQualter JL, Brouard N, Williams B, et al. Endogenous fibroblastic progenitor cells in the adult mouse lung are highly enriched in the sca-1 positive cell fraction. Stem Cells 2009;27:623–33.
42. Herzog EL, Chai L, Krause DS. Plasticity of marrow-derived stem cells. Blood 2003;102:3483–93.
43. Liebler JM, Lutzko C, Banfalvi A, et al. Retention of human bone marrow-derived cells in murine lungs following bleomycin-induced lung injury. Am J Physiol Lung Cell Mol Physiol 2008;295:L285–92.
44. Rojas M, Xu J, Woods CR, et al. Bone marrow-derived mesenchymal stem cells in repair of the injured lung. Am J Respir Cell Mol Biol 2005;33:145–52.
45. Kotton DN, Fine A. Lung stem cells. Cell Tissue Res 2008;331:145–56.
46. Neuringer IP, Randell SH. Stem cells and repair of lung injuries. Respir Res 2004;5:6.
47. Thebaud B, Abman SH. Bronchopulmonary dysplasia—where have all the vessels gone? Roles of angiogenic growth factors in chronic lung disease. Am J Respir Crit Care Med 2007;175:978–85.
48. Alvarez DF, Huang L, King JA, et al. Lung microvascular endothelium is enriched with progenitor cells that exhibit vasculogenic capacity. Am J Physiol Lung Cell Mol Physiol 2008;294:L419–30.
49. Alphonse RS, Vadivel A, Waszak P, et al. Existence, functional impairment and therapeutic potential of endothelial colony forming cells (ECFCS) in oxygen-induced arrested alveolar growth. Am J Respir Crit Care Med 2011;183:A1237.
50. Balasubramaniam V, Mervis CF, Maxey AM, et al. Hyperoxia reduces bone marrow, circulating, and lung endothelial progenitor cells in the developing lung: implications for the pathogenesis of bronchopulmonary dysplasia. Am J Physiol Lung Cell Mol Physiol 2007;292:L1073–84.
51. Irwin D, Helm K, Campbell N, et al. Neonatal lung side population cells demonstrate endothelial potential and are altered in response to hyperoxia-induced lung simplification. Am J Physiol Lung Cell Mol Physiol 2007;293:L941–51.
52. van Haaften T, Byrne R, Bonnet S, et al. Airway delivery of mesenchymal stem cells prevents arrested alveolar growth in neonatal lung injury in rats. Am J Respir Crit Care Med 2009;180:1131–42.
53. Tropea KA, Leder E, Aslam M, et al. Bronchoalveolar stem cells increase after mesenchymal stromal cell treatment in a mouse model of bronchopulmonary dysplasia. Am J Physiol Lung Cell Mol Physiol 2012;302(9):L829–37.
54. Popova AP, Bozyk PD, Bentley JK, et al. Isolation of tracheal aspirate mesenchymal stromal cells predicts bronchopulmonary dysplasia. Pediatrics 2010;126:e1127–33.

55. Hennrick KT, Keeton AG, Nanua S, et al. Lung cells from neonates show a mesenchymal stem cell phenotype. Am J Respir Crit Care Med 2007;175: 1158–64.

56. Popova AP, Bozyk PD, Goldsmith AM, et al. Autocrine production of TGF-beta1 promotes myofibroblastic differentiation of neonatal lung mesenchymal stem cells. Am J Physiol Lung Cell Mol Physiol 2010;298:L735–43.

57. Pierro M, Thebaud B. Mesenchymal stem cells in chronic lung disease: culprit or savior? Am J Physiol Lung Cell Mol Physiol 2010;298:L732–4.

58. Baker CD, Ryan SL, Ingram DA, et al. Endothelial colony-forming cells from preterm infants are increased and more susceptible to hyperoxia. Am J Respir Crit Care Med 2009;180:454–61.

59. Borghesi A, Massa M, Campanelli R, et al. Circulating endothelial progenitor cells in preterm infants with bronchopulmonary dysplasia. Am J Respir Crit Care Med 2009;180:540–6.

60. Paviotti G, Fadini GP, Boscaro E, et al. Endothelial progenitor cells, bronchopulmonary dysplasia and other short-term outcomes of extremely preterm birth. Early Hum Dev 2011;87:461–5.

61. Dominici M, Le Blanc K, Mueller I, et al. Minimal criteria for defining multipotent mesenchymal stromal cells. The International Society for Cellular Therapy position statement. Cytotherapy 2006;8:315–7.

62. Helmy KY, Patel SA, Silverio K, et al. Stem cells and regenerative medicine: accomplishments to date and future promise. Ther Deliv 2010;1: 693–705.

63. Horwitz EM, Prockop DJ, Fitzpatrick LA, et al. Transplantability and therapeutic effects of bone marrow-derived mesenchymal cells in children with osteogenesis imperfecta. Nat Med 1999;5:309–13.

64. Vats A, Bielby RC, Tolley NS, et al. Stem cells. Lancet 2005;366:592–602.

65. Agostini C. Stem cell therapy for chronic lung diseases: hope and reality. Respir Med 2010;104(Suppl 1):S86–91.

66. Blaisdell CJ, Gail DB, Nabel EG. National Heart, Lung, and Blood Institute perspective: lung progenitor and stem cells—gaps in knowledge and future opportunities. Stem Cells 2009;27:2263–70.

67. Sueblinvong V, Weiss DJ. Stem cells and cell therapy approaches in lung biology and diseases. Transl Res 2010;156:188–205.

68. Lee JW, Gupta N, Serikov V, et al. Potential application of mesenchymal stem cells in acute lung injury. Expert Opin Biol Ther 2009;9:1259–70.

69. Weiss DJ, Bertoncello I, Borok Z, et al. Stem cells and cell therapies in lung biology and lung diseases. Proc Am Thorac Soc 2011;8:223–72.

70. Aslam M, Baveja R, Liang OD, et al. Bone marrow stromal cells attenuate lung injury in a murine model of neonatal chronic lung disease. Am J Respir Crit Care Med 2009;180:1122–30.

71. Zhang X, Wang H, Shi Y, et al. The role of bone marrow-derived mesenchymal stem cells in the prevention of hyperoxia-induced lung injury in newborn mice. Cell Biol Int 2012;36(6):589–94.

72. Chang YS, Choi SJ, Sung DK, et al. Intratracheal transplantation of human umbilical cord blood derived mesenchymal stem cells dose-dependently attenuates hyperoxia-induced lung injury in neonatal rats. Cell Transplant 2011. [Epub ahead of print].

73. Chang YS, Oh W, Choi SJ, et al. Human umbilical cord blood-derived mesenchymal stem cells attenuate hyperoxia-induced lung injury in neonatal rats. Cell Transplant 2009;18:869–86.

74. Balasubramaniam V, Ryan SL, Seedorf GJ, et al. Bone marrow-derived angiogenic cells restore lung alveolar and vascular structure after neonatal hyperoxia in infant mice. Am J Physiol Lung Cell Mol Physiol 2010;298: L315–23.

75. Vosdoganes P, Hodges RJ, Lim R, et al. Human amnion epithelial cells as a treatment for inflammation-induced fetal lung injury in sheep. Am J Obstet Gynecol 2011;205:156.e26–33.

76. Till JE, McCulloch E. A direct measurement of the radiation sensitivity of normal mouse bone marrow cells. Radiat Res 1961;14:213–22.

77. Northway WH Jr, Rosan RC, Porter DY. Pulmonary disease following respirator therapy of hyaline-membrane disease. Bronchopulmonary dysplasia. N Engl J Med 1967;276:357–68.

78. Ling TY, Kuo MD, Li CL, et al. Identification of pulmonary Oct-4+ stem/progenitor cells and demonstration of their susceptibility to SARS coronavirus (SARS-CoV) infection in vitro. Proc Natl Acad Sci U S A 2006;103:9530–5.

79. Wang D, Morales JE, Calame DG, et al. Transplantation of human embryonic stem cell-derived alveolar epithelial type II cells abrogates acute lung injury in mice. Mol Ther 2010;18:625–34.

80. Kumamoto M, Nishiwaki T, Matsuo N, et al. Minimally cultured bone marrow mesenchymal stem cells ameliorate fibrotic lung injury. Eur Respir J 2009;34: 740–8.

81. Ortiz LA, Dutreil M, Fattman C, et al. Interleukin 1 receptor antagonist mediates the antiinflammatory and antifibrotic effect of mesenchymal stem cells during lung injury. Proc Natl Acad Sci U S A 2007;104:11002–7.

82. Moodley Y, Atienza D, Manuelpillai U, et al. Human umbilical cord mesenchymal stem cells reduce fibrosis of bleomycin-induced lung injury. Am J Pathol 2009; 175:303–13.

83. Aguilar S, Scotton CJ, McNulty K, et al. Bone marrow stem cells expressing keratinocyte growth factor via an inducible lentivirus protects against bleomycin-induced pulmonary fibrosis. PLoS One 2009;4:e8013.

84. Murphy S, Lim R, Dickinson H, et al. Human amnion epithelial cells prevent bleomycin-induced lung injury and preserve lung function. Cell Transplant 2011;20:909–23.

85. Gupta N, Su X, Popov B, et al. Intrapulmonary delivery of bone marrow-derived mesenchymal stem cells improves survival and attenuates endotoxin-induced acute lung injury in mice. J Immunol 2007;179:1855–63.

86. Iyer SS, Torres-Gonzalez E, Neujahr DC, et al. Effect of bone marrow-derived mesenchymal stem cells on endotoxin-induced oxidation of plasma cysteine and glutathione in mice. Stem Cells Int 2010;2010:868076.

87. Xu J, Woods CR, Mora AL, et al. Prevention of endotoxin-induced systemic response by bone marrow-derived mesenchymal stem cells in mice. Am J Physiol Lung Cell Mol Physiol 2007;293:L131–41.

88. Yang KY, Shih HC, How CK, et al. IV delivery of induced pluripotent stem cells attenuates endotoxin-induced acute lung injury in mice. Chest 2011;140: 1243–53.

89. Mei SH, McCarter SD, Deng Y, et al. Prevention of LPS-induced acute lung injury in mice by mesenchymal stem cells overexpressing angiopoietin 1. PLoS Med 2007;4:e269.

90. Xu J, Qu J, Cao L, et al. Mesenchymal stem cell-based angiopoietin-1 gene therapy for acute lung injury induced by lipopolysaccharide in mice. J Pathol 2008;214:472–81.

91. Kim ES, Chang YS, Choi SJ, et al. Intratracheal transplantation of human umbilical cord blood-derived mesenchymal stem cells attenuates *Escherichia coli*-induced acute lung injury in mice. Respir Res 2011;12:108.

92. Chien MH, Bien MY, Ku CC, et al. Systemic human orbital fat-derived stem/stromal cell transplantation ameliorates acute inflammation in lipopolysaccharide-induced acute lung injury. Crit Care Med 2012;40:1245–53.

93. Lam CF, Roan JN, Lee CH, et al. Transplantation of endothelial progenitor cells improves pulmonary endothelial function and gas exchange in rabbits with endotoxin-induced acute lung injury. Anesth Analg 2011;112:620–7.

94. Sun J, Han ZB, Liao W, et al. Intrapulmonary delivery of human umbilical cord mesenchymal stem cells attenuates acute lung injury by expanding CD4+CD25+ Forkhead Boxp3 (FOXP3)+ regulatory T cells and balancing anti- and pro-inflammatory factors. Cell Physiol Biochem 2011;27:587–96.

95. Gao X, Chen W, Liang Z, et al. Autotransplantation of circulating endothelial progenitor cells protects against lipopolysaccharide-induced acute lung injury in rabbit. Int Immunopharmacol 2011;11:1584–90.

96. Curley GF, Hayes M, Ansari B, et al. Mesenchymal stem cells enhance recovery and repair following ventilator-induced lung injury in the rat. Thorax 2012;67(6): 496–501.

97. Baber SR, Deng W, Master RG, et al. Intratracheal mesenchymal stem cell administration attenuates monocrotaline-induced pulmonary hypertension and endothelial dysfunction. Am J Physiol Heart Circ Physiol 2007;292: H1120–8.

98. Kanki-Horimoto S, Horimoto H, Mieno S, et al. Implantation of mesenchymal stem cells overexpressing endothelial nitric oxide synthase improves right ventricular impairments caused by pulmonary hypertension. Circulation 2006; 114:I181–5.

99. Raoul W, Wagner-Ballon O, Saber G, et al. Effects of bone marrow-derived cells on monocrotaline- and hypoxia-induced pulmonary hypertension in mice. Respir Res 2007;8:8.

100. Umar S, de Visser YP, Steendijk P, et al. Allogenic stem cell therapy improves right ventricular function by improving lung pathology in rats with pulmonary hypertension. Am J Physiol Heart Circ Physiol 2009;297:H1606–16.

101. Zhao YD, Courtman DW, Deng Y, et al. Rescue of monocrotaline-induced pulmonary arterial hypertension using bone marrow-derived endothelial-like progenitor cells: efficacy of combined cell and eNOS gene therapy in established disease. Circ Res 2005;96:442–50.

102. Takahashi M, Nakamura T, Toba T, et al. Transplantation of endothelial progenitor cells into the lung to alleviate pulmonary hypertension in dogs. Tissue Eng 2004; 10:771–9.

103. Cho KS, Park HK, Park HY, et al. IFATS collection: immunomodulatory effects of adipose tissue-derived stem cells in an allergic rhinitis mouse model. Stem Cells 2009;27:259–65.

104. Park HK, Cho KS, Park HY, et al. Adipose-derived stromal cells inhibit allergic airway inflammation in mice. Stem Cells Dev 2010;19:1811–8.

105. Firinci F, Karaman M, Baran Y, et al. Mesenchymal stem cells ameliorate the histopathological changes in a murine model of chronic asthma. Int Immunopharmacol 2011;11:1120–6.

106. Ou-Yang HF, Huang Y, Hu XB, et al. Suppression of allergic airway inflammation in a mouse model of asthma by exogenous mesenchymal stem cells. Exp Biol Med (Maywood) 2011;236:1461–7.

107. Ionescu LI, Alphonse RS, Arizmendi N, et al. Airway delivery of soluble factors from plastic-adherent bone marrow cells prevents murine asthma. Am J Respir Cell Mol Biol 2012;46:207–16.

108. Nemeth K, Keane-Myers A, Brown JM, et al. Bone marrow stromal cells use TGF-beta to suppress allergic responses in a mouse model of ragweed-induced asthma. Proc Natl Acad Sci U S A 2010;107:5652–7.

109. Huh JW, Kim SY, Lee JH, et al. Bone marrow cells repair cigarette smoke-induced emphysema in rats. Am J Physiol Lung Cell Mol Physiol 2011;301:L255–66.

110. Zhen G, Liu H, Gu N, et al. Mesenchymal stem cells transplantation protects against rat pulmonary emphysema. Front Biosci 2008;13:3415–22.

111. Shigemura N, Okumura M, Mizuno S, et al. Lung tissue engineering technique with adipose stromal cells improves surgical outcome for pulmonary emphysema. Am J Respir Crit Care Med 2006;174:1199–205.

112. Shigemura N, Okumura M, Mizuno S, et al. Autologous transplantation of adipose tissue-derived stromal cells ameliorates pulmonary emphysema. Am J Transplant 2006;6:2592–600.

113. Katsha AM, Ohkouchi S, Xin H, et al. Paracrine factors of multipotent stromal cells ameliorate lung injury in an elastase-induced emphysema model. Mol Ther 2011;19:196–203.

114. Hegab AE, Kubo H, Fujino N, et al. Isolation and characterization of murine multipotent lung stem cells. Stem Cells Dev 2010;19:523–36.

Brain Injury in Chronically Ventilated Preterm Neonates
Collateral Damage Related to Ventilation Strategy

Kurt H. Albertine, PhD[a,b,c,*]

KEYWORDS

- White matter injury • Gray matter injury • Bronchopulmonary dysplasia
- Neonatal chronic lung disease

KEY POINTS

- Brain injury is a frequent comorbidity in chronically ventilated preterm infants. However, the molecular basis of the brain injury remains incompletely understood.
- This article focuses on the subtle (diffuse) form of brain injury that has white matter and gray matter lesions, without germinal matrix hemorrhage–intraventricular hemorrhage, posthemorrhagic hydrocephalus, or cystic periventricular leukomalacia.
- This article synthesizes data that suggest that diffuse lesions to white matter and gray matter are collateral damage related to ventilator strategy.
- Evidence is introduced from the 2 large-animal, physiologic models of evolving neonatal chronic lung disease that suggest that an epigenetic mechanism may underlie the collateral damage.

INTRODUCTION

The brain of chronically ventilated preterm infants is vulnerable to injury during the days, weeks, or months of ventilation support with oxygen-rich gas that are necessary to keep them alive.[1] Familiar lesions are germinal matrix hemorrhage–intraventricular hemorrhage, posthemorrhagic hydrocephalus, or periventricular leukomalacia, particularly with parenchymal cysts.[2] These gross histopathologic lesions are not the focus of this article. This article focuses on more subtle diffuse lesions that lead to abnormal neural function and subsequent suboptimal neurodevelopmental outcome.

Portions of this work were supported by NIH grants HL062875 and HL110002.
Dr Albertine has no conflicts of interest to disclose.
[a] Department of Pediatrics, University of Utah School of Medicine, Salt Lake City, UT 84158, USA; [b] Department of Medicine, University of Utah School of Medicine, Salt Lake City, UT 84158, USA; [c] Department of Neurobiology & Anatomy, University of Utah School of Medicine, Salt Lake City, UT 84158, USA
* Department of Pediatrics, University of Utah, PO Box 581289, Williams Building, Salt Lake City, UT 84158-1289.
E-mail address: kurt.albertine@hsc.utah.edu

Diffuse lesions to white matter and gray matter are recognized among chronically ventilated preterm infants.[3] Diffuse white matter lesions within the first week of life are characterized histopathologically at autopsy as palely stained and soft regions of degeneration of white matter and thinning of the corpus callosum. Gray matter lesions also occur.[4] Gray matter lesions are characterized by diffuse neuronal loss in deeper cerebral cortical layers, the hippocampus, thalamus, globus pallidus, and cerebellar Purkinje cell layers in the dentate nucleus.[4] A mixture of diffuse white and gray matter lesions presumably contributes to subtler delays and/or deficits in neurodevelopment and impairments in motor skills, learning disabilities, attention deficit/hyperactivity disorders, and/or anxiety disorders in former preterm children.[3,5]

Subtler adverse neurodevelopmental outcomes affect the health and quality of life of the survivors and their families. The outcomes also increase the cost for health care borne by the families and society. Therefore, diffuse brain injury in chronically ventilated preterm neonates is a significant national public health issue.

In spite of increasing recognition of diffuse lesions to white matter and gray matter in chronically ventilated preterm infants, the molecular basis of the lesions remains incompletely understood. This article synthesizes data that suggest that ventilator strategy leads to collateral white and gray matter lesions. Evidence is introduced later to suggest that an epigenetic mechanism may underlie the collateral damage.

PREMATURITY AS THE SETTING FOR COLLATERAL DAMAGE TO THE BRAIN

Prematurity contributes to about a third of all infant deaths in the United States.[6] Mortality is greatest among infants born at or before 25 weeks of gestation (http://www.nichd.nih.gov/about/org/cdbpm/pp/prog_epbo/epbo_case.cfm).

Infants born prematurely are at risk of acute respiratory distress or failure because the future gas-exchange regions of the lung are not developed structurally. The relative or absolute absence of surfactant contributes to collapse of the distal airspaces (atelectasis), which contributes to functional mismatch of ventilation and perfusion that impairs gas exchange.[7]

Two treatments are used routinely for anticipated preterm birth and subsequent respiratory distress. One treatment is antenatal corticosteroid administration to the mother who is in premature labor. The objective of administering antenatal corticosteroids is to stimulate production of endogenous surfactant in the fetus.[8] The other treatment is postnatal surfactant replacement to the preterm infant.[9] The intended consequence of these treatments is to reduce surface tension and thereby increase lung compliance and gas exchange.[10–13] Preterm infants with larger surfactant pools are likely to be supported by nasal continuous positive airway pressure (nasal CPAP). The rationale for using nasal CPAP is to avoid or minimize endotracheal intubation and positive pressure ventilation support.[14–17] However, when nasal CPAP is insufficient, the remedy is endotracheal intubation and positive pressure ventilation using an oxygen-rich gas mixture. High inflation pressure and mean airway pressure may be necessary to recruit the collapsed distal airspaces to achieve ventilation and oxygenation targets. Infants who do not recover from acute respiratory distress and require prolonged positive pressure ventilation with oxygen-rich gas are predisposed to develop neonatal chronic lung disease (also called bronchopulmonary dysplasia [BPD] or the so-called "new" BPD).[18,19]

VULNERABILITY OF THE IMMATURE BRAIN IN CHRONICALLY VENTILATED PRETERM NEONATES

Vulnerability for collateral damage to the brain is related in part to the width of the developmental window and the types of developmental processes that occur within the window. The developmental window of vulnerability is 22 to 36 weeks of gestation (**Table 1**). The types of developmental processes during this window include proliferation, differentiation, and migration of neurons and glia. During the same period, neuronal circuits develop as synapses form and synaptic connections are optimized through a process of synaptic stabilization. Functional circuits become evident as spontaneous electroencephalographic bursts.[20–25] A structural manifestation of these processes occurs in the subplate layer of neurons, which attains maximal thickness around the 36th week of gestation. Cortical folding also occurs during this developmental window. From 28 weeks of gestation to postnatally after term gestation, the earlier exuberant proliferation of neurons and glia is pruned by apoptosis to optimize their numbers. Myelination occurs from the 36th week of gestation to 2 to 3 years postnatally.

Details regarding development of the cerebral circulation are incomplete. The cerebral circulation expands during the period of 22 to 36 weeks of gestation (see **Table 1**). However, blood vessel formation lags in deep regions, including the germinal matrix, periventricular white matter, corpus callosum, and deep gray matter structures such as the basal ganglia and hippocampus.[26] The lag in blood vessel formation in deep regions of the brain is part of the basis of the watershed explanation of vulnerability of germinal matrix, periventricular white matter, and deep cortical gray matter. Developmental immaturity of the blood-brain barrier also creates vulnerability for circulating toxic molecules to access the brain parenchyma.[25,27]

Table 1
Timing of structural development of the human brain

Time from Conception	Developmental Process	References
3–4 wk	Formation of neuroectoderm	77
3–4 wk	Primary neurulation	77–79
5–10 wk	Formation of prosencephalon and hemispheres	77
5–10 wk, potentially to years postnatally	Cerebral angiogenesis and formation of the blood-brain barrier	80
7–10 wk	Generation of the subplate layer of neurons (from germinal matrix)	81
10–15 wk, potentially to years postnatally	Neurogenesis	77
12–24 wk	Neuronal migration	77,82–86
16–24 wk	Blood vessel density in subcortical white matter is low	87
20 wk, potentially to years postnatally	Synaptogenesis and synaptic stabilization	43,44,88
20 wk, potentially to years postnatally	Gliogenesis	77,89–91
22–36 wk	Maximal thickness of the subplate layer of neurons (from germinal matrix) is reached	81
23–29 wk	Cortical folding and spontaneous EEG bursts; δ brushes	20–24
28–36 wk	Blood vessel density in deep white matter is low	87,92
28 wk, potentially to years postnatally	Neuronal and glial apoptosis	77
36 wk, potentially to years postnatally	Myelination	77,89

The immature brain is vulnerable to fluctuations in systemic blood pressure.[28–30] Fluctuations are dangerous because of the immaturity of autoregulation, which may expose the brain to increased or decreased blood pressure, a characteristic that is said to be pressure passive. For example, systemic hypotension combined with a pressure-passive cerebral circulation may lead to hypoxic ischemia (hypoperfusion) of white matter and/or gray matter.[31–33] A subsequent vulnerability may be reperfusion injury, particularly in association with systemic hypertension.[3,6,28,29,34–42] Another cerebrovascular vulnerability is increased intrathoracic pressure in preterm infants who are intubated and ventilated or who develop a pneumothorax. Increased intrathoracic pressure may affect cerebral perfusion pressure and/or flow.[43,44]

Molecules that participate in brain injury are numerous. Inflammatory cytokines and chemokines, with or without infection, are participants.[45–48] Their participation, in part, is mediated by platelet and neutrophil adhesion in cerebral blood vessels.[49,50] Other molecular participants are reactive species of oxygen or nitrogen that are generated during reperfusion following hypoxia-ischemia.[49,51] In addition, expression of growth factors is reduced, notably insulin-like growth factor-1 (IGF-1).[52,53] IGF-1 is emphasized here because its regulation of expression is relevant to an epigenetic hypothesis that is proposed later in this article.

Developmental processes that are vulnerable in the brain are summarized in **Table 2**. The vulnerabilities include germinal matrix injury, diffuse white matter injury, and diffuse gray matter injury.

COLLATERAL DAMAGE TO THE BRAIN RELATED TO VENTILATION STRATEGY: AN EPIGENETIC HYPOTHESIS

A trend in the last decade is the initial use of nasal CPAP or early extubation to nasal CPAP. The rationale is to reduce the primary injury to the preterm infant's lungs and

Table 2
Vulnerability of the brain of preterm neonates

Time from Conception	Developmental Process	Vulnerability	References
10–15 wk, potentially to years postnatally	Neurogenesis		
12–24 wk	Neuronal migration		
16–24 wk	Low vessel density in subcortical white matter	Germinal matrix injury	91,93,94
20 wk, potentially to years postnatally	Synaptogenesis and synaptic stabilization		
20 wk, potentially to years postnatally	Gliogenesis		
22–36 wk	Maximal thickness of the subplate layer of neurons (from germinal matrix) is reached	Diffuse white matter lesions (periventricular leukomalacia)	5,87,92,93,95–102
28–36 wk	Blood vessel density in deep white matter is low		
28 wk, potentially to years postnatally	Neuronal and glial apoptosis		
36 wk, potentially to years postnatally	Myelination	Diffuse gray matter lesions	93,103,104

secondary injury to other organs, notably the brain. However, the impact of ventilation strategy on mechanisms of pathogenesis of brain injury in preterm neonates remains uncertain. To this end, insights are being gained using large-animal, physiologic models of neonatal chronic lung disease in which brain injury is an accompaniment. The models share the common feature of brain injury without intraventricular hemorrhage or cystic periventricular leukomalacia.

Preterm Baboon Model

Brain injury occurs in preterm baboons that have evolving neonatal chronic lung disease. An experiment compared brain injury outcomes when the preterm baboons were weaned from mechanical ventilation to nasal CPAP.[54] One group was weaned at 24 hours of life (early nasal CPAP); the other starting at 5 days of life (delayed nasal CPAP). The principal results showed brain injury in both nasal CPAP groups compared with fetal lambs that were not ventilated. In both groups, brain injury was diffuse, without hemorrhage or cystic infarction, and affected white matter and gray matter. The results secondarily showed that injury severity was less in the early nasal CPAP group compared with the delayed nasal CPAP group. The latter result suggests that duration of mechanical ventilation is directly related to brain injury. The molecular mechanisms of these pathologic changes were not part of the study.

Preterm Lamb Model

We use chronically ventilated preterm lambs to identify molecular mechanisms that are involved in injury to multiple organs, notably the lung and brain. Our studies led us to propose an epigenetic hypothesis for the pathogenesis of neonatal chronic lung disease and its associated comorbidities, including brain injury.

We focus on epigenetics because of their role in fetal and perinatal adaptation.[55,56] Epigenetic regulation of gene expression in the perinatal period is associated with readjustment in gene expression in response to changes in environment.[57] For example, intrauterine growth restriction, which predisposes to preterm labor and delivery, is associated with reduced levels of IGF-1 in the liver of rat pups.[58] In addition, many of the affected epigenetic characteristics persist postnatally, in conjunction with persistently less IGF-1 mRNA and protein levels. Does the same hold true in chronically ventilated preterm lambs? Before answering that question, concepts about epigenetics are provided.

Epigenetic regulation of gene expression uses modifications to chromatin, the unit of which is the nucleosome. Nucleosomes have 146 bp of DNA wrapped around an octomeric core of histone proteins.[59] The modifications constitute an epigenetic code for regulation of gene expression by directing interactions between transcription complexes with DNA. Because the interactions are dynamic, transcriptional levels of proteins are adjusted and readjusted over time, including long term (lifelong).

Epigenetic regulation of gene expression can use several mechanisms, including histone modifications, DNA methylation, microRNAs, and nucleosome positioning.[60,61] Histone modifications consist of acetylation, methylation, phosphorylation, and ubiquitination. Enzymes that add histone modifications include histone acetylases and methyltransferases.[62] Enzymes that take away histone modifications include histone deacetylases (HDACs) and demethylases. DNA methylation occurs on a cytosine base where cytosine precedes, and is linked to a guanosine by phosphate. Therefore, the modification is referred to as methylation of CpG. Methylation involves DNA methyltransferases.[60] Methyl-cytosine demethylation involves the ten-eleven translocation (Tet) gene family.[63,64] These enzymatic processes seem biologically to be coordinated dynamically.[65] MicroRNAs, short RNA molecules that do not code for a protein, silence target genes by binding to their 3′ untranslated regions.[66] Nucleosome positioning regulates gene transcription by exposing or not exposing transcription start sites to transcription complexes and RNA polymerase, as described later in this article. Understanding how these processes are regulated and dysregulated is necessary to identify their roles in health and disease.

The dynamic nature of epigenetics is complex, making generalizations difficult when comparing one cell type with another, one organ with another, one species with another, along the continuum of developmental processes, and among diseases. Difficulty is even greater in the in vivo context, in which interplay among epigenetic, genetic, physiologic, and pathophysiologic processes occurs dynamically in the setting of a whole organism.[67] Although daunting, testing epigenetic hypotheses in vivo, using large-animal models of human disease, and in humans, is necessary to translate epigenetic concepts and principles to understand the epigenetic basis of human health and disease.

Our recent work suggests that epigenetic characteristics in the brain are affected in chronically ventilated preterm lambs with evolving neonatal chronic lung disease (unpublished data). Highlights of some of these studies are summarized from 2 perspectives of epigenetic characteristics: (1) genome-wide and (2) candidate-gene–specific epigenetic characteristics. Comparative results are highlighted for the brain and lung from the same preterm lambs.

Genome-wide epigenetic characteristics

Some clinical evidence suggests that nasal CPAP reduces the risk for premature infants to develop neonatal chronic lung disease and its comorbidities.[17] However, the biologic basis for the different outcomes is not known. To address this unknown, we are pursuing studies in chronically ventilated preterm lambs. One study is assessing genome-wide epigenetic characteristics in the brain (and lung) of preterm lambs that are supported by either positive pressure ventilation or a version of bubble nasal CPAP that delivers high-frequency ventilation (HFV) at the level of the nose (nasal HFV).[68]

We measure levels of several histone modifications in homogenates of brain and lung tissue. For example, lower levels of genome-wide acetylation of histone 3 lysine 14 (H3K14ac) occurred in the brain and lung of mechanically ventilated preterm lambs compared with preterm lambs supported by nasal HFV. Another histone modification that we measured is trimethylated H3K36 (H3K36me^3). Lower levels of H3K36me^3 are detected in the mechanically ventilated group compared with the nasal HFV group. These initial results suggest that ventilation strategy affects genome-wide histone covalent modifications.

Gene-specific epigenetic characteristics

A limitation of our studies is that the results do not identify an epigenetically regulated gene as a molecular culprit. An alternative approach is to test the participation of a candidate gene in vivo.

Our current research efforts are focusing on IGF-1 as a prototypic, epigenetically regulated gene.[57,58] Our rationale is a follows. First, IGF-1 is involved in brain and lung development.[69] Second, IGF-1 expression is increased in the lung of preterm infants who died during acute respiratory distress or neonatal chronic lung disease.[70] Whether IGF-1 expression is affected in the brain of chronically ventilated preterm infants remains to be determined. IGF-1 expression is decreased in the brain in other models of perinatal insult in which growth is disrupted and adverse long-term neurodevelopmental outcomes are detected.[71,72] Together, these characteristics make the

IGF-1 gene a candidate to study in the context of brain vulnerability to injury in chronically ventilated preterm lambs.

Our initial results suggest that IGF-1 expression is affected in the brain and lung of ventilated preterm lambs. For example, the brain of mechanically ventilated preterm lambs seems to have lower IGF-1 protein levels compared with preterm lambs supported by nasal HFV. Lower levels of IGF-1 protein in the brain are consistent with the reduction that occurs in other models of perinatal insult, such as intrauterine growth restriction.[58,71] In the same preterm lambs, the lung seems to have higher levels of IGF-1 protein in the mechanically ventilated group compared with the nasal HFV group. Increased IGF-1 in the lung of the mechanically ventilated preterm lambs is consistent with results obtained at autopsy of preterm infants who died with respiratory failure.[70]

Finding less IGF-1 protein in the brain, and more in the lung, in mechanically ventilated preterm lambs prompted us to ask how the changes may occur. As a start, we are determining the pattern of histone modifications (the histone code) along the length of the IGF-1 gene locus in sheep. The rationale for assessing the histone code is that its pattern plays a prominent role in regulating gene transcription.[57,58,71] Chromatin is condensed in the heterochromatic state. When chromatin is condensed, access of transcription complexes to transcription start sites is blocked physically by close packing of nucleosomes (**Fig. 1**A). For transcription to be initiated, the chromatin has to open, forming euchromatin. Opening chromatin, and therefore permitting transcription, is mediated in part by acetylation of histones. As acetylation occurs, open space is created upstream of a transcription start site or sites by unraveling a nucleosome, creating a nucleosome-free zone (see **Fig. 1**B). The open space provides access for transcription complexes to bind to the exposed transcription start site. The converse is that eventual silencing to reduce or stop transcription occurs when other histones are methylated, especially trimethylated. A consequence of increasing trimethylation of histones is decreasing acetylation of histones. This reciprocal shift is thought to help condense the chromatin along the body of the gene to prevent inappropriate transcription initiation from occurring downstream of the designated transcription start site.

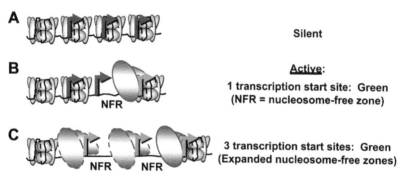

A   **Silent**

B   <u>**Active**</u>:
                                         1 transcription start site: Green
                          NFR   **(NFR = nucleosome-free zone)**

C   **3 transcription start sites: Green**
                  NFR   NFR   **(Expanded nucleosome-free zones)**

Fig. 1. Transcription start sites in a promoter region. (*A*) Transcriptionally silent promoter. Transcription start sites are shown in red because they are covered by nucleosomes and therefore are not accessible to transcription complexes. (*B*) Transcriptionally active promoter. A nucleosome-free region (NFR) is shown, where a nucleosome is displaced, exposing a transcription start site (*green*). A transcription complex (*ovals*) is shown immediately upstream to the exposed (*green*) transcription start site, where access is available for RNA polymerase. (*C*) Transcription is potentially enhanced by expanded nucleosome-free zones, which expose 3 transcription start sites to RNA polymerase.

With the aforementioned outline of the process of epigenetic regulation of gene expression in mind, what might be the explanation for the results in the brain and lung of preterm lambs, depending on ventilation strategy? First, the scenario is hypothetical. That is, we do not have direct cause-and-effect evidence. Taking into account that epigenetic regulation is organ specific and that every cell has the same genetic information, but each organ develops uniquely, we hypothesize that uniqueness is conferred by cell-specific or cell-specific and organ-specific epigenetic regulation. We specifically hypothesize that genome-wide hypoacetylation in the brain shifts the balance toward more apoptosis, and less proliferation of astrocytes and oligodendrocytes (Alvord, unpublished data). Reduced numbers of both types of glia would decrease IGF-1 locally in the brain because astrocytes and oligodendrocytes synthesize and secrete IGF-1.[73-76]

How might more IGF-1 in the lung of the same chronically ventilated preterm lambs be explained, given that the lung also has genome-wide histone hypoacetylation? We propose that lung-specific epigenetic mechanisms may lead to more expression of pulmonary IGF-1. One mechanism is that the source of IGF-1 mRNA and protein in the lung is mesenchymal cells.[70] We showed that mesenchymal cell proliferation exceeds apoptosis in the walls of the distal airspaces of preterm lambs that are supported by mechanical ventilation compared with nasal HFV.[68] Another possibility is that mechanical ventilation may lead to promiscuous transcription of IGF-1 in the lung. To explain this hypothesis, attention is drawn again to **Fig. 1**. **Fig. 1**C depicts several transcription start sites that are uncovered because numerous nucleosomes are absent (nucleosome-free zones). We have new preliminary data to suggest that ventilation of preterm lambs exposes multiple transcription start sites for IGF-1 in the lung. By comparison, only 1 site seems to be used in the lung of fetal lambs that are not allowed to breathe. We propose that exposure of more transcription start sites across a longer length of the gene locus upstream of promoter 1 may contribute to more IGF-1 transcription in the lung of chronically ventilated preterm lambs. Other epigenetic mechanisms may also influence gene expression, such as regulation of elongation and/or termination of transcription. Such potential epigenetic mechanisms need to be investigated.

A hypothesis that remains to be tested is whether early changes in the histone code provide a survival advantage (adaptation) in the short run but also exact a cost later in life, the cost being vulnerability to subsequent insults and/or the onset of adult diseases. Testing this hypothesis will be important because survival advantage in the short term may create vulnerability to disease (eg, tumor formation), to subsequent insults later in life (eg, recurrent respiratory tract infections), and/or to adult-onset diseases (eg, obesity, diabetes, cardiovascular disease). To this end, our newest studies use a modified protocol whereby preterm lambs are weaned from ventilation support and fostered for the equivalent of 2 years or 6 to 8 years of postnatal life in humans. The intention of these new studies is to correlate epigenetic characteristics of gene regulation with long-term neurodevelopmental delays and deficits among former preterm, ventilated lambs.

A histone modification–specific transgene construct will be necessary to definitively show that a specific epigenetic modification causes a specific phenotype.

SUMMARY

Structural and functional immaturity of a preterm neonate's lung necessitates the use of antenatal steroids, postnatal surfactant replacement therapy, postnatal ventilation support with oxygen-rich gas, and other measures to keep the neonate alive. Acute lung injury often ensues. If recovery from acute lung injury does not happen, endotracheal intubation and prolonged positive pressure ventilation support with oxygen-rich gas may be necessary, leading to neonatal chronic lung disease. A frequent comorbidity of evolving neonatal chronic lung disease is brain injury. However, the molecular basis of the brain injury remains incompletely understood. This void is addressed by the use of large-animal, physiologic models of brain injury in the setting of evolving neonatal chronic lung disease. An advantage of the chronically ventilated preterm baboon and lamb models is that the setting of preterm birth is uncomplicated by antenatal conditions, such as intrauterine infection or asphyxia, that may potentiate brain injury. Also, neither chronic model is associated with intraventricular hemorrhage or cystic lesions of periventricular white matter, so drawing mechanistic conclusions is more straightforward. However, the less complicated setting for the large-animal models may be thought to be a disadvantage because the models lack antenatal conditions that may potentiate injury to the lung and brain. Nonetheless, new mechanistic insights are being provided by the chronic animal models. In particular, involvement of epigenetics in the pathogenesis of lung and brain injury creates new scope for mechanistic studies that may provide opportunities for interventions. Endotracheal intubation with prolonged positive pressure ventilation support and oxygen-rich gas seems to change epigenetic determinants of gene expression. Such ventilation support seems to scramble the histone code, at least based on results for IGF-1. This effect does not seem to occur when nasal HFV is used. A caveat is whether altering epigenetic regulatory patterns provides short-term adaptations that improve survival during the neonatal period, but creates unintended consequences later in life. This caveat makes it a high-risk/high-potential-benefit pursuit for understanding and improving the health and outcomes of chronically ventilated preterm infants.

ACKNOWLEDGMENTS

Appreciation is expressed to Dr Robert McKnight, Dr Ronald Bloom, Dr Robert H. Lane, and Dr Lisa Joss-Moore for their invaluable input.

REFERENCES

1. Walsh MC, Morris BH, Wrage LA, et al. Extremely low birthweight neonates with protracted ventilation: mortality and 18-month neurodevelopmental outcomes. J Pediatr 2005;146:798–804.
2. Banker BQ, Larroche JC. Periventricular leukomalacia of infancy. A form of neonatal anoxic encephalopathy. Arch Neurol 1962;7:386–410.
3. Perlman JM. Neurobehavioral deficits in premature graduates of intensive care–potential medical and neonatal environmental risk factors. Pediatrics 2001;108:1339–48.
4. Pierson CR, Folkerth RD, Billiards SS, et al. Gray matter injury associated with periventricular leukomalacia in the premature infant. Acta Neuropathol 2007; 114:619–31.
5. Taylor HG, Burant CJ, Holding PA, et al. Sources of variability in sequelae of very low birth weight. Child Neuropsychol 2002;8:163–78.
6. Mathews TJ, MacDorman MF. Infant mortality statistics from the 2007 period linked birth/infant death data set. Natl Vital Stat Rep 2011;59:1–30.
7. Avery ME, Mead J. Surface properties in relation to atelectasis and hyaline membrane disease. Am J Dis Child 1959;97:517–23.
8. Liggins GC, Howie RN. A controlled trial of antepartum glucocorticoid treatment for prevention of the respiratory distress syndrome in premature infants. Pediatrics 1972;50:515–20.

9. Merritt TA, Hallman M, Bloom BT, et al. Prophylactic treatment of very premature infants with human surfactant. N Engl J Med 1986;315:785–90.

10. Enhorning G, Shennan A, Possmayer F, et al. Prevention of neonatal respiratory distress syndrome of tracheal instillation of surfactant: a randomized clinical trial. Pediatrics 1985;76:145–53.

11. Husain AN, Siddiqui NH, Stocker JT. Pathology of arrested acinar development in postsurfactant bronchopulmonary dysplasia. Hum Pathol 1988;29:710–7.

12. Jobe AH. Pulmonary surfactant therapy. NEJM 1993;328:861–8.

13. Kwong MS, Egan EA, Notter RH, et al. Double-blind clinical trial of calf lung surfactant extract for the prevention of hyaline membrane disease in extremely premature infants. Pediatrics 1985;76:585–92.

14. Avery ME, Tooley WH, Keller JB, et al. Is chronic lung disease in low birth weight infants preventable? A survey of eight centers. Pediatrics 1987;79:26–30.

15. Dani C, Bertini G, Pezzati M, et al. Early extubation and nasal continuous positive airway pressure after surfactant treatment for respiratory distress syndrome among preterm infants <30 weeks' gestation. Pediatrics 2004;113:e560–3.

16. Gregory GA, Kitterman JA, Phibbs RH, et al. Treatment of the idiopathic respiratory-distress syndrome with continuous positive airway pressure. NEJM 1971;284:1333–40.

17. Van Marter LJ, Allred EN, Pagano M, et al. Do clinical markers of barotrauma and oxygen toxicity explain interhospital variation in rates of chronic lung disease? The Neonatology Committee for the Developmental Network. Pediatrics 2000;105:1194–201.

18. Albertine KH, Pysher TJ. Impaired lung growth after injury in premature lung. In: Polin RA, Fox WW, Abman S, editors. Fetal and neonatal physiology. 4th edition. New York: Elsevier Science; 2011. p. 1039–47.

19. Northway WH Jr, Rosan RC, Porter DY. Pulmonary disease following respirator therapy of hyaline-membrane disease. Bronchopulmonary dysplasia. NEJM 1967;276:357–68.

20. Biagioni E, Frisone MF, Laroche S, et al. Maturation of cerebral electrical activity and development of cortical folding in young very preterm infants. Clin Neurophysiol 2007;118:53–9.

21. Flores Guevara R, Giannuzzi R, de Oliveira Nosralla M, et al. Positive slow waves in the EEG of premature infants between 24 and 36 weeks of conceptional age. Clin Neurophysiol 2008;119:180–9.

22. Katz LC, Crowley JC. Development of cortical circuits: lessons from ocular dominance columns. Nat Rev Neurosci 2002;3:34–42.

23. Khazipov R, Sirota A, Leinekugel X, et al. Early motor activity drives spindle bursts in the developing somatosensory cortex. Nature 2004;432:758–61.

24. Milh M, Kaminska A, Huon C, et al. Rapid cortical oscillations and early motor activity in premature human neonate. Cereb Cortex 2007;17:1582–94.

25. Mirro R, Leffler CW, Armstead WM, et al. Positive-pressure ventilation alters blood-to-brain and blood-to-CSF transport in neonatal pigs. J Appl Physiol 1991;70:584–9.

26. Hambleton G, Wigglesworth JS. Origin of intraventricular haemorrhage in the preterm infant. Arch Dis Child 1976;51:651–9.

27. Stonestreet BS, McKnight AJ, Sadowska G, et al. Effects of duration of positive-pressure ventilation on blood-brain barrier function in premature lambs. J Appl Physiol 2000;88(5):1672–7.

28. Hagberg H, Peebles D, Mallard C. Models of white matter injury: comparison of infectious, hypoxic-ischemic, and excitotoxic insults. Ment Retard Dev Disabil Res Rev 2002;8:30–8.

29. Mallard C, Welin AK, Peebles D, et al. White matter injury following systemic endotoxemia or asphyxia in the fetal sheep. Neurochem Res 2003;28:215–23.
30. Perlman JM, Volpe JJ. Cerebral blood flow velocity in relation to intraventricular hemorrhage in the premature newborn infant. J Pediatr 1982;100:956–9.
31. Funato M, Tamai H, Noma K, et al. Clinical events in association with timing of intraventricular hemorrhage in preterm infants. J Pediatr 1992;121:614–9.
32. Osborn DA, Evans N, Kluckow M. Hemodynamic and antecedent risk factors of early and late periventricular/intraventricular hemorrhage in premature infants. Pediatrics 2003;112:33–9.
33. Watkins AM, West CR, Cooke RW. Blood pressure and cerebral haemorrhage and ischaemia in very low birthweight infants. Early Hum Dev 1989;19:103–10.
34. Ando M, Takashima S, Mito T. Endotoxin, cerebral blood flow, amino acids and brain damage in young rabbits. Brain Dev 1988;10:365–70.
35. Gilles FH, Averill DR, Kerr CS. Neonatal endotoxin encephalopathy. Ann Neurol 1977;2:49–56.
36. Kaiser JR, Gauss CH, Williams DK. Surfactant administration acutely affects cerebral and systemic hemodynamics and gas exchange in very-low-birth-weight infants. J Pediatr 2004;144:809–14.
37. Lou HC, Lassen NA, Friis-Hansen B. Impaired autoregulation of cerebral blood flow in the distressed newborn infant. J Pediatr 1979;94:118–21.
38. Marlow N, Wolke D, Bracewell MA, et al. Neurologic and developmental disability at six years of age after extremely preterm birth. NEJM 2005;352:9–19.
39. Pryds O, Andersen GE, Friis-Hansen B. Cerebral blood flow reactivity in spontaneously breathing, preterm infants shortly after birth. Acta Paediatr Scand 1990;79:391–6.
40. Pryds O, Greisen G, Lou H, et al. Heterogeneity of cerebral vasoreactivity in preterm infants supported by mechanical ventilation. J Pediatr 1989;115:638–45.
41. Tsuji M, Saul JP, du Plessis A, et al. Cerebral intravascular oxygenation correlates with mean arterial pressure in critically ill premature infants. Pediatrics 2000;106:625–32.
42. Yoshioka H, Goma H, Sawada T. Cerebral hypoperfusion and leukomalacia. No To Hattatsu 1996;28:128–9 [in Japanese].
43. Coughtrey H, Rennie JM, Evans DH. Variability in cerebral blood flow velocity: observations over one minute in preterm babies. Early Hum Dev 1997;47:63–70.
44. Perlman J, Thach B. Respiratory origin of fluctuations in arterial blood pressure in premature infants with respiratory distress syndrome. Pediatrics 1988;81:399–403.
45. Dommergues MA, Patkai J, Renauld JC, et al. Proinflammatory cytokines and interleukin-9 exacerbate excitotoxic lesions of the newborn murine neopallium. Ann Neurol 2000;47:54–63.
46. Eklind S, Mallard C, Leverin AL, et al. Bacterial endotoxin sensitizes the immature brain to hypoxic–ischaemic injury. Eur J Neurosci 2001;13:1101–6.
47. Hedtjarn M, Leverin AL, Eriksson K, et al. Interleukin-18 involvement in hypoxic-ischemic brain injury. J Neurosci 2002;22:5910–9.
48. Rezaie P, Dean A. Periventricular leukomalacia, inflammation and white matter lesions within the developing nervous system. Neuropathology 2002;22:106–32.
49. Hudome S, Palmer C, Roberts RL, et al. The role of neutrophils in the production of hypoxic-ischemic brain injury in the neonatal rat. Pediatr Res 1997;41:607–16.
50. Liu XH, Kwon D, Schielke GP, et al. Mice deficient in interleukin-1 converting enzyme are resistant to neonatal hypoxic-ischemic brain damage. J Cereb Blood Flow Metab 1999;19:1099–108.

51. Palmer C, Menzies SL, Roberts RL, et al. Changes in iron histochemistry after hypoxic-ischemic brain injury in the neonatal rat. J Neurosci Res 1999;56: 60–71.

52. Barres BA, Hart IK, Coles HS, et al. Cell death in the oligodendrocyte lineage. J Neurobiol 1992;23:1221–30.

53. Guan J, Bennet L, Gluckman PD, et al. Insulin-like growth factor-1 and post-ischemic brain injury. Prog Neurobiol 2003;70:443–62.

54. Loeliger M, Inder T, Cain S, et al. Cerebral outcomes in a preterm baboon model of early versus delayed nasal continuous positive airway pressure. Pediatrics 2006;118:1640–53.

55. Mathers JC, McKay JA. Epigenetics - potential contribution to fetal programming. Adv Exp Med Biol 2009;646:119–23.

56. Zeisel SH. Epigenetic mechanisms for nutrition determinants of later health outcomes. Am J Clin Nutr 2009;89:1488S–93S.

57. Joss-Moore LA, Albertine KH, Lane RH. Epigenetics and the developmental origins of lung disease. Mol Genet Metab 2011;104:61–6.

58. Fu Q, Yu X, Callaway CW, et al. Epigenetics: intrauterine growth retardation (IUGR) modifies the histone code along the rat hepatic IGF-1 gene. FASEB J 2009;23:2438–49.

59. Luger K, Mader AW, Richmond RK, et al. Crystal structure of the nucleosome core particle at 2.8 A resolution. Nature 1997;389:251–60.

60. Kouzarides T. Chromatin modifications and their function. Cell 2007;128: 693–705.

61. Roth DM, Balch WE. Modeling general proteostasis: proteome balance in health and disease. Curr Opin Cell Biol 2011;23:126–34.

62. Marmorstein R, Trievel RC. Histone modifying enzymes: structures, mechanisms, and specificities. Biochim Biophys Acta 2009;1789:58–68.

63. Ito S, D'Alessio AC, Taranova OV, et al. Role of Tet proteins in 5mC to 5hmC conversion, ES-cell self-renewal and inner cell mass specification. Nature 2010;466:1129–33.

64. Tahiliani M, Koh KP, Shen Y, et al. Conversion of 5-methylcytosine to 5-hydroxymethylcytosine in mammalian DNA by MLL partner TET1. Science 2009;324:930–5.

65. Cedar H, Bergman Y. Linking DNA methylation and histone modification: patterns and paradigms. Nat Rev Genet 2009;10:295–304.

66. Sato F, Tsuchiya S, Meltzer SJ, et al. MicroRNAs and epigenetics. FEBS J 2011; 278:1598–609.

67. Aagaard-Tillery KM, Grove K, Bishop J, et al. Developmental origins of disease and determinants of chromatin structure: maternal diet modifies the primate fetal epigenome. J Mol Endocrinol 2008;41:91–102.

68. Reyburn B, Li M, Metcalfe DB, et al. Nasal ventilation alters mesenchymal cell turnover and improves alveolarization in preterm lambs. Am J Respir Crit Care Med 2008;178:407–18.

69. Lallemand AV, Ruocco SM, Joly PM, et al. In vivo localization of the insulin-like growth factors I and II (IGF I and IGF II) gene expression during human lung development. Int J Dev Biol 1995;39:529–37.

70. Chetty A, Andersson S, Lassus P, et al. Insulin-like growth factor-1 (IGF-1) and IGF-1 receptor (IGF-1R) expression in human lung in RDS and BPD. Pediatr Pulmonol 2004;37:128–36.

71. Ke X, Lei Q, James SJ, et al. Uteroplacental insufficiency affects epigenetic determinants of chromatin structure in brains of neonatal and juvenile IUGR rats. Physiol Genomics 2006;25:16–28.

72. Woods KA, Camacho-Hubner C, Barter D, et al. Insulin-like growth factor I gene deletion causing intrauterine growth retardation and severe short stature. Acta Paediatr Suppl 1997;423:39–45.
73. Barkho BZ, Song H, Aimone JB, et al. Identification of astrocyte-expressed factors that modulate neural stem/progenitor cell differentiation. Stem Cells Dev 2006;15:407–21.
74. Gluckman P, Klempt N, Guan J, et al. A role for IGF-1 in the rescue of CNS neurons following hypoxic-ischemic injury. Biochem Biophys Res Commun 1992;182:593–9.
75. Mozell RL, McMorris FA. Insulin-like growth factor I stimulates oligodendrocyte development and myelination in rat brain aggregate cultures. J Neurosci Res 1991;30:382–90.
76. Ye P, Li L, Richards RG, et al. Myelination is altered in insulin-like growth factor-I null mutant mice. J Neurosci 2002;22:6041–51.
77. Volpe JJ. Overview: normal and abnormal human brain development. Ment Retard Dev Disabil Res Rev 2000;6:1–5.
78. Colas JF, Schoenwolf GC. Towards a cellular and molecular understanding of neurulation. Dev Dyn 2001;221:117–45.
79. Smith JL, Schoenwolf GC. Neurulation: coming to closure. Trends Neurosci 1997;20:510–7.
80. Mollgard K, Saunders NR. The development of the human blood-brain and blood-CSF barriers. Neuropathol Appl Neurobiol 1986;12:337–58.
81. Kostovic I, Judas M. Correlation between the sequential ingrowth of afferents and transient patterns of cortical lamination in preterm infants. Anat Rec 2002; 267:1–6.
82. Gressens P. Mechanisms and disturbances of neuronal migration. Pediatr Res 2000;48:725–30.
83. Gressens P, Richelme C, Kadhim HJ, et al. The germinative zone produces the most cortical astrocytes after neuronal migration in the developing mammalian brain. Biol Neonate 1992;61:4–24.
84. Rakic P. Developmental and evolutionary adaptations of cortical radial glia. Cereb Cortex 2003;13:541–9.
85. Rakic P. Specification of cerebral cortical areas. Science 1988;241:170–6.
86. Sidman RL, Rakic P. Neuronal migration, with special reference to developing human brain: a review. Brain Res 1973;62:1–35.
87. Miyawaki T, Matsui K, Takashima S. Developmental characteristics of vessel density in the human fetal and infant brains. Early Hum Dev 1998;53:65–72.
88. Changeux JP, Danchin A. Selective stabilisation of developing synapses as a mechanism for the specification of neuronal networks. Nature 1976;264:705–12.
89. Battin MR, Maalouf EF, Counsell SJ, et al. Magnetic resonance imaging of the brain in very preterm infants: visualization of the germinal matrix, early myelination, and cortical folding. Pediatrics 1998;101:957–62.
90. Childs AM, Ramenghi LA, Evans DJ, et al. MR features of developing periventricular white matter in preterm infants: evidence of glial cell migration. AJNR Am J Neuroradiol 1998;19:971–6.
91. Volpe JJ. Neurobiology of periventricular leukomalacia in the premature infant. Pediatr Res 2001;50:553–62.
92. Inage YW, Itoh M, Takashima S. Correlation between cerebrovascular maturity and periventricular leukomalacia. Pediatr Neurol 2000;22:204–8.
93. McQuillen PS, Sheldon RA, Shatz CJ, et al. Selective vulnerability of subplate neurons after early neonatal hypoxia-ischemia. J Neurosci 2003;23:3308–15.

94. Volpe JJ. Brain injury in premature infants: a complex amalgam of destructive and developmental disturbances. Lancet Neurol 2009;8:110–24.

95. Dommergues MA, Plaisant F, Verney C, et al. Early microglial activation following neonatal excitotoxic brain damage in mice: a potential target for neuroprotection. Neuroscience 2003;121:619–28.

96. Haynes RL, Folkerth RD, Trachtenberg FL, et al. Nitrosative stress and inducible nitric oxide synthase expression in periventricular leukomalacia. Acta Neuropathol 2009;118:391–9.

97. Kadhim H, Tabarki B, Verellen G, et al. Inflammatory cytokines in the pathogenesis of periventricular leukomalacia. Neurology 2001;56:1278–84.

98. Merrill JE, Ignarro LJ, Sherman MP, et al. Microglial cell cytotoxicity of oligodendrocytes is mediated through nitric oxide. J Immunol 1993;151:2132–41.

99. Perlman JM. White matter injury in the preterm infant: an important determination of abnormal neurodevelopment outcome. Early Hum Dev 1998;53:99–120.

100. Rezaie P, Male D. Colonisation of the developing human brain and spinal cord by microglia: a review. Microsc Res Tech 1999;45:359–82.

101. Smith ME, van der Maesen K, Somera FP. Macrophage and microglial responses to cytokines in vitro: phagocytic activity, proteolytic enzyme release, and free radical production. J Neurosci Res 1998;54:68–78.

102. Volpe JJ. Cerebral white matter injury of the premature infant-more common than you think. Pediatrics 2003;112:176–80.

103. Tanaka F, Ozawa Y, Inage Y, et al. Association of osteopontin with ischemic axonal death in periventricular leukomalacia. Acta Neuropathol 2000;100:69–74.

104. Volpe JJ. Subplate neurons–missing link in brain injury of the premature infant? Pediatrics 1996;97:112–3.

Index

Note: Page numbers of article titles are in **boldface** type.

Clin Perinatol 39 (2012) 741–752
http://dx.doi.org/10.1016/S0095-5108(12)00080-2
0095-5108/12/$ – see front matter © 2012 Elsevier Inc. All rights reserved.

perinatology.theclinics.com

Moving?

Make sure your subscription moves with you!

To notify us of your new address, find your **Clinics Account Number** (located on your mailing label above your name), and contact customer service at:

Email: journalscustomerservice-usa@elsevier.com

800-654-2452 (subscribers in the U.S. & Canada)
314-447-8871 (subscribers outside of the U.S. & Canada)

Fax number: 314-447-8029

Elsevier Health Sciences Division
Subscription Customer Service
3251 Riverport Lane
Maryland Heights, MO 63043

Printed and bound by CPI Group (UK) Ltd, Croydon, CR0 4YY

03/10/2024

01040449-0010